Ethical Issues in
Clinical Research:
A Practical Guide

Ethical Issues in Clinical Research: A Practical Guide

Bernard Lo, MD, FACP

Professor of Medicine
Director, Program in Medical Ethics
University of California, San Francisco
Attending Physician, Moffitt-Long Hospital
San Francisco, California

Wolters Kluwer | Lippincott Williams & Wilkins
Health
Philadelphia • Baltimore • New York • London
Buenos Aires • Hong Kong • Sydney • Tokyo

Acquisitions Editor: Sonya Seigafuse
Managing Editor: Kerry Barrett
Associate Production Manager: Kevin Johnson
Manufacturing Manager: Benjamin Rivera
Marketing Manager: Kim Schonberger
Design Coordinator: Stephen Druding
Production Service: Maryland Composition/ASI

Printed in The People's Republic of China

Library of Congress Cataloging-in-Publication Data

Lo, Bernard.
  Ethical issues in clinical research: a practical guide / Bernard Lo.
    p. ; cm.
  Includes bibliographical references and index.
  ISBN 978-0-7817-8817-5
  1. Clinical trials—Moral and ethical aspects. 2. Medicine—Research—Moral and ethical aspects. I. Title.
  [DNLM: 1. Ethics, Research. 2. Patient Rights—ethics. 3. Researcher-Subject Relations—ethics.
  4. Scientific Misconduct—ethics. 5. Vulnerable Populations. W 20.5 L795e 2009]
  R853.C55L6 2009
  615.5072′4—dc22

                                                                                              2008052577

Care has been taken to confirm the accuracy of the information presented and to describe generally accepted practices. However, the authors, editors, and publisher are not responsible for errors or omissions or for any consequences from application of the information in this book and make no warranty, expressed or implied, with respect to the currency, completeness, or accuracy of the contents of the publication. Application of the information in a particular situation remains the professional responsibility of the practitioner.

The authors, editors, and publisher have exerted every effort to ensure that drug selection and dosage set forth in this text are in accordance with current recommendations and practice at the time of publication. However, in view of ongoing research, changes in government regulations, and the constant flow of information relating to drug therapy and drug reactions, the reader is urged to check the package insert for each drug for any change in indications and dosage and for added warnings and precautions. This is particularly important when the recommended agent is a new or infrequently employed drug.

Some drugs and medical devices presented in the publication have Food and Drug Administration (FDA) clearance for limited use in restricted research settings. It is the responsibility of the health care provider to ascertain the FDA status of each drug or device planned for use in their clinical practice.

To purchase additional copies of this book, call our customer service department at (800) 638-3030 or fax orders to (301) 223-2320. International customers should call (301) 223-2300.

Visit Lippincott Williams & Wilkins on the Internet: at LWW.com. Lippincott Williams & Wilkins customer service representatives are available from 8:30 am to 6 pm, EST.

10 9 8 7 6 5 4 3 2 1

RRS0903

For Laurie, Aaron, and Maya

CONTENTS

SECTION V   ETHICAL ISSUES IN SPECIFIC TYPES OF RESEARCH

PREFACE

C linical research is the wellspring of better tests and treatments to benefit patients. During my career as a physician, new therapies, such as statins for elevated cholesterol, beta-blockers in myocardial infarction, antibiotics for peptic ulcer disease, and new cancer therapies, have been proven effective through clinical trials. Research with medical records has shown that disparities in access to care leads to poorer health outcomes and that preventive services reduce morbidity and mortality. Furthermore, research using existing biological specimens helped establish that smoking causes lung cancer and led to the use of Pap smears to detect cervical cancer.

Ethical issues are unavoidable when research is carried out with human participants. In a research study, the benefits are unknown and participants undergo risks primarily to benefit future patients. Informed consent, assessment of risk and benefit, protection of confidentiality, and payment to participants commonly pose ethical dilemmas. New types of research, such as genomic sequencing and clinical trials in resource-poor countries, present novel ethical concerns. In some recent studies, egregious ethical problems have occurred, including failure to publish negative findings from clinical trials, authorship by persons who did not make substantial intellectual contributions to a manuscript and project, and outright fabrication and falsification of data.

This book presents a comprehensive and practical analysis of the common ethical dilemmas that scientists face when conducting research with human participants. The first chapters address fundamental topics such as the ethical and regulatory framework, assessment of risks and benefits, consent, and confidentiality. The next group of chapters addresses the researcher-participant relationship, covering issues such as recruitment of participants and payment. Next are chapters on responsible conduct of research. In addition to chapters on misconduct and authorship, there are chapters on patents and conflicts of interest. The following chapters are on vulnerable research subjects including children, ethnic and cultural minorities, and persons in resource-poor countries. The final group of chapters cover ethical dilemmas in common types of research studies including research with existing data and materials, clinical trials, and genomics research. Taken together, the chapters provide in-depth coverage of common topics in research ethics.

This book grew out of a course I teach on ethical issues in clinical research for postdoctoral fellows and junior faculty members who are starting their research careers. These students are simultaneously taking a course in which they design a research project. The goal of the course is not only to help trainees understand the ethical issues in their specific project but also to present an approach to ethical issues they are likely to face in future research. Several years ago when preparing the course syllabus, I realized that there was no book on research ethics targeted to this audience; this book is intended to meet that gap. The book therefore is suitable for courses in research ethics, for example, those developed in conjunction with NIH Clinical and Translational Sciences Awards.

My experience with ethical dilemmas in actual research projects has also shaped this book. At UCSF, through the Center for AIDS Prevention Studies and the Clinical and Translational Sciences Institute, I provide consultation on ethical issues to researchers. This book addresses the common issues that students and researchers have brought to me in these consultations.

The book provides practical advice. In addition to analyzing these ethical issues, it gives specific suggestions on how to address or resolve them. Several features are intended to help readers learn how to apply the recommendations to specific research projects. Numerous case studies illustrate ethical issues arising in clinical research and show how to resolve them. These studies are visually set off from the chapter text, but are integrated with the discussion in the text. Tables and take-home points at the end of each chapter will also help readers grasp the main points. An annotated bibliography and extensive references at the end of each chapter point readers to additional in-depth reading.

I am grateful to the many colleagues and friends who have shared with me their clear thinking, common sense, and expertise. Over the years, Nancy Dubler and Robert Steinbrook have been extraordinary friends and colleagues, from whom I have learned a tremendous amount. Rick Wagner, Lisa Voss, Geoff Lomax, and Alta Charo have helped me understand the intracacies of research regulations. I owe thanks to Leslie Wolf, Steve Morin, Mark Barnes, Baruch Brody, Jim Childress, Pat King, Deborah Grady, Arnold Kriegstein, Doug White, and John Witte for thoughtful and stimulating discussions. I have been fortunate to work with splendid colleagues at the Greenwall Foundation Faculty Scholars Program, the Institute of Medicine, the California Institute of Regenerative Medicine, and various data and safety monitoring boards. Lindsay Parham, Chris Broom, and Patti Zettler have been expert research assistants. I thank the Greenwall Foundation, the Roadmap for Medical Research program at National Center for Research Resources (NCRR), and the National Institute of Mental Health for supporting the work that formed the basis of this book.

To my family, I owe my greatest thanks. I am ever grateful that my parents, C.P. and Lucy Lo, and my aunt, Edith Chu, provided a model of love of learning and integrity. My wife, Laurie Dornbrand, is both my best friend and my toughest critic, who unfailingly helps fix muddled passages. Our son Aaron copyedited a draft of the book and made many helpful suggestions, particularly on how to make the main points stand out more clearly. Our daughter Maya can always be counted on to enliven us with a fresh perspective.

Bernard Lo, MD, FACP
Professor of Medicine
Director, Program in Medical Ethics
University of California, San Francisco
Attending Physician, Moffitt-Long Hospital
San Francisco, California

Ethical and Regulatory Background

1

Historical Perspective

Research with human participants has revolutionized our understanding and ability to treat serious diseases. During the past 20 years, the dangers of second-hand cigarette smoke, the etiology of peptic ulcer disease, and the epidemiology of HIV infection have been clarified through research involving human participants, their medical records, and stored biological materials. Furthermore, clinical trials have demonstrated dramatic advances in the treatment of coronary artery disease, peptic ulcer disease, breast cancer, and HIV infection. However, research with human participants raises ethical concerns because volunteers accept risks to advance scientific knowledge and help future patients. Moreover, the exact risks and benefits of research are uncertain—by definition, research projects involve questions whose answers are unknown. In several highly publicized cases, serious ethical lapses have occurred in clinical research and participants have suffered grievous harm. The usual response to these egregious cases is to enact regulations. However, the resulting regulatory system is flawed; it is burdensome for researchers and research institutions, and it still may not effectively protect participants and the public. If researchers wish to avoid additional regulations, they need to take more responsibility for ensuring the integrity of the research and protecting the research participants.

HISTORICAL BACKGROUND

NAZI "EXPERIMENTS"

During World War II, Nazi physicians intentionally inflicted serious, even fatal, harm on inmates of concentration camps or mental institutions who gave no consent. In some projects, "researchers" intentionally immersed prisoners in ice tanks and deprived them of oxygen to simulate hypothermia and hypoxia suffered by downed pilots, infected prisoners with typhus to try to develop a vaccine, and tried to develop efficient methods to induce sterility (1). In response to these atrocities, the Declaration of Helsinki of 1964 required researchers to obtain voluntary and informed consent from research subjects, and established the need to balance the risks and benefits of a study (2).

THE TUSKEGEE STUDY

The Tuskegee study of the natural history of syphilis, which was conducted by the U.S. government, was intended to document the natural history and long-term manifestations of untreated syphilis (3,4). Researchers deceived impoverished, poorly educated African-American men into believing that they were receiving treatment for syphilis. For example, lumbar punctures done for research purposes were misrepresented as "special free treatments." Furthermore, researchers took steps to withhold treatments as they became available. In response to the Tuskegee study, in 1974 the federal government issued regulations on human-subjects research that required informed consent to be obtained from subjects and created institutional review boards (IRBs) to review federally sponsored human research. These federal regulations form the basis for government oversight of clinical research today.

DEATH OF JESSE GELSINGER

In 1999, 18-year-old Jesse Gelsinger, an asymptomatic volunteer, died from liver failure during a Phase I gene transfer trial (5,6). In retrospect, investigators did not pay sufficient heed to animal data indicating the possibility of adenovirus-induced liver failure, and also overlooked abnormalities in Gelsinger's liver function tests on the day the investigational intervention was administered. The principal investigator had founded the biotechnology company that produced that adenovirus vector used in the study and thus had a significant financial interest in the success of the clinical trial. The researchers in this study also failed to use the IRB-approved consent form and did not report instances of mild liver toxicity in previous participants as adverse events. The tragic outcome in this highly publicized case led to additional federal regulations regarding conflicts of interest, educating investigators in protection of human participants, and reporting adverse events.

DEATH OF ELLEN ROCHE

In 2001, 24-year-old Ellen Roche volunteered to participate in a study on the pathophysiology of asthma (7). Investigators administered hexamethonium to participants to study their airway relaxation. Ms. Roche developed adult respiratory distress syndrome and multi-organ failure and died after 4 weeks in the intensive care unit. Both a National Institutes of Health (NIH) study section and the IRB had approved the study. However, a federal investigation found serious problems with the study. Although hexamethonium was described as a "medication" in the consent form, it is not approved by the Food and Drug Administration (FDA) for use in humans and is sold as a laboratory reagent. The researchers failed to respond appropriately to previous adverse events in the study. The first volunteer in the study had developed a cough and shortness of breath, which was ascribed to an upper respiratory tract infection. However, the researchers changed how the hexamethonium was prepared, without informing the IRB. In addition, the research subject was a technician in the asthma and allergy center where the study was conducted, raising concerns about undue influence. An external review termed the use of employees and students as research participants a "culture of possible coercion."

A federal investigation found serious problems with IRB reviews at the university. The IRB did not follow federal regulations regarding research on children, expedited review, waiver of informed consent, or research with prisoners. It approved studies when no IRB members with pertinent expertise were present. For example, it approved a cancer clinical trial without an oncologist present, even though one IRB member suggested that such expertise would be helpful. Although the university is one of the largest recipients of NIH funding, it had only two IRBs, which was judged to be inadequate to review the number of protocols submitted. The minutes of IRB meetings were lacking for extended periods. The investigation concluded that the IRB failed in its charge to protect human participants. As a result of this investigation, all federally funded research at the university was suspended.

Public outrage at such cases is understandable. Participants cannot appreciate the risks and potential benefits of a research study as well as investigators, peer reviewers, and IRBs do. Participants depend on these professionals to ensure that the risks of the study are acceptable and minimized. If there is misrepresentation during the consent process or the study entails excessive risk, participants and the public may feel betrayed. A common response to egregious or tragic cases is a demand for more rigorous regulation.

NIH-funded research has also been temporarily suspended at other leading academic health centers (8). These suspensions shocked other universities, which began to allocate more resources for IRB staffing and set up additional IRB committees.

However, other consequences of the Roche case have been more controversial. There has been increased emphasis on documentation of IRB decisions, which some have criticized as elevating form over substance. Reporting of adverse events was expanded, but the reporting requirements have been criticized as redundant and counterproductive. Many IRBs and researchers complain that the administrative burdens of compliance with federal regulations have greatly increased, without increasing protection for research participants (9,10).

WITHHOLDING INFORMATION ABOUT ADVERSE EVENTS IN CLINICAL TRIALS

In several recent major clinical trials sponsored by industry, negative findings were allegedly withheld from publications or were not submitted for peer-reviewed abstract presentations or publications until long after conclusion of the trial. These incidents involved several drug manufacturers and types of drugs. Table 1.1 summarizes these incidents.

Incomplete or selective reporting of data undermines the integrity of the conclusions and constitutes scientific misconduct, as discussed in Chapter 12. Ideally, scientific inquiry should be guided by a search for the truth, which requires presenting data completely and honestly.

TABLE 1.1	Failure to Publish Serious Adverse Events in Industry-Sponsored Clinical Trials
Drug	**Incident**
Celecoxib (11)	In a pivotal trial of celecoxib, only 6-month data on outcomes were presented, even though the original protocol called for a longer duration of the trial and outcomes at 12 months were available when the manuscript was submitted. The 6-month outcomes showed an advantage for the study drug, but the 12-month outcomes showed no advantage compared to control drugs.
Rofecoxib (12)	Myocardial infarctions in the arm receiving the study drug were underreported in the journal article, even though the correct number was reported to the FDA.
Selective serotonin reuptake inhibitors (SSRIs) (13)	Although published trials suggest that SSRIs are beneficial in children with depression, when unpublished data are considered, the risks appear to outweigh the benefits for all but one drug in this class.
Paroxetine (14)	Results of trials of paroxetine showing an increased risk of teenage suicide or lack of efficacy were released (on manufacturer's website) only after a lawsuit was brought against the manufacturer.
Ezetimibe plus a statin (15)	Results of clinical trial showing no benefit on carotid artery wall thickness were not published until 2 years after the conclusion of the trial.
PolyHeme, a blood substitute (16,17)	Results from a clinical trial showing increased mortality were not released (on manufacturer's website) until 5 years after the trial was stopped by the sponsor.
Implantable cardioverter-defibrillator (18)	The manufacturer of an implantable cardioverter-defibrillator allegedly failed to report critical, potentially fatal design defects for more than 3 years.
Immunologic modulator for treatment of HIV infection (19)	Manufacturer/sponsor refused to provide a complete data set to investigators in a randomized clinical trial that showed that the study agent was ineffective, and tried to block publication. Results were published by the principal investigator after data were collected from the site principal investigators.
Brand-name thyroid hormone (20,21)	Manufacturer/sponsor tried to block the publication of a pharmacologic study showing that a generic thyroid replacement had similar bioavailability.

TAKE HOME POINTS

1. Scandals have eroded public trust in research and led to new government regulations. However, the resulting regulations have been criticized as burdensome and ineffective.
2. The ethical integrity and judgment of the investigators are crucial protections for research participants, particularly in situations where the regulations are silent, ambiguous, or controversial.
3. If researchers do not fulfill their ethical obligations when designing and carrying out clinical research, the public may press for stricter government oversight, which might delay important research or impose burdens on investigators and IRBs without strengthening protections for participants.

ANNOTATED BIBLIOGRAPHY

Emanuel EJ, Grady C, Crouch RA, et al, eds. *The Oxford Textbook of Clinical Research Ethics*. New York: Oxford University Press; 2008.
    Multi-authored comprehensive book with excellent chapters on history of research ethics.
Krumholz HM, Ross JS, Presler AH, et al. What have we learnt from Vioxx? *BMJ* 2007;334:120–123.
    Lucid analysis of internal drug company documents obtained during patient lawsuits, which reveal ethical problems with the conduct of clinical trials.

REFERENCES

1. Weindling PJ. The Nazi medical experiments. In: Emanuel EJ, Grady C, Crouch RA, et al, eds. *The Oxford Textbook of Clinical Research Ethics*. New York: Oxford University Press; 2008:18–30.
2. World Medical Association. Declaration of Helsinki, 2004. Available at: http://www.wma.net/e/ethicsunit/helsinki.htm. Accessed August 30, 2008.
3. Federman DD, Hanna KE, Rodriguez LL, eds. *Preserving Public Trust: Accreditation and Human Participant Research Protection Programs*. Washington, DC: National Academies Press; 2001.
4. Jones JH. The Tuskegee syphilis experiment. In: Emanuel EJ, Grady C, Crouch RA, et al, eds. *Oxford Textbook of Research Ethics*. New York: Oxford University Press; 2008.
5. Lo B, Wolf LE. Ethical issues in clinical research: an issue for all internists. *Am J Med* 2000;109:82–85.
6. Steinbrook R. The Gelsinger case. In: Emanuel EJ, Grady C, Crouch RA, et al, eds. *The Oxford Textbook of Clinical Research Ethics*. New York: Oxford University Press; 2008:110–120.
7. Steinbrook R. Protecting research subjects—the crisis at Johns Hopkins. *N Engl J Med* 2002;346:716–720.
8. Steinbrook R. Improving protection for research subjects. *N Engl J Med* 2002;346:1425–1430.
9. National Bioethics Advisory Commission. *Ethical and Policy Issues in Research Involving Human Participants*. Rockville, MD: National Bioethics Advisory Commission; 2001.
10. Federman DD, Hanna KE, Rodriguez LL, eds. *Responsible Research: A Systems Approach to Protecting Research Participants*. Washington, DC: National Academies Press; 2002.
11. Wright JM, Perry TL, Bassett KL, et al. Reporting of 6-month vs 12-month data in a clinical trial of celecoxib. *JAMA* 2001;286:2398–2400.
12. Krumholz HM, Ross JS, Presler AH, et al. What have we learnt from Vioxx? *BMJ* 2007;334:120–123.
13. Whittington CJ, Kendall T, Fonagy P, et al. Selective serotonin reuptake inhibitors in childhood depression: systematic review of published versus unpublished data. *Lancet* 2004;363:1341–1345.
14. Gibson L. GlaxoSmithKline to publish clinical trials after US lawsuit. *BMJ* 2004;328:1513.
15. Kastelein JJ, Akdim F, Stroes ES, et al. Simvastatin with or without ezetimibe in familial hypercholesterolemia. *N Engl J Med* 2008;358:1431–1443.
16. Burton TM. Amid alarm bells, a blood substitute keeps pumping. *Wall Street Journal* 2006 February 22.
17. Northfield Laboratories. Northfield Laboratories releases summary observations from its elective surgery trial. Available at: http://phx.corporate-ir.net/phoenix.zhtml?c=91374&p=irol-newsArticle&ID=833808&highlight=. Accessed April 25, 2008.
18. Hauser RG, Maron BJ. Lessons from the failure and recall of an implantable cardioverter-defibrillator. *Circulation* 2005;112:2040–2042.
19. Kahn JO, Cherng DW, Mayer K, et al. Evaluation of HIV-immunogen, an immunologic modifier, administered to patients infected with HIV having 300 to 549×10^6/L CD4 cell counts. *JAMA* 2000;284:2193–2202.
20. Dong BJ, Hauck WW, Gambertoglio JG, et al. Bioequivalence of generic and brand-name levothyroxine products in the treatment of hypothyroidism. *JAMA* 1997;277:1205–1213.
21. Rennie D, Flanagin A. Thyroid storm. *JAMA* 1997;277:1238–1243.

2

An Ethical Framework for Research

A fundamental ethical tension arises in human subjects research because the persons who benefit from research generally are not those who suffer its risks. Research participants experience risks, including inconvenience, intrusions on privacy and confidentiality, and, in some studies, medical complications. The risks may be greater than anticipated, or the benefits less than expected. However, research is not intended primarily to benefit participants; rather, it is meant to benefit future patients by generating new scientific knowledge. By definition, research poses questions whose answers are not known until after the study is completed.

Because of these unavoidable ethical concerns, several questions need to be addressed in all research with human participants:

- Are the risks to research participants excessive in light of the potential benefits?
- Have the participants given informed and voluntary consent to participate in the research?
- Are the burdens of the research distributed fairly, and will people have equitable access to the benefits of the research?

A number of research studies have caused moral outrage because of excessive risk, lack of informed and voluntary consent, or exploitation of vulnerable participants (see Chapter 1). The ethical challenge is to allow research that may lead to improved medical care to proceed while also protecting research participants.

WHAT IS RESEARCH?

The federal regulations for human subjects research define *research* as a "systematic investigation designed to develop or contribute to generalizable knowledge" (1). Classifying an activity as research means that federal requirements for IRB review and informed consent may be applicable. Conversely, if an activity is not considered research, IRB review and special provisions for informed consent are not required.

In the definition of research, the concept of *generalizable knowledge* has two components (2). First, the study must be scientifically rigorous so that the findings will be valid. If no valid knowledge will be generated, no inconvenience or risks to subjects can be justified. Second, the findings must be disseminated in order for other scientists, practicing physicians, and future patients to take advantage of them. Many IRBs operationalize the concept of generalizable knowledge by asking whether the investigator plans or hopes to publish the findings or present them at a professional meeting. If so, the activity is considered research.

It may be difficult to decide whether some activities should be classified as research, as the following examples indicate.

INNOVATIVE CLINICAL CARE

Research needs to be distinguished from innovative clinical care whose goal is to benefit an individual patient. According to the Common Rule, the design of the project is crucial because research is designed to produce generalizable knowledge. Not every new, different, or unproven medical activity is considered research. For example, when treating an individual patient, a physician may use higher-than-usual doses of a medication or use it for an indication that has not been approved by the FDA. Similarly, a surgeon may modify a surgical procedure to try to improve it or to take into account individual anatomical variation. Because such innovative clinical care is designed or intended to improve the individual patient's health, it is not considered research. No IRB oversight is required.

In practice, however, the distinction between research and innovative clinical care is blurred. The design of the project does not fully capture all the relevant ethical considerations.

STUDY 2.1   **Laparoscopic cholecystectomy.**

A surgeon has helped to develop new laparoscopic surgical techniques. After practicing with animal models, he tries the procedure on human patients. He makes modifications and improvements in technique after each of the first 20 cases. He presents his work to a joint conference for the teaching hospitals affiliated with the medical school.

After the surgeon has operated on 100 patients using essentially the same technique, he prepares a retrospective case series for presentation at a national meeting and for publication.

In Study 2.1, it is helpful to separate the different phases of this project: starting an innovative clinical intervention, improving the quality of the surgical procedure, and assessing its benefits and risks through a case series. Are these activities research?

Federal regulations focus on the design of the project, and often this is interpreted as the intent of the surgeon. However, the design of the project or the intent of the surgeon may change as the project evolves. A physician may start intending to provide benefit to an individual patient or a few patients, but later realize that other physicians and patients would benefit if the new surgical procedure were developed more fully and its effectiveness established. Whether Study 2.1 is considered research or not, the surgeon has an ethical responsibility to address the following questions.

Is the Risk Acceptable?

To show that the risk of the new surgical procedure is acceptable, it may be necessary to first carry out experiments with animals. Laparoscopic cholecystectomy, one of the first laparoscopic procedures to be developed, was sufficiently different from open cholecystectomy that extensive animal research was required. For minor variations of standard surgical procedures, animal studies may not be necessary.

Should the Procedure be Reviewed by Peers?

Peer review can suggest ways to reduce the risks or enhance the benefits of a new procedure, such as by excluding persons who are at greatly increased risk. Many surgeons might consider peer review of an innovative procedure burdensome. Developing a new surgical procedure requires a series of modifications in technique. Requirements to write a formal protocol may be thought to stifle improvements in the procedure and impose premature standardization. The challenge is to keep the burdens of oversight from discouraging innovation.

Should Patients be Informed About the Innovative Nature of the Procedure?

The potential benefits and risks of the innovative procedure should be discussed in comparison with standard care when obtaining informed consent for surgery. Patients should be informed that it is innovative and not established therapy, and offered the option of standard therapy. The extent of discussion will vary with the situation. At one extreme, if the physician is planning to use a highly innovative procedure on all her patients, they should be offered the option to seek care from another surgeon. At the other extreme, minor changes in technique, such as changes in suturing materials, need not be discussed with patients.

Should Outcomes of the New Procedure be Evaluated?

If a major new surgical procedure, such as laparoscopy, is introduced, the referring physicians and their patients will want to know how the outcomes of the new procedure compare with those of current approaches to care. To answer this question, outcome information needs to be collected systematically. Often this is done in a retrospective case series, as we discuss next.

ANALYZING A CASE SERIES

After introducing an innovation in clinical care, a physician or clinical group may want to review the outcomes of the new approach. The review might be presented at a teaching conference. If the findings will not be disseminated beyond the clinical unit, many IRBs would not consider the project research. However, if the findings will be presented at a conference or published, the project generally would be considered generalizable knowledge and hence research.

In a retrospective case series, a physician reviews medical records that have already been recorded as part of clinical care. Because tests or treatments have already been carried out, the review involves no physical risks, and the only risk is a breach of confidentiality. As discussed in Chapter 23, a retrospective review of medical records may be exempt from IRB review if the investigator records data in a manner that does not allow participants to be identified.

Some case series have a prospective component, as in the following continuation of Study 2.1.

STUDY 2.1   (Continued).

The case series in Study 1 revealed an unexpectedly high number of cases of bile duct injury. To monitor more carefully for biliary tract complications, the surgeon plans to add CT scans of the biliary tract to the liver function tests routinely done during follow-up visits. If he can obtain funding for a research assistant, he will carry out another case series, taking advantage of these additional outcomes data.

The surgeon may intend to both improve care for specific patients and strengthen the knowledge gained from another case series. If the surgeon would perform additional tests even if the outcomes study could not be done, the additional tests could be considered enhancements in care that do not require IRB review. In pragmatic terms, the issue is whether the surgeon would order the CT scans even if he knows there is no research funding and the second case series is unlikely.

Some physicians may complain that it is burdensome to have to submit to the IRB a project to carry out tests that are clinically appropriate at a follow-up visit. Indeed, routinely ordering this imaging test might be characterized as quality improvement (QI), which ordinarily also does not require IRB review, as we discuss next.

QUALITY IMPROVEMENT

QI projects are designed to improve patient outcomes while posing very little risk to patients. For example, QI projects commonly try to reduce medical errors or increase adherence to evidence-based practice guidelines, such as guidelines for cancer prevention and screening.

A recent QI project raised fears that important QI projects may be stifled by literal application of the federal research regulations (3), and illustrates the controversy about the line between QI projects and research.

STUDY 2.2   Project to decrease catheter-related infections.

A university and a consortium of 67 community hospitals carried out a QI project to reduce the incidence of catheter-related bloodstream infections in intensive-care units (ICUs). The intervention included five procedures that had been shown in previous studies to reduce such infections and were recommended by the Centers for Disease Control: hand washing, using barrier precautions, cleaning the skin with chlorhexidine, avoiding femoral lines, and removing unnecessary catheters. Additional features of the project included establishment of team leaders, education of clinicians, a checklist of these infection-control practices, and feedback to site teams on the rate of catheter-related infections at their institution compared to others. The project used a before/after design and measured the incidence of catheter-related bloodstream infections. Each ICU collected data on the number of catheter days and infections, and deidentified data were reported to the university for analysis.

The university IRB determined that this QI project was exempt from federal human subjects regulations because the investigators received only deidentified data.

After 3 months, the mean rate of infections decreased from 2.7 per 1000 catheter days at baseline to zero; this decrease was sustained for the entire 18 months of the project. These results were published in a major peer-reviewed journal.

Responding to an anonymous complaint after the study was published, the Office of Human Research Protections (OHRP) ruled that the project was research and was not exempt, and that the university IRB had failed to implement the federal regulations regarding informed consent. Furthermore, an IRB at each hospital needed to review and approve the project. OHRP noted that the project was characterized as research in grant applications and on the IRB review form. Because the data were being collected prospectively, the exemption for use of existing data and records did not apply. Later, OHRP stated that the project qualified for expedited review and waiver of informed consent.

In many QI projects, the interventions are small-scale changes in the process of care, and the effects of these changes are closely monitored (4). These interventions are designed to improve patient outcomes in specific settings, not to produce generalizable knowledge. Other QI projects, such as Study 2.2, use broader interventions such as staff education, individual feedback to providers, and the use of checklists, standardized orders, and clinical algorithms, which have been shown to be beneficial in other clinical settings and have minimal risk compared to standard care (5,6). QI projects often aim to increase adherence to evidence-based practice guidelines that have been shown to improve patient outcomes. Indeed, interventions to achieve these goals may be implemented administratively in health care institutions without any consent from individual patients or health care workers, and without IRB review (5). It makes little sense to allow these interventions but not the systematic collection and analysis of data to determine whether the project is effective in a range of settings. Compared to the alternatives of not trying to improve care, or instituting interventions without measuring their impact on patient outcomes, QI poses minimal risk and indeed may well provide more benefit than risk (5). QI does involve some risk of breaches of privacy and confidentiality in the collection of outcomes data, but this risk can be minimized if adequate confidentiality precautions are taken.

Is the Project Research?

Study 2.2 was designed to produce generalizable knowledge that will be applicable to many institutions. Moreover, project leaders applied for research grants and planned to publish the results. Thus, many IRBs would determine that it meets the regulatory definition of research. Depending on their design, other QI projects may not be research, may not be human subjects research, or may be exempt from the Common Rule (see Fig. 6.1 for how to determine these issues). If the study can be defined as research, the burdens of regulatory compliance would be decreased.

Critics of the OHRP's rulings in Study 2.2 argue that the vast majority of QI projects are simply part of good patient care. In this view, physicians and health care institutions have an ethical obligation to try to improve the quality of care as part of their obligation to act in the best interest of patients. The Joint Commission, which accredits hospitals and other health care organizations, requires institutions seeking accreditation to have QI programs. Furthermore, in agreeing to health care, patients implicitly consent to minimal risk QI projects (5).

From this perspective, the knowledge gained from QI is so valuable and the risks are so small that the costs and burdens of IRB oversight do far more harm than good. The current regulatory system does not provide meaningful protections to participants in QI projects and in fact is often counterproductive, delaying or deterring projects that offer a high likelihood of improving patient outcomes with very little risk compared to ordinary clinical care. In this view, such QI projects deserve an exception to the Common Rule.

To be sure, caution is indicated because some projects termed QI are not based on evidence-based interventions and may involve unacceptable risks to patients. For example, projects may be designated QI but have as a goal administrative efficiency, such as shorter inpatient lengths of stay (7). Furthermore, some projects should be considered both research and QI, such as projects that test interventions that go beyond current science and experience, that involve researchers who have no long-term commitment to improving the quality of care at an institution, or that receive funding from external sources, particularly agencies that fund research (5).

Should Informed Consent be Required?

Critics argue that there is little to be gained by obtaining informed consent in QI interventions such as Study 2.2, which pose no more than a minimal increase in risk compared to standard clinical care, do not violate patient autonomy, and cannot be separated from clinical care. Furthermore, data on catheter infections would be collected even for clinical purposes even if the QI project were not carried out. Thus, a requirement for informed consent would provide no additional protection to patients (6). Some writers argue that QI is a legitimate exception to the requirement of informed consent, similar to the exception for emergency research (6) (see Chapter 19). Others argue that consent for QI is implicit in consent for medical care (5).

Should the Project Receive Independent Review?

Critics charge that IRB review results in more burdens than benefits for participants in many QI projects (6,8). Participants gain little protection because they are already protected against unacceptable risk in other ways. QI projects should be approved by clinicians who lead clinical units, such as the ICU leaders in Study 2.2. Thus oversight of QI should be part of accountability for clinical care (5).

IRB review also may be burdensome and may delay or deter useful projects. Most QI projects that meet the regulatory definition of research should qualify for expedited review (6). Even expedited review, however, may not be feasible in community hospitals or clinics that lack IRBs. It is better for such institutions to join a larger project where they can learn from QI experts and obtain feedback comparing their performance with that of other sites. Obtaining approval from multiple IRBs is daunting and may delay or discourage valuable QI projects. Although Study 2.2 had a consortium of hospitals that might serve as the IRB of record for all sites in the study, this arrangement is not available for many other projects.

PUBLIC HEALTH PRACTICE

Public health officials are required by law to investigate and control outbreaks of certain diseases, to carry out surveillance, and to conduct contact tracing. For these activities, informed consent is not required for interviews, examinations, testing, and, in some circumstances, prophylaxis or treatment. Public health officials argue that requirements for IRB review and informed consent do not make sense because the government has mandated these public health activities (9). Thus, just as regulations for research are not applied to innovative clinical practices designed primarily to benefit an individual patient, they should also not be applied when innovative methods are employed primarily to investigate and control a threat to the public health. Although this distinction between public health practice and research may seem clear in the abstract, in practice the line is often blurred (10).

The study described below illustrates how public health practice needs to keep pace with new threats. Novel scientific methods may be needed to understand emerging infections, new patterns of infection, or bioterrorism threats. Furthermore, these new methods need to be validated and then disseminated through presentations and publications.

Tuberculosis (TB) control has been complicated by the spread of multidrug-resistant strains and extensively drug-resistant (XDR) strains, and by coinfection with HIV. The following study pioneered the novel technique of molecular fingerprinting by restriction-fragment-length polymorphism (RFLP), a laboratory technique, to identify cases caused by the same strain of the TB bacterium (11). Patients who shared the same RFLP formed a cluster with the same strain of bacterium, strongly suggesting person-to-person transmission within the cluster.

STUDY 2.3   **Molecular epidemiology in outbreak investigation.**

Traditional contact tracing identified connections between patients in only 4% of TB cases investigated in San Francisco during 1991 and 1992. However, 40% of the patients were found to share an RFLP pattern with at least one other patient. Conventional contact tracing therefore identified only 10% of the patients in clusters and thus greatly underestimated the extent of transmission. In this city about one-third of new cases resulted from transmission from another patient with active TB rather than from reactivation of latent infection.

Patients who had AIDS, were Black or Hispanic, and who resided in a high-poverty area were more likely to be part of a cluster. In the largest clusters, many patients did not live or work with anyone else in the cluster. Several were linked only by receiving medical care in the same hospital ward or same clinic. Some members of the same cluster had no apparent connections with each other. Each presumptive index case in large cluster outbreaks had positive smears and was poorly compliant with therapy. Because Study 1 was carried out with data and samples collected as part of an outbreak investigation, the IRB exempted it from review and did not require informed consent. Funding from the NIH and the Howard Hughes Institute allowed university faculty to carry out RFLP analyses of isolates identified on cultures.

Study 2.3 illustrates how using novel methodologies in basic public health activities can generate knowledge that has significance beyond the setting where the work was carried out. The unexpected finding that many new TB cases are the result of recent infections provides strong support for attention to compliance with therapy and aggressive contact tracing.

Is the Project Research?

Regulatory definitions. Under HIPAA, protected health information can be disclosed to or used by public health officials without authorization for public health purposes. The HIPAA regulations do not define what constitutes public health. Under the Common Rule, an activity is not research if it is not designed "to develop or contribute to generalizable knowledge." However, this definition of research may be difficult to apply to particular public health projects.

Design or intent of a project. The Common Rule defines research in terms of the design of a project. The primary goal of public health is to prevent or control disease and improve the health of communities, not to discover generalizable knowledge. However, Study 2.3 was also designed to assess the value of molecular epidemiology in investigations of TB outbreaks. The implication was that the finding that molecular epidemiology can identify connections between cases that seemed unrelated after a conventional outbreak investigation would generalize to other cities.

IRBs often operationalize the regulatory definition of research by asking whether the results of an empirical project will be published. The investigators in Study 2.3 clearly planned to do so, hence by this criterion it would be considered research.

Methodology. Some argue that public health may be distinguished from research because it involves the implementation of standard or proven strategies and interventions rather than the discovery of new ones (12). However, as illustrated in Study 2.3, it may be useful for public health officials to try novel methods during outbreak investigations.

Views of stakeholders. From the point of view of the funding agencies, Study 2.3 was a research project. The NIH and Howard Hughes Institute fund research; they do not support public health practice. Medical journals view themselves as publishing research and therefore commonly require that every submitted study have IRB approval or a waiver.

Thus, different criteria yield different conclusions, but it would be reasonable to conclude that the project has characteristics of both public health practice and research. Note that if the project were considered research, it would not be considered human subjects research if the identity of the participants could not be readily ascertained by the investigators (see Chapter 6).

Should Informed Consent be Required?

As noted above, public health officials have the power when carrying out epidemiologic investigations of reported diseases to require persons to be interviewed, examined, and evaluated, and to provide specimens for testing. Even if Study 2.3 were considered research, informed consent would not be required because the data and specimens are not identifiable.

Should the Project Receive Independent Review?

If Study 2.3 were deemed to be public health practice and not research, it would not require IRB review. However, some projects designated as public health practice are so ethically sensitive that it may still be desirable to have some type of external ethical review. Public health officials should clarify ethical principles for public health practice. Regardless of whether an activity is regarded as public health practice or research, public health officials need to address the ethical concerns in public health practice. Ethical standards should include minimizing risks to persons from whom data are collected, protecting confidentiality, treating subjects with respect, and applying public health regulations fairly across subgroups of the population (9,13,14).

Some types of public health practice, such as surveillance, outbreak investigations, and field epidemiology may share characteristics with research (10). These activities may use the same methodologies as research, such as interviews and laboratory testing, and raise similar ethical concerns regarding privacy and confidentiality. Whether an activity is regarded as public health practice or research, ethical standards should be followed, including minimizing risks, protecting confidentiality, and treating subjects with respect.

OTHER ACTIVITIES

Research is also distinguished from other activities in which information is gathered from individuals, such as news reporting and public opinion polls. These activities produce information about a specific event or time, but do not generate generalizable knowledge. Furthermore, these activities are very low risk. They pose little threat to the participants' autonomy because they are a familiar part of daily life and can easily be refused or terminated.

WHAT ETHICAL PRINCIPLES SHOULD GUIDE HUMAN PARTICIPANTS RESEARCH?

The 1979 Belmont Report identified three ethical principles to guide research with human participants (15):

Respect for persons requires researchers to "give weight to autonomous persons' considered opinions and choices." Autonomous individuals who are capable of deliberating about personal goals and acting upon them "should be given the opportunity to choose what shall or shall not happen to them." Hence, research participants must give informed and voluntary consent. Chapter 6 discusses informed consent in detail.

However, not all people are capable of self-determination, such as children, persons whose mental faculties are incapacitated by illness, or prisoners whose liberty is severely restricted. However, persons who lack decision-making capacity must still be respected; researchers should protect them by honoring their objections and by seeking the permission of appropriate surrogates. The degree of protection needed will depend on the risk of harm and the likelihood of benefit. Chapter 16 discusses research with persons whose decision-making capacity is impaired.

Beneficence requires researchers to protect the participants' well-being. Often participants will be exposed to risks during research projects. The ethical dilemma is "to decide when it is justifiable to seek certain benefits despite the risks involved, and when the benefits should be foregone because of the risks." More specifically, researchers should ensure that the risks and likelihood of benefit are proportionate and should minimize the risks of research. Both the probability and magnitude of harm and benefits need to be considered. Chapter 5 discusses how to assess the benefits and risks of research.

Justice requires that the benefits and burdens of research be fairly distributed. Certain vulnerable persons, such as ethnic minorities, poor or uninsured persons, or persons confined to institutions, should not be systematically selected as research participants simply because they are readily available or easy to manipulate. Also research participants should not be selected primarily from populations that are highly unlikely to receive the therapeutic benefits anticipated from the research. Some studies carried out in resource-poor countries have prompted allegations of exploitation. In response, some have urged researchers to provide fair benefits to the communities where research participants are recruited. Chapters 20 and 22 discuss how researchers should address concerns about justice when carrying out research with ethnic or minority populations or in resource-poor countries.

Subsequent chapters specify how these general ethical principles should be applied and interpreted in various research situations.

EMERGING ETHICAL ISSUES

Emerging ethical issues will require the attention of investigators and oversight bodies.

THE SHIFT FROM PROTECTION TO ACCESS

Historically, participants in clinical research have been viewed as serving as guinea pigs, undergoing risky procedures without personal benefit (see Chapter 1). Recently, however, some patients with serious medical conditions have begun to view clinical trials as a means of gaining access to promising new therapies. Early in the HIV epidemic, the only way to get antiretrovirals was through clinical trials. Rather than wanting to be protected from the risks of research, many patients want to gain greater access to research and newer medications. Similarly, patients who have received an organ transplant may press to join clinical trials of new immunosuppressive drugs that might be more effective or less toxic than the current therapy. Under these circumstances, justice is viewed not as preventing exploitation of vulnerable groups but as providing equitable access to the benefits of research.

This new perspective on clinical trials means that investigators and IRBs may be under pressure from patients and their advocates to move new drugs into clinical trials more rapidly. There is an ethical tension between carrying out important clinical trials expeditiously and rushing into a clinical trial without appropriate evidence of safety and proof of principle.

THE CHANGING LOCATION OF CLINICAL TRIALS

The location of clinical trials has dramatically changed in the past decade. The site of clinical trials has shifted away from academic health centers (AHCs) to contract research organizations (CROs). In 2003, CROs played a substantial role in 64% of clinical trials (compared to 28% in 1993) (16).

The majority of clinical trials now are being conducted by CROs, for-profit companies to whom pharmaceutical companies outsource clinical trials. Typically, the sponsor writes the protocol and the CRO finds sites, enrolls participants, carries out the trial, and sends the data to the sponsor for analysis. CROs are usually more efficient at running clinical trials than AHCs, which reduces the cost and duration of clinical trials. CROs may subcontract with site-management organizations (SMOs) to recruit practice-based physicians to clinical trials and to provide administrative support to help physicians enroll participants and collect data. SMOs also are typically for-profit organizations.

Clinical trials also have increasingly moved away from the United States to overseas sites. In 2008, 45% of clinical trials registered on the website www.ClinicalTrials.gov were conducted outside the United States. This shift is driven by lower costs and faster recruitment of trial participants in China, India, and Eastern Europe.

These changes in the location of clinical trials raise ethical concerns regarding the quality of informed consent and IRB review, as well as conflicts of interest. Many resource-poor countries lack both a tradition of informed consent in clinical care and an infrastructure of experienced IRBs. A U.S. IRB may have little sense of the actual conditions in the host country and hence may be in a poor position to assess the recruitment and consent process. Thus, a clinical trial conducted overseas may not receive rigorous IRB review. Furthermore, clinical trials designed by drug manufacturers and carried out by CROs may not receive the same independent scientific peer review as they would at an AHC; however, there are no empirical studies on this issue.

Many private research sponsors follow the Guidelines for Good Clinical Practice of the International Conference of Harmonization, which require informed consent and review by an IRB. However, these international guidelines have no provisions regarding conflicts of interest or training investigators on human subjects protection.

CONCERNS ABOUT CONFLICTS OF INTEREST IN CLINICAL RESEARCH

Currently, about 40% of clinical trials registered with www.ClinicalTrials.gov are sponsored by industry. In a number of recent major clinical trials sponsored by pharmaceutical manufacturers, negative findings have been withheld from publication or delayed until long after the trial concluded (see Chapter 1). In some cases, the university-based researchers who were leading the trial did not have access to complete data or faced restrictions when they sought to publish unfavorable results.

CRITICISMS OF RESEARCH OVERSIGHT IN THE U.S.

A variety of specific criticisms of IRBs have been raised (17). Faced with an increasing number of studies to be reviewed, many IRBs lack the resources and personnel to carry out their tasks. IRB members, who for the most part are volunteers, are hard-pressed to find time to carry out reviews. Deficiencies in policies, procedures, and record-keeping raise further concerns that IRB reviews will be inconsistent. In response to such criticisms, many academic medical centers have increased the number of IRBs and the resources allocated to them. At the same time, investigators complain that IRBs overemphasize bureaucratic requirements, such as documentation and forms, rather than concentrating on serious ethical issues raised by the research. Researchers and research sponsors complain that excessive requirements significantly delay research, waste scarce research dollars, and slow the introduction of new therapies. OHRP responds that without explicit policies and procedures and careful record-keeping, IRBs are open to charges of inconsistent and biased review.

A SYSTEMS APPROACH TO RESEARCH OVERSIGHT

IRBs are sometimes regarded as being solely responsible for protecting research participants. In fact, no single individual or body bears total responsibility for the ethical integrity of research. IRBs cannot oversee day-to-day research activities. Independent data and safety monitoring boards (DSMBs) and institutional compliance officials are in a better position to determine whether a protocol approved by the IRB is being implemented appropriately. Other important actions to protect participants are also outside the scope of IRBs, including training in research ethics and management of conflicts of interest. All of these task bodies should be coordinated (18). Investigators have the ultimate responsibility for ensuring the quality and ethical integrity of their research.

TAKE HOME POINTS

1. Research with human subjects may be hard to distinguish from innovative clinical care, QI, and public health practice.
2. The ethical principles of respect for persons, beneficence, and justice should guide research with human participants.
3. New ethical issues will require attention from investigators and oversight bodies.

ANNOTATED BIBLIOGRAPHY

Fairchild AL, Bayer R. Public health. Ethics and the conduct of public health surveillance. *Science* 2004;303:631–632.
    Analysis of ethical issues in public health surveillance.
Lynn J, Baily MA, Bottrell M, et al. The ethics of using quality improvement methods in health care. *Ann Intern Med* 2007;146:666–673.
    Consensus recommendations on ethical issues regarding quality improvement.

REFERENCES

1. Protection of Human Subjects. 45 CFR 46 (2005). Available at: http://www.hhs.gov/ohrp/humansubjects/guidance/45cfr46.htm. Accessed August 29, 2008.
2. Committee on the Role of Institutional Review Boards in Health Services Research Data Privacy Protection. *Protecting Data Privacy in Health Services Research.* Washington, DC: National Academies Press; 2000:51–70.
3. Pronovost P, Needham D, Berenholtz S, et al. An intervention to decrease catheter-related bloodstream infections in the ICU. *N Engl J Med* 2006;355:2725–2732.
4. Berwick DM. Developing and testing changes in delivery of care. *Ann Intern Med* 1998;128:651–656.
5. Lynn J, Baily MA, Bottrell M, et al. The ethics of using quality improvement methods in health care. *Ann Intern Med* 2007;146:666–673.
6. Miller FG, Emanuel EJ. Quality-improvement research and informed consent. *N Engl J Med* 2008;358:765–767.
7. Lo B, Groman M. Oversight of quality improvement: focusing on benefits and risks. *Arch Intern Med* 2003;163:1481–1486.
8. Kass N, Pronovost PJ, Sugarman J, et al. Controversy and quality improvement: lingering questions about ethics, oversight, and patient safety research. *Jt Comm J Qual Patient Saf* 2008;34:349–353.
9. Fairchild AL, Bayer R. Public health. Ethics and the conduct of public health surveillance. *Science* 2004;303:631–632.
10. Coughlin SS. Ethical issues in epidemiologic research and public health practice. *Emerg Themes Epidemiol* 2006;3:16.
11. Small PM, Hopewell PC, Singh SP, et al. The epidemiology of tuberculosis in San Francisco. A population-based study using conventional and molecular methods. *N Engl J Med* 1994;330:1703–1709.
12. Taylor HA, Johnson S. Ethics of population-based research. *J Law Med Ethics* 2007;35:295–299.
13. Fairchild AL, Gable L, Gostin LO, et al. Public goods, private data: HIV and the history, ethics, and uses of identifiable public health information. *Public Health Rep* 2007;122 Suppl 1:7–15.

14. Myers J, Frieden TR, Bherwani KM, et al. Ethics in public health research: privacy and public health at risk: public health confidentiality in the digital age. *Am J Public Health* 2008;98:793–801.

15. National Commission for the Protection of Human Subjects of Biomedical and Behavioral Research. *The Belmont Report: Ethical Principles and Guidelines for the Protection of Human Subjects of Biomedical and Behavioral Research.* Washington, DC: U.S. Government Printing Office; 1979.

16. Shuchman M. Commercializing clinical trials—risks and benefits of the CRO boom. *N Engl J Med* 2007;357: 1365–1368.

17. Federman DD, Hanna KE, Rodriguez LL, eds. *Responsible Research: A Systems Approach to Protecting Research Participants.* Washington, DC: National Academies Press; 2002.

18. Institute of Medicine. *Responsible Research: A Systems Approach to Protecting Research Participants.* Washington, DC: National Academies Press; 2003.

CHAPTER 3

Federal Regulations on Human Participants Research

F ederal regulations for the protection of human subjects, which were first issued in 1974, are intended to ensure that such research is conducted ethically and that research participants are protected (1). These regulations are technical and complex. This chapter describes their key features, namely, informed consent and review by an institutional review board (IRB). Subsequent chapters discuss in detail how to apply them to specific research studies.

Although the regulations refer to human "subjects," the term "participants" is generally preferred today. Subpart A of the regulations, known as the Common Rule, has been adopted by 17 other federal agencies, including the Department of Health and Human Services (HHS, which includes the National Institutes of Health [NIH] and the Centers for Disease Control [CDC]), the Department of Defense (DOD), the Environmental Protection Agency (EPA), and Housing and Urban Development (HUD). Subparts B, C, and D, which deal with vulnerable populations, have been officially adopted by only HHS and several other agencies. Subpart B deals with research involving pregnant women and fetuses, Subpart C pertains to prisoners, and Subpart D deals with children.

Researchers also need to understand additional federal regulations on health privacy, issued in accordance with the Health Insurance Portability and Accountability Act (HIPAA). These regulations, which are discussed in Chapter 7, require researchers to obtain authorization from patients to use or disclose identifiable health information in research (2–4).

THE COMMON RULE

WHAT RESEARCH IS SUBJECT TO THE COMMON RULE?

The Common Rule applies to research involving human participants that is:

- Funded by or carried out by federal agencies that have adopted the Common Rule.
- Conducted by institutions that have promised that *all* research on human subjects will comply with the Common Rule, including research privately funded or conducted off-site. Almost all universities have agreed to this condition.
- To be submitted to the Food and Drug Administration (FDA) in support of an investigational new drug or device application. FDA regulations are very similar to the Common Rule.

A good deal of human participants research is not subject to the Common Rule (5), such as research that is conducted with private funding at for-profit institutions. However, researchers and institutions may voluntarily comply with the federal regulations even though they are not required to.

TABLE 3.1	Criteria for IRB Review

The IRB must determine that the following criteria are satisfied before it approves a study:

- The risks of the study are minimized.
- Risks are reasonable in relation to the anticipated benefits.
- Selection of participants is equitable.
- Informed consent is obtained.
- Confidentiality is maintained.
- Data are adequately monitored.

HOW IS HUMAN SUBJECTS RESEARCH DEFINED IN THE FEDERAL REGULATIONS?

Activities that fall outside the definition of human subjects research are not subject to the federal regulations and therefore do not require IRB approval or informed consent. Table 3.1 provides a systematic approach to answer this question. Investigators need to understand how the Common Rule defines such key terms such as "research," "identifiable," and "human subjects."

Is the Activity Research?

The Common Rule defines *research* as "a systematic investigation . . . designed to develop or contribute to generalizable knowledge" (1). IRBs often operationalize this definition by asking whether there are plans to disseminate the findings through publications or presentations at professional meetings. Chapter 2 discusses in more detail how human subjects research differs from activities such as innovative clinical care, public health practice, and quality improvement, which are not subject to these regulations.

Does the Research Involve Human Subjects?

Research using data that cannot be linked to individual participants is not human subjects research and thus not subject to the Common Rule.

Human subjects are living individuals about whom an investigator obtains either "data through intervention or interaction with the individual" or "identifiable private information." Interventions include both physical procedures to collect data (for example, venipuncture or questionnaires) and manipulations of subjects or their environment for research purposes (for example, assigning participants to control and intervention groups in a clinical trial). Researchers who collect identifiable information from a review of medical records are conducting human subjects research, even though they never meet or interact with the patients they are studying. Note that dead persons are not considered research subjects.

Private information comprises (i) information that a person can reasonably expect is not being observed or recorded, and (ii) information that has been provided for specific purposes and that "the individual can reasonably expect will not be made public (for example, a medical record)."

Information or specimens are *identifiable* if "the identity of the subject is or may be readily ascertained by the investigator or associated with the information." Suppose a researcher receives coded data or specimens from a health care institution, insurer, biobank, or tissue repository (that is, the researcher knows the participants only as 001, 002, etc.). These data and specimens are not considered individually identifiable if:

- the key that deciphers the code (i.e., links data or specimens to identifying information about the persons being studied) is destroyed before the research begins, or
- the key will not be released to the investigators. For example, the investigators and the holder of the key may agree to this condition, or the institution providing the data or specimens may have a policy prohibiting release of the key to the investigators.

The ethical justification for excluding research that does not involve human subjects from the protections of the Common Rule is that no one can be harmed by the research. The requirements of the Common Rule—IRB approval and informed consent—would impose regulatory burdens without providing any meaningful protection to participants. However, the researcher may still need to submit some information to the IRB. Many institutions do not allow researchers to simply decide for themselves whether their study is human subjects research, but instead require them to provide sufficient information to the IRB to document that their project meets the regulatory criteria. There is another reason why investigators may need to submit information to the IRB about research that does not involve human subjects. Many journals require manuscripts to state that the IRB either approved the project or determined that review was not required.

WHAT RESEARCH IS EXEMPT FROM THE COMMON RULE?

Clinical investigators may wish to avoid an IRB review because it would delay low-risk projects. Thus it is important to understand the situations in which the Common Rule allows exceptions to IRB review.

STUDY 3.1   Questionnaire study.
A neurologist is planning a multisite study to examine the risk factors for poor control of seizures among patients with epilepsy. She has developed a questionnaire and wishes to pilot test it at several of the sites. The questionnaire asks about such issues as the frequency of seizures, adherence to medications, alcohol use, and substance abuse. The researcher wants to carry out this questionnaire study as quickly as possible so that she can gather preliminary information to submit a grant to fund the major study. Because of possible delays in obtaining approval from IRBs at several sites, she asks whether the preliminary study to administer the questionnaire is exempt from IRB review.

Certain types of low-risk human subjects research are exempt from the federal regulations. Therefore, IRB review and consent may not be required. These activities include the following:

Research involving surveys, interviews, observation of public behavior, or educational tests, unless the researcher records information in a manner that allows the subjects to be identified and any disclosure of the subjects' responses "could reasonably place the subjects at risk of criminal or civil liability or be damaging to the subjects' financial standing, employability, or reputation." Hence, questionnaires on such issues as drug addiction, depression, HIV risk behaviors, or illegal immigration would not be exempt.

Research involving existing data, records, or specimens, provided that these are either publicly available or the investigator records information in such a manner that subjects cannot be identified either directly or through identifiers. In Chapter 23, we discuss research involving existing medical records and biological materials in more detail.

Research in educational settings, including research on the effectiveness of instructional techniques or curricula. Examples include research on teaching methods or curricula, such as a study of how students' test scores changed after the curriculum was reformed.

Evaluations of public benefit or service programs that are conducted by or approved by a federal department or agency. This includes studies of procedures for obtaining benefits or services under programs such as Medicaid or Medicare, or studies of changes in methods or levels of payment for benefits.

The implicit rationale for exempting these activities from the Common Rule is that they present such low risks that regulation would be unnecessary and burdensome, while doing little to protect research participants.

STUDY 3.1   (Continued).

The questionnaire in Study 3.1 does not qualify for an exemption from the Common Rule because it asks about use of illegal drugs. If the researcher omitted these questions and any other questions that might cause tangible psychosocial risks if confidentiality were breached, the study would be exempt. Thus the researcher needs to decide how to balance the scientific value of the information obtained from the questionnaire with the time needed to obtain IRB review.

Note that other strategies to avoid IRB review would not be applicable in this study. The researcher could make the responses anonymous, so that no identifiable data are collected. However, the questionnaire would still be research because she interacts with the respondents.

As we discuss later in this chapter, even though the study requires IRB review, it does qualify for expedited review, which might reduce the time needed to gain IRB approvals.

Because obtaining approval from the IRBs at each site may be very time-consuming, the researcher may decide to pilot test only at sites where the IRB review is efficient.

IS INFORMED CONSENT REQUIRED?

A common question is whether a project requires informed consent. Chapter 6 discusses this topic in detail, and Chapter 23 discusses it with regard to research with existing data and specimens.

WHAT MUST INSTITUTIONS DO TO OVERSEE RESEARCH?

The Common Rule establishes several general requirements for institutions that carry out research involving human participants.

First, an institution must establish an IRB to review all research studies involving human participants. Before approving a protocol, the IRB must determine that it meets the criteria discussed below, which include informed consent and assessment of risks and benefits. Chapter 5 discusses risks and benefits, and Chapter 6 discusses informed consent.

Second, the IRB must have written procedures for initial and continuing review, and for reporting to the IRB changes in a research protocol, unanticipated problems involving risks to subjects, and cases in which investigators fail to comply with IRB requirements or federal policies.

Third, the institution must submit a written "assurance of compliance" to the Office of Human Research Protection (in HHS), to comply with the Common Rule and ethical principles. Almost all institutions agree to apply the federal regulations to all research carried out by faculty and staff, even if the research is not funded by a federal agency.

Fourth, the institution must provide to the federal government a list of IRB members and their relationship to the institution.

THE IRB

WHAT IS THE RATIONALE FOR IRBs?

The purpose of IRBs is to protect research participants. A committee that is independent of the research team might identify ethical concerns that the researchers overlooked, or suggest modifications to reduce risks or strengthen informed consent. Furthermore, independent review bolsters public confidence that research is being carried out under careful oversight. The requirement for IRB review does not imply that researchers are unethical or not to be trusted. It is simply human nature that someone with fresh eyes might notice issues that are not evident to people closely involved in a project.

IRBs should be sensitive to local values, expectations, and concerns. The IRB should appreciate whether participants in the study are likely to be vulnerable. For example, participants who have low health literacy may have difficulty reading and understanding consent forms. Also, the IRB should understand what recruitment procedures and levels of payment would be considered acceptable in the communities where participants are recruited. For instance, a city may have established a "living wage" or set the minimum wage higher than federal standards. Moreover, the IRB should pay attention to the investigator's competence and conscientiousness (6).

WHAT ARE THE CRITERIA FOR IRB APPROVAL?

To approve a study, the IRB must determine that it meets all of the criteria summarized in Table 3.1. These issues are discussed in more detail in subsequent chapters.

Risks are Minimized

Research procedures may not unnecessarily expose participants to risk. For example, when possible, the research should use procedures that are already being performed on participants for diagnostic or therapeutic purposes, such as collecting blood samples for a research project during a venipuncture procedure already required for clinical care.

Risks are Reasonable in Relation to the Anticipated Benefits

The risks posed to participants must be reasonable in relation to any anticipated benefits to the participants and to the importance of the knowledge that researchers expect to gain from the research. IRBs may only consider risks and benefits resulting from research procedures, not from interventions that the participant would receive as part of clinical care even if they did not participate in the research. Chapter 5 discusses risks and benefits.

Selection of Participants is Equitable

The IRB must pay particular attention to research involving "vulnerable populations, such as children, . . . mentally disabled persons, or economically or educationally disadvantaged persons." If some or all of the participants are "likely to be vulnerable to coercion or undue influence," the study must have additional safeguards to protect them. Chapter 8 discusses equitable selection of participants.

Informed Consent is Obtained

Each participant, or the legally authorized representative of participants who lack decision-making capacity, must give consent. State law determines who may serve as the legally authorized representative for participants who lack the capacity to give informed consent; generally, this is the person who can legally make clinical decisions for such persons. Informed consent must also be appropriately documented. Chapter 6 discusses informed consent.

Confidentiality is Maintained

Adequate provisions must be made to protect the privacy of the participants and maintain the confidentiality of the data. Chapter 7 discusses confidentiality.

Data are Adequately Monitored

When appropriate, there must be an adequate plan for monitoring the data as it is collected, to ensure the safety of subjects.

WHEN MAY A STUDY RECEIVE EXPEDITED REVIEW?

Under expedited review, a protocol is reviewed by the IRB chair or someone designated by the chair, rather than by the full IRB. An expedited review, as the name suggests, usually takes less time than a full IRB committee review.

STUDY 3.2	Study involving magnetic resonance imaging (MRI).

A researcher is studying the diagnostic value of MRI in patients with shoulder pain. The multisite study will enroll consecutive patients presenting to emergency departments or acute-care clinics with a chief complaint of shoulder pain. The investigators will review clinical data from the medical record. In addition, all patients will receive an MRI examination to look for abnormalities not detected on history and physical exam. The research project will pay for the cost of the MRI exam. The principal investigator, concerned about delays in getting IRB approval at multiple sites, wishes to apply for expedited review. The researcher says, "Everything we're doing has minimal risk and is widely used in clinical care. It's ridiculous to have to wait several months for IRBs to approve the study."

To be eligible for expedited review, a study may present only minimal risk and all study procedures must be in the categories listed in Table 3.2.

The regulatory definition of "minimal risk" is not equivalent to routine clinical care. MRI scans, which are commonly ordered in clinical care, may not qualify as minimal risk (7).

STUDY 3.2	(Continued).

Many physicians might agree with the researcher that this research project involves very low risk and that little is to be gained from full IRB review. According to the federal Office for Human Research Protections (OHRP), MRIs, which do not involve radiation, qualify for expedited review. However, because some people experience anxiety or claustrophobia inside a closed MRI scanner, physicians commonly write orders for mild sedation if needed. Research involving sedation is not considered minimal risk and therefore must receive full IRB review. This example illustrates that some measures researchers propose to reduce risks to participants ironically may make the review process more complicated.

MONITORING OF ONGOING STUDIES BY THE IRB

The IRB needs to know about adverse events occurring during a research project that may change their assessment of the benefits and risks of the study.

WHAT ADVERSE EVENTS MUST BE REPORTED TO THE IRB?

Unanticipated Problems

Investigators must promptly report "unanticipated problems involving risks to subjects or others" to the IRB. Sometimes investigators mistakenly believe that they must report all adverse events in the study to the IRB, resulting in unnecessary paperwork for themselves and the IRB. To reduce regulatory burdens, the federal Office for Human Research Protections has defined unanticipated problems as:

- unexpected, AND
- related or possibly related to participation in research, AND
- suggesting that the risk to subjects is greater than previously known or recognized.

Only events that have all three characteristics need to be reported. These unanticipated problems also need to be reported to any federal agency funding the research and, if the IRB is not at the research institution where the adverse event occurred, to that institution.

TABLE 3.2	Procedures Eligible for Expedited IRB Review
Collection of blood samples by venipuncture	Restrictions related to the health and age of subjects. Collection of blood by finger stick, heel stick, or ear stick also permitted.
Noninvasive collection of specimens	Includes urine, feces, saliva, and buccal swab.
Noninvasive procedures routinely employed in clinical practice	Includes electrocardiograms, echocardiography, and ultrasound. X-rays, sedation, and general anesthesia or sedation are not considered minimal risk.
Research involving data, documents, records, or specimens collected solely for nonresearch purposes	Includes data and samples collected for clinical care. May also qualify for exemption from the Common Rule.
Survey, interview, or focus-group research	Includes other low-risk behavioral science. May also qualify for exemption from the Common Rule.
Collection of voice or video recordings	
Continuing review of previously approved research	Study must be in the data-analysis phase or have completed enrollment and interventions, with only long-term follow-up remaining.
Minor changes in approved protocols	

Responses to Reports

The investigator and IRB might take a number of steps to modify the protocol in response to unanticipated problems, such as modifying the inclusion and exclusion criteria for the study, monitoring participants more closely, changing the consent process for new participants, providing additional information to participants already enrolled in the study, modifying study procedures, or suspending or terminating the study.

Adverse Events

Adverse events are untoward or unfavorable medical outcomes, which may or may not be related to participation in research. In clinical trials, "adverse events" must be reported to the FDA, Data and Safety Monitoring Boards (DSMBs), study sponsors, and, in many studies, to a designated study monitor who tracks adverse events. However, not all adverse events need to be reported to the IRBs—just unanticipated ones related to the research project. The vast majority of adverse events in research are anticipated, such as known side effects of drugs or complications of procedures. Many adverse events are not related to the research, including those caused by progression of the participant's disease or condition. Anticipated adverse events do not need to be reported because the IRB has already taken them into account in reviewing the study.

Some unanticipated problems that must be reported to IRBs are not adverse events. Examples include protocol violations, drug administration errors that cause no adverse consequences, and breaches of confidentiality, such as the theft of a computer containing identifiable information about participants.

MONITORING OF DATA

The Common Rule requires that the research plan "make adequate provision[s] for monitoring the data collected to ensure the safety of subjects." Generally, the IRB is not the appropriate body to monitor data because it cannot determine the frequency of adverse events and, in randomized trials, does not know whether the adverse event occurred in the active or control arm. Thus the IRB cannot judge whether changes to the protocol or the consent process are needed. Depending on the nature of the research, data monitoring may be carried out by the principal investigator, the study sponsor, the coordinating or statistical center, an independent medical monitor, a data monitoring committee (DMC), or a DSMB.

Plans for data monitoring need to be tailored to the nature of the research study. In a minimal risk study, no formal monitoring plan may be needed. However, for a large multicenter clinical trial, a DSMB is usually appropriate, and the protocol should specify what data will be monitored, who will carry out the monitoring, when monitoring will occur, what criteria or stopping rules will trigger responses by the monitoring body, and how regulatory reporting requirements will be carried out. Chapter 26 discusses the analysis of interim data and statistical stopping rules in more detail.

In clinical trials, the study sponsor or the manufacturer of the drug or device being tested might consider information about adverse events to be confidential trade secrets. The nature of the drugs under study or the populations under study may provide valuable information to competitors that would reduce the manufacturer's competitive advantage. However, because unanticipated adverse events can be serious or even fatal, protecting research participants by reporting adverse events should take priority over protecting the interests of sponsors and manufacturers.

MULTICENTER CLINICAL TRIALS

In some multicenter studies, adverse events from other study sites have been reported to the IRB of the principal investigator, resulting in excessive paperwork without advancing the goal of protecting research participants. OHRP has clarified that such reporting is not required. The central DSMB or DMC is the appropriate body to receive adverse event reports. If this central monitoring agency judges that an adverse event was unanticipated and that the risks are greater than previously appreciated, it should report the event to IRBs at all study sites and to the IRB of the principal investigator.

CONTINUING REVIEW

The IRB must review research protocols at least annually to decide whether the balance of benefits and risks has changed significantly, and therefore whether the consent process or protocols need to be changed. The IRB should review unanticipated problems from the study, as well as pertinent articles in the literature, that could alter their assessment of risks to subjects.

Continuing reviews may be expedited in certain circumstances. If the original protocol qualified for expedited review, the annual review may also be expedited. Expedited review also is permitted for studies in their final phases if the remaining activities are limited to data analysis or to long-term follow-up of subjects after all participants have been enrolled and all research interventions have been completed.

PRACTICAL SUGGESTIONS FOR IRB SUBMISSION AND REVIEW

KNOW WHAT YOUR IRB REQUIRES

Each IRB has its own procedures, policies, and forms. Generally, these are available on the IRB website. IRBs may have policies that are stricter than the Common Rule. Investigators should be familiar with and follow these local requirements.

ANTICIPATE IRB CONCERNS

The IRB application needs to be written for a general audience. Some members of the IRB are not scientists, and few will be specialists in the area of research. Thus, acronyms and specialist terms need to be defined. Furthermore, the context of the study needs to be explained.

In certain situations, the IRB can be predicted to ask certain questions or raise specific concerns. For example, in a placebo-controlled, randomized clinical trial, the IRB will want a clear justification for the use of placebo and randomization. If an effective treatment for the condition is available, the justification for using a placebo will be particularly scrutinized. Similarly, if the trial is being carried out with vulnerable persons, such as people who are poor or have low health literacy, the targeting of such participants needs to be carefully justified.

ASK THE IRB STAFF QUESTIONS

Experienced IRB staff can help investigators understand what issues and concerns IRB members are likely to raise, what additional information they might require, and how similar cases have been handled in the past. Investigators should enlist the aid of IRB staff to prepare the strongest and most complete application possible, rather than submit an application that is likely to be returned because of insufficient information or unconvincing justification of the study design.

Some investigators fear that if they ask IRB staff questions, their submission will be flagged for heightened scrutiny. They might worry that asking questions will make it more difficult or take longer to receive IRB approval. These fears are seldom warranted; IRB staff have an interest in ensuring that complete and strong submissions are presented to the committee.

GET IT RIGHT THE FIRST SUBMISSION

Having to resubmit a protocol will lengthen the time needed to gain IRB approval. Some principal investigators have the project coordinator or research staff complete the IRB forms and get personally involved only if they need to respond to questions or concerns that the IRB raises. Although delegating responsibility is important, the investigator needs to take responsibility for ensuring that the staff has sufficient training and experience for the materials submitted in their name. If the submission seems sloppy, it may give a bad impression to IRB members with whom the investigator may need to work in other situations. Different parts of the application need to be consistent. There should be no discrepancies between the consent form and the methods section of the protocol. In a clinical trial, the names of the study interventions and study groups should be the same throughout the protocol.

TAKE HOME POINTS

1. The Common Rule generally requires IRB review and informed consent from participants. However, IRB review and informed consent are not required for activities that are not human subjects research or for research that is exempt.
2. Some research qualifies for expedited IRB review.
3. Researchers must report unanticipated problems to the IRB.

ANNOTATED BIBLIOGRAPHY

Gostin LO, Nass S. *Beyond the HIPAA Privacy Rule: Enhancing Privacy, Improving Health Through Research.* Washington, DC: National Academies Press; 2009.
> Consensus report on the impact of the federal health privacy (HIPAA) regulations. Contains a conceptual overview of privacy and confidentiality. Can be accessed through http://www.nap.edu/.

Protection of Human Subjects. 45 CFR 46 (2005). Available at: http://www.hhs.gov/ohrp/humansubjects/guidance/45cfr46.htm. Accessed August 29, 2008.
> Federal regulations on human subjects research, also known as the Common Rule.

REFERENCES

1. Protection of Human Subjects. 45 CFR 46 (2005). Available at: http://www.hhs.gov/ohrp/humansubjects/guidance/45cfr46.htm. Accessed August 29, 2008.
2. Department of Health and Human Services. 45 CFR Parts 160 and 164. Standards for Privacy of Individually Identifiable Health Information. Available at: http://www.hhs.gov/ocr/hipaa/finalreg.html. Accessed December 2, 2008.
3. National Institutes of Health. Protecting personal health information in research: understanding the HIPAA Privacy Rule. 2003. Available at: http://privacyruleandresearch.nih.gov/. Accessed July 28, 2008.
4. Gunn PP, Fremont AM, Bottrell M, et al. The Health Insurance Portability and Accountability Act Privacy Rule: a practical guide for researchers. *Med Care* 2004;42:321–327.
5. National Bioethics Advisory Commission. Ethical and policy issues in research involving human participants. Rockville, MD: National Bioethics Advisory Commission; 2001.
6. Macklin R. How independent are IRBs? *IRB* 2008;30:15–19.
7. Marshall J, Martin T, Downie J, et al. A comprehensive analysis of MRI research risks: in support of full disclosure. *Can J Neurol Sci* 2007;34:11–17.

CHAPTER 4

IRB Review of Human Participants Research

IRB review is a key component of research oversight. Chapter 3 discusses the federal regulations concerning human subjects research, including the standards that a research study must meet to be approved by an IRB. That chapter explains to investigators how the IRB will review their studies. This chapter discusses IRB structure and function, and will be of more interest to IRB members. Several monographs describe in more detail how an IRB should function.

IRB COMPOSITION

As a group, IRB members must have the expertise, experience, and diversity of backgrounds needed to review the typical types of research conducted at an institution. Diversity of backgrounds should include not only areas of scientific or professional expertise but also culture, race, and gender.

At least one IRB member must be concerned primarily with scientific topics. The IRB needs to understand the science underlying the studies it reviews to determine whether the study will yield valid, generalizable knowledge, and whether less risky approaches could be used without compromising the science. Typically, most IRB members are researchers who are familiar with the kinds of research reviewed by the committee.

At least one IRB member must be concerned primarily with nonscientific topics. At least one IRB member must also be otherwise unaffiliated with the institution. These nonaffiliated and nonscientific members are expected to represent the concerns of research participants. According to one study, nonaffiliated and nonscientific members view their role as addressing concerns about consent forms, the safety of participants, vulnerable participants, and recruitment (1). Most reported having positive interactions with scientist IRB members, but most also had some negative experiences, such as when a scientist disrespected them or did not take them seriously. Many nonaffiliated and nonscientific members sometimes felt intimidated in interactions with scientific members of the IRB. These members believed that more training and education in research ethics would allow them to perform their roles more effectively.

IRBs that deal frequently with vulnerable participants should consider including members who are "knowledgeable about and experienced in working with" such persons and issues (2). Such members can help determine whether the proposed recruitment and consent procedures are acceptable and whether psychosocial risks have been identified and minimized.

When the IRB needs additional expertise to address special issues, it may appoint nonvoting ad hoc members.

CRITICISMS OF IRBs

IRBs have received a number of criticisms for their performance (3,4), as discussed later.

IRBs PLACE UNDUE EMPHASIS ON CONSENT FORMS

IRBs allegedly spend an inordinate amount of time reviewing and revising consent forms, without increasing protection for participants. Model consent forms on IRB websites are usually written at or above the 10th-grade reading level, the level that the IRBs themselves usually recommend (5). Many consent forms used in actual projects are written at the reading level of a college graduate (6). In addition, revisions of consent forms by IRBs may actually reduce readability (7). In multisite trials, different IRBs may make inconsistent changes in the wording of consent forms.

IRBs FAIL TO ADDRESS IMPORTANT ETHICAL ISSUES

A review of the scientific merit of the research is usually beyond the expertise of the IRB and is left to the funding agency. Projects funded internally or by for-profit sponsors may not receive any scientific review. IRBs do not typically check whether research is actually carried out in accordance with the approved protocols.

IRBs IMPOSE EXCESSIVE BUREAUCRATIC REQUIREMENTS

Investigators must complete an application form for continuing review, even if the researchers have completed all interactions with participants and are only analyzing data, and no unanticipated problems have occurred. In this situation, there is little to be gained from continuing review, even expedited review. Arguably, it would be a better use of resources for investigators to certify that the conditions have been met to receive an exemption from review; the IRB could then focus on research that poses substantial risks to participants.

IRBs DELAY RESEARCH

Extensive delays in IRB review have been documented in several large multimember studies (8). Furthermore, IRBs vary greatly in the time required to review the same protocol. In one multisite clinical trial involving 39 IRBs, the median time to approval was 104 days, with a range of 31–346 days (7). Similarly, in a genetic epidemiology study involving 31 IRBs, the median time to approval was 92 days, with a range of 13–252 days (9).

REVIEW OF MULTISITE RESEARCH STUDIES IS INCONSISTENT

Carrying out a research study at multiple sites is desirable because it results in shorter, more efficient trials and more generalizable findings. Also, if pivotal trials are conducted in several countries simultaneously, the sponsor can apply to license a new drug in those countries at the same time. However, multicenter trials also present many additional challenges in terms of oversight.

Each local IRB implements federal regulations using its own forms, procedures, and guidelines, and there is no appeal to a higher body. There is considerable variation in the review process from one IRB to another (8). The same study may require full committee review at some sites, but be exempted or receive expedited review at others. Local IRBs differ widely in their assessments of risk and benefit in clinical research (9). Inconsistent reviews by different IRBs lead to delays in finalizing a common protocol (9). Moreover, full review by multiple local IRBs requires duplication of effort, leads to few substantive changes, and places an unnecessary burden on sites that enroll few participants (10).

CONFLICTS OF INTEREST

IRB members should not participate in a review of studies in which they have a conflicting interest, and should expect to provide background information to the committee. The regulations do not define what constitutes a conflict of interest.

A recent survey found that IRB members frequently have conflicts of interest (11); over one-third of the respondents had at least one financial relationship with the pharmaceutical industry during the previous year. Most believed that these relationships were beneficial for reviewing protocols;

15% said that during the past year the IRB had reviewed at least one protocol that was sponsored either by a company with which they had a financial relationship or by a competitor. Responses to conflicts of interest were varied: only 58% of respondents who had such conflicts disclosed them all the time, and 23% never disclosed them. Only 64% said they never voted in such a situation, and 19% said they always voted. The study did not distinguish between different types of relationships. *De minimus* relationships, such as participating in a single meeting or conference, differ markedly from holding a management position in industry.

These findings suggest that IRBs need to clarify what constitutes a conflict of interest. At a minimum, conflicts of interest need to be disclosed to the institution and to other members of the IRB. Furthermore, voting on a protocol sponsored by a company with which the IRB member has an ongoing substantial financial relationship violates the federal prohibition on conflicts of interest.

There may be institutional conflicts of interest in addition to conflicts of interest by individual members (12). A university or research institution has a vested interest in continuing to carry out research, and IRB members may feel a pressure to approve large research projects and to allow colleagues to carry out their work. We next discuss conflicts of interest that occur when for-profit IRBs are concerned about retaining clients.

NEW DEVELOPMENTS

INDEPENDENT IRBs

Some IRBs are not affiliated with a single research institution and have many different research institutions as clients (12). These for-profit IRBs, which charge for their review and pay their members, offer faster review than IRBs at academic health centers, which are less efficient. Compared to academic IRBs, for-profit IRBs have larger staffs, meet more frequently (every week or even more often), have more extensive pre-reviews of protocols by IRB staff, and use more electronic forms.

For-profit IRBs have been criticized for having a fundamental conflict of interest. However, others point out that there is no empirical evidence that independent IRBs provide poorer-quality reviews than IRBs at academic health centers (13). In fact, several for-profit IRBs are fully accredited, and a number of academic health centers outsource some protocol reviews to for-profit IRBs. The Office for Human Research Protections (OHRP) has also asked an independent IRB to re-review studies from academic institutions where OHRP had suspended research.

ACCREDITATION OF IRBs

Accreditation of IRBs may be a less burdensome and more effective and flexible alternative to increased government regulation (4). Accreditation stimulates quality improvement programs and is an indicator of excellence in human subjects protection. A quality improvement approach may focus attention on improving outcomes of the oversight system rather than on complying with regulations for their own sake. The challenge is to devise outcome measures that are appropriate and practical. The Association for the Accreditation of Human Research Protection Programs (AAHRPP) carries out voluntary accreditation of IRBs. This program requires self-assessment, site visits, and evaluation. As of August 2008, over 150 organizations had achieved full accreditation.

SUGGESTIONS

IRBs can take several steps to improve the quality of their protocol reviews and reduce unnecessary burdens on researchers.

USE ELECTRONIC FORMS

Electronic forms reduce paperwork and can expedite the IRB review process. Structured forms can highlight pertinent ethical issues for different types of research and help ensure that an IRB has adequate information for its review. Structured forms can also decrease the likelihood that the IRB will return the application to the investigator for further information. For example, if a waiver of consent or expedited review is requested, the submission form to the IRB could require the investigator to document that the study satisfies each of the regulatory requirements.

REDUCE DUPLICATIVE REVIEWS

In multisite projects, one IRB can take the lead in the review so that other institutions can choose not to carry out a full review. By reducing duplicative reviews, IRBs can shorten the review process without compromising the safety of participants. The OHRP and FDA have both clarified that federal regulations permit joint review, reliance on another IRB, and similar arrangements to avoid duplicative review.

Central IRBs

The National Cancer Institute (NCI) Centralized IRB Initiative (CIRB) reviews multisite clinical trials carried out by cooperative cancer groups. The CIRB provides facilitated reviews. A national IRB whose members have appropriate ethical, legal, and scientific expertise carries out in-depth reviews. For a particular study, local IRBs can download a Facilitated Review Packet that contains the detailed CIRB review, minutes, and correspondence with investigators. With this information, the local IRB may choose to require full local IRB review for any study, or it may accept CIRB review. Local IRBs always maintain a role in determining whether the local context requires minor changes in the protocol or consent form, and in ensuring that the local researchers are qualified to carry out the research and receive adequate training in human subjects protection. If CIRB review is accepted, the local IRB may still make additions to the consent form or minor changes in wording, but may not delete parts of the consent form. As of December 2006, over 4300 protocols had been submitted by the CIRB to local IRBs. A similar centralized IRB system introduced in the United Kingdom faced procedural difficulties, mostly because local research ethics committees were unwilling to defer to a centralized authority (14). More information on the CIRB is available on its website: http://www.ncicirb.org/CIRB_Project.asp.

The Biomedical Research Alliance of New York (BRANY) was started by the New York Academy of Medicine to facilitate review of multisite clinical trials. It includes over 160 hospitals and practices nationwide. The IRB is drawn from the chairs and vice-chairs of IRBs at academic centers and meets every week.

Cooperative Arrangements

One IRB in a multicenter trial may take the lead in reviewing the protocol, with other IRBs deferring to its review while retaining the ability to address local concerns. The Multicenter Academic Clinical Research Organization (MACRO) is a consortium of five academic health centers that have agreed to cooperate in IRB review of clinical trials.

INCREASE COMMUNITY REPRESENTATION ON IRBs

Greater representation of nonscientists and community members on IRBs may help ensure that the perspectives and concerns of research participants and vulnerable communities are appropriately considered (15). Lay and noninstitutional IRB members may identify unappreciated risks in the study and problems with the consent process, as well as suggest how to ameliorate them. Having a larger number of community representatives on an IRB may help them overcome a sense of isolation and thus more effectively articulate their concerns. Experience with Community Advisory Boards in international HIV prevention trials has demonstrated that representatives from low-income communities can be trained to understand complicated research protocols and can provide constructive suggestions (16).

ENSURE HIGH-QUALITY REVIEWS

IRB reviews can be made more rigorous in several ways (12). IRBs can discourage "IRB shopping," in which investigators whose protocols have been rejected by one IRB resubmit it to another IRB rather than making the required changes. In addition, IRBs should take into account the competence, conscientiousness, and record of the investigators. It makes sense to give more careful review to protocols submitted by researchers whose work has raised concerns in the past. Finally, IRBs should ensure that the science has been reviewed by peers. If there is no scientific merit in the study or the study design will not yield valid results, it is hard to justify any risk or inconvenience to participants.

TAKE HOME POINT

1. IRBs need to address the concerns raised by critics and try to reduce administrative burdens on researchers while focusing on their mission to protect research participants.

ANNOTATED BIBLIOGRAPHY

Emanuel EJ, Lemmens T, Elliot C. Should society allow research ethics boards to be run as for-profit enterprises? *PLoS Med* 2006;3:e309.
   Pro and con articles on independent IRBs.
Macklin R. How independent are IRBs? *IRB* 2008;30:15–19.
   Analyzes different ways in which the independence of IRBs can be compromised.

REFERENCES

1. Sengupta S, Lo B. The roles and experiences of nonaffiliated and non-scientist members of institutional review boards. *Acad Med* 2003;78:212–218.
2. Department of Health and Human Services. Protection of Human Subjects. 45 CFR Part 46 (1991).
3. Office of the Inspector General. Institutional Review Boards: Their Role in Reviewing Approved Research. Washington, DC: Department of Health and Human Services; 1998.
4. Federman DD, Hanna KE, Rodriguez LL, eds. Preserving Public Trust: Accreditation and Human Participant Research Protection Programs. Washington, DC: National Academies Press; 2001.
5. Paasche-Orlow MK, Taylor HA, Brancati FL. Readability standards for informed-consent forms as compared with actual readability. *N Engl J Med* 2003;348:721–726.
6. Advisory Committee on Human Radiation Experiments. Final Report. New York: Oxford University Press; 1998.
7. Burman W, Breese P, Weis S, et al. The effects of local review on informed consent documents from a multicenter clinical trials consortium. *Control Clin Trials* 2003;24:245–255.
8. Greene SM, Geiger AM. A review finds that multicenter studies face substantial challenges but strategies exist to achieve institutional review board approval. *J Clin Epidemiol* 2006;59:784–790.
9. McWilliams R, Hoover-Fong J, Hamosh A, et al. Problematic variation in local institutional review of a multicenter genetic epidemiology study. *JAMA* 2003;290:360–366.
10. Christian MC, Goldberg JL, Killen J, et al. A central institutional review board for multi-institutional trials. *N Engl J Med* 2002;346:1405–1408.
11. Campbell EG, Weissman JS, Vogeli C, et al. Financial relationships between institutional review board members and industry. *N Engl J Med* 2006;355:2321–2329.
12. Macklin R. How independent are IRBs? *IRB* 2008;30:15–19.
13. Emanuel EJ, Lemmens T, Elliot C. Should society allow research ethics boards to be run as for-profit enterprises? *PLoS Med* 2006;3:e309.
14. Tully S. The party's over. *Fortune* 2000;26:156.
15. National Bioethics Advisory Commission. *Ethical and Policy Issues in Research Involving Human Participants.* Rockville, MD: National Bioethics Advisory Commission; 2001.
16. Morin SF, Maiorana A, Koester KA, et al. Community consultation in HIV prevention research: a study of community advisory boards at 6 research sites. *J Acquir Immune Defic Syndr* 2003;33:513–520.

CHAPTER 5

Assessment of Risks and Benefits

Risks and benefits must be acceptably balanced in human participants research. Although the assessment of risks and benefits is important in clinical care, it is even more critical in research. Clinical care has safeguards to protect patients from unacceptable risks. The treating physician plays the role of acting in the patient's best interests and ensuring that the benefits of an intervention outweigh the risks. Furthermore, the patient who assumes the risks personally benefits from care. These safeguards are not present in research. Researchers are primarily trying to obtain generalizable knowledge, not acting in the individual participant's best interests. Moreover, the outcomes of research are unknown.

The Common Rule requires that risks must be minimized and appropriate in light of the anticipated benefits of research. The nature, probability, and magnitude of both benefits and risks need to be assessed. Because value judgments are inevitable, researchers, participants, and the public may disagree on how to assess the risks and benefits of a study.

BENEFITS OF CLINICAL RESEARCH

The following study illustrates how people may disagree over how to characterize the benefits of a study (1).

STUDY 5.1   Phase I cancer trial.

In a multicenter Phase I study, researchers are studying a new experimental cytotoxic agent for glioblastoma. To be eligible, participants must have failed front-line therapy for this cancer. Expected side effects include nausea, vomiting, and bone marrow suppression. Twelve participants will be enrolled. The initial dose is the equivalent of 50% of the target dose, which is the maximally tolerated dose in animal models, adjusted for body size. If the first three patients do not experience dose-limiting toxicity, the dose will be increased to 75% of the projected target dose. If the second cohort of three participants also experiences no dose-related toxicity, the third cohort will receive 100% of the target dose. The dose for the fourth cohort will be 125% of the target dose. If at any level one participant experiences dose-related toxicity, an additional participant will receive that dose. If at any dose two participants experience toxicity as a result of the study, the trial will terminated and that dose will be considered the dose for a Phase II study.

The IRB at one site approved a consent form that stated, "Personal benefit cannot be guaranteed. The hope is that we can improve your symptoms and prolong your life with this treatment." A consent form approved by an IRB at another site stated, "You should not expect to gain any benefit from taking part in this study. We hope the information learned from

STUDY 5.1   (Continued).

this study will benefit future patients with a malignant brain tumor."
Study 5.1 raises several issues:

- What are the benefits and risks of a clinical trial?
- How should these benefits and risks be described to participants?

Phase I trials are needed to determine the safety and appropriate dosing of new drugs. However, Phase I cancer trials raise several ethical questions regarding risks and benefits.

WHAT ARE THE BENEFITS AND RISKS OF PHASE I CANCER TRIALS?

Several questions will help investigators and IRBs evaluate the benefits and risks of Phase I cancer clinical trials.

What is the Magnitude and Scope of Benefits and Risks?

Some types of Phase I trials offer participants a small probability of direct benefit. Overall, 10.6% of participants in recent Phase I cancer trials had a complete or partial response to the drug (2). The response rate varied by the type of investigational agent administered. With a single new cytotoxic agent, the overall response rate was 4.4%. With a combination of investigational and FDA-approved agents, the overall response rate was higher: 16.4%. For other types of investigational agents, the response rate was somewhat lower: 3.2% for receptor or signal transduction agents administered as a single agent, 3.4% for vaccines, and 3.9% for single antiangiogenesis agents. The overall toxic death rate in Phase I cancer trials was 0.49%.

What is the Clinical Significance of the Prospective Benefits?

Phase I cancer clinical trials commonly evaluate whether the size of a tumor has decreased (the so-called "objective response"). In some studies, stabilization of the tumor size may also be considered a response. An objective response may be partial or complete, long lasting, or short-lived. A short-term partial response in a Phase I clinical trial may be sufficient evidence to justify further clinical trials. However, it might not be associated with a clinically meaningful outcome, such as a decrease in symptoms or prolongation of survival. The limited nature of these benefits is particularly significant because most participants in Phase I cancer trials overestimate them.

How do the Risks and Benefits Vary in Different Treatment Groups?

The dose of a new cytotoxic agent that produces the optimal biologic response is likely to be close to the maximum tolerated dose. In many Phase I studies of new cytotoxic drugs, as in Study 5.1, the first several participants receive doses well below the maximum tolerated dose. These early participants who receive the lowest dose have less likelihood of toxicity, but also less likelihood of benefit.

What are Appropriate Comparison Interventions?

Because participants have decided to continue disease-oriented treatments rather than seek solely palliative care, the appropriate comparison is with off-label uses of FDA-approved cancer therapy (3). One review concluded that "it is difficult to argue convincingly that the risks and direct benefits of phase I trials are unfavorable when compared with those of the relevant alternatives" (3). Furthermore, participants enrolled in clinical trials commonly have better outcomes than patients receiving the same regimen in ordinary clinical care. Although this may be a result of the closer attention paid to dosage and monitoring, it may also be a "volunteer effect," that is, participants in clinical trials may have better outcomes than persons who are eligible but do not enroll, because the participants have better functional status or more active and effective coping styles.

TYPES OF BENEFIT
Direct Benefits

These are benefits to participants that are intended by the study design. For example, a Phase II/III clinical trial is designed to determine whether an experimental intervention has greater effectiveness, fewer adverse effects, more convenience, or less cost than the control intervention. Thus participants in the trial have a prospect of direct benefit. To be sure, not all participants will receive the study intervention. However, if the arms of the trial are in equipoise, there is no conclusive evidence that one arm is superior to the other, and there is uncertainty or serious disagreement over which arm is superior (see Chapter 17). Thus it cannot be said at the onset of an ethically designed randomized controlled trial (RCT) that participants in the active arm are more or less likely to receive direct benefit than individuals in the control arm.

In some types of research, such as survey research and research with existing medical records and outcomes research, there is no direct benefit to participants.

Collateral Benefits

Participants can receive collateral benefits by taking part in a study, whether or not they receive the experimental intervention (4). They are also called inclusion benefits or indirect benefits. Examples include more personal attention, closer follow-up and monitoring, or greater attention paid to the timing and dosage of therapies, which might lead to improved clinical outcomes even if the study intervention is no more effective than standard care (5,6). Another collateral benefit might be screening tests to determine eligibility or additional or more frequent tests to determine outcomes. However, more tests may not necessarily be a clinical benefit even though they might unexpectedly reveal a serious condition; if they would not be recommended in ordinary care, there are problems with false-positive results and low predictive value (7).

Collateral benefits must be considered carefully when evaluating the balance of benefits and risks in a research study (4). Although it is desirable for researchers to spend time with participants and give them close attention, it is ethically problematic if the amount of time and attention in ordinary clinical care is deficient. Furthermore, a high level of collateral benefits should not be used to justify significant risks that have not been minimized. Moreover, many alleged inclusion "benefits" may not be regarded as beneficial by some participants who consider extra monitoring and study visits intrusive or burdensome.

Hope and Other Psychosocial Rewards

Hope is another potential benefit of clinical trials, particularly for patients for whom no effective therapy is available. Hope is always desirable in medicine, but unrealistic hope can lead to uninformed decisions to participate in clinical trials. Ideally, a participant would realize that although the probability of a meaningful response in a Phase I trial is low, he could still hope, despite long odds, that he would obtain such a response (1,8). Another psychosocial benefit of research is the satisfaction of acting altruistically by contributing to scientific knowledge that might benefit future patients.

Payments

Payments to participants can include reimbursement for out-of-pocket expenses (such as transportation), compensation for time or risk, or an incentive to enroll in the study. IRBs are not permitted to consider payments as a benefit when assessing the risks and benefits of the study.

THERAPEUTIC MISCONCEPTION

Biomedical research has produced dramatic therapeutic advances in cancer, heart attacks, AIDS, and organ transplantation. Moreover, public and disease advocacy groups sometimes view clinical research as a way to gain access to new therapies. Participation in biomedical research may no longer be viewed as serving as a "guinea pig," but rather as an opportunity to receive new treatments (9).

Participants often do not understand how research differs from clinical care. Often they misunderstand the purpose of clinical trials, mistakenly believe that the trial will benefit them personally, and incorrectly believe that the choice of interventions will be based on their individualized needs. This widespread misconception that clinical research is intended to provide direct benefits to participants has been termed the *therapeutic misconception* (10–12). Chapter 6 discusses the therapeutic misconception in more detail.

STUDY 5.1   **(Continued).**

The experimental cytotoxic agent has a small chance of producing a decrease in the size of the tumor. The duration and clinical significance of any response is uncertain. Early participants who receive lower doses should not be expected to have a response.

In summary, the benefits of research are unknown. Most research studies are not intended to provide direct benefits to participants. Researchers must take care not to overstate the benefits of clinical research.

RISKS OF CLINICAL RESEARCH

PHYSICAL HARM

Clinical research sometimes can cause serious harm, even in studies that are believed to be low risk.

STUDY 5.2   **Death of a healthy volunteer in research study.**

Ellen Roche, a healthy 24-year-old volunteer, died during an NIH-funded study on the pathogenesis of asthma. Investigators had healthy volunteers inhale hexamethonium, a ganglionic neural blocker.

The day after Ms. Roche was administered hexamethonium, she began to cough. She developed respiratory failure and required mechanical ventilation in the intensive care unit. She then developed multiorgan failure, and she died after 24 days in the hospital.

An earlier subject in this study had developed cough and mild shortness of breath, which resolved and was attributed to a viral upper respiratory infection. However, the investigators changed the acidity of the solution containing hexamethonium, without informing the IRB. After Ms. Roche was hospitalized, an additional literature search revealed that hexamethonium had been reported to cause pulmonary toxicity.

Hexamethonium was described in the consent form as "a medication that has been given during surgery." However, it is no longer approved by the FDA. The preparation administered in the study was labeled "For laboratory use only. Not for drug, household, or other use." The consent form also understated the risks of the study.

This tragedy and the subsequent suspension of all clinical research at one of the leading medical centers in the country shocked researchers and research institutions (13). This study, which offered no direct benefit to participants, illustrates that serious unanticipated risks may occur in research. Review by appropriate scientific and ethical committees does not guarantee there will be no serious complications. This study was approved in accordance with the rigorous NIH review process. In retrospect, the occurrence of cough in the first participant should not have been attributed to a concurrent viral infection, but should have stimulated the more detailed literature review that found that hexamethonium could cause pulmonary toxicity. It is prudent to consider every unexpected adverse event in the organ system being studied to be a result of the research intervention until proven otherwise.

PSYCHOSOCIAL HARM

In addition to physical risks, research participants may also suffer significant psychosocial risks.

STUDY 5.3   **Epidemiology of hepatitis C.**

After the hepatitis C virus was characterized, researchers proposed a prospective cohort study to determine risk factors and incidence. Persons at high risk for infections transmitted by blood or other bodily fluids, such as injection drug users and persons with multiple sexual partners, would be eligible for this study. Every 6 months, blood samples would be collected for liver function tests, viral hepatitis serologies, and HIV testing. Participants would complete a questionnaire asking about risk factors for liver disease, blood-borne infections, and sexually transmitted infections, such as alcohol use, injection drug use, and sexual behaviors. Participants would receive counseling about substance abuse and HIV prevention, with referrals to services agencies provided as needed.

In Study 5.3, venipuncture presents very little medical risk. Completing a questionnaire also poses very little physical risk. However, the questionnaire will ask about highly private or illegal activities. In a prospective cohort study, identifiers need to be retained to link new data to previous data about a participant. If the confidentiality of such sensitive information is violated, participants might suffer a range of nonphysical harms, including:

- Psychological harm, such as shame or embarrassment.
- Social harm, such as disruption of relationships with friends or relatives, stigmatization, or discrimination.
- Economic harm, such as loss of employment.
- Legal harm, such as prosecution for illegal behaviors such as illicit drug use or commercial sex work.

WEIGHING THE RISKS AND BENEFITS

How can an overall assessment of the risks and benefits of a research study be made? One approach is to classify the study as a whole as either "therapeutic" or "nontherapeutic." Intuitively, it can seem that more risks are acceptable if a research project is "therapeutic" for participants. However, these terms are logically incoherent and best avoided. It makes little sense to classify an entire research project as therapeutic or nontherapeutic because many projects contain elements of each. If the entire study is classified as "therapeutic," some interventions whose sole purpose is to answer the research question may be accepted even though they are inappropriately risky. A better approach is "component analysis," which we discuss next.

COMPONENT ANALYSIS

In any research study, research interventions can be roughly divided into two categories (14). Some components of the protocol may be characterized as being for therapeutic purposes (15) or as having the prospect of providing a direct personal health benefit to participants. Other components may be carried out only to answer scientific questions (15). The risks and benefits of these two components of the research should be analyzed separately.

| STUDY 5.4 | Trial of a new cholesterol-lowering drug. |

A randomized controlled Phase II trial studied whether a new drug to lower LDL cholesterol prevents the progression of coronary artery disease. The experimental drug was compared with a drug currently licensed for elevated cholesterol. Baseline and follow-up coronary angiograms would be obtained. The primary endpoint in this study was progression of disease on angiography. Secondary endpoints were progression of ischemia as assessed by exercise nuclear imaging, and a combined clinical endpoint of coronary death plus myocardial infarction. The study was powered to detect differences in the primary endpoint, not the combined clinical endpoint. Study 5.4 raises several ethical issues:

- *How may invasive procedures that would not be acceptable in clinical care be justified in clinical research?*
- *How can the risks and benefits of different components of a research study be combined into an overall evaluation of the risks and benefits of the study?*

Study 5.4 illustrates several dilemmas regarding the risks and benefits of a research project. Angiography would not be indicated in ordinary clinical care to monitor a patient started on a cholesterol-lowering drug; instead, the patient would be monitored simply by obtaining a repeat cholesterol level. Thus, in this study, angiography was carried out solely to measure outcomes in a rigorous manner. Can an invasive procedure that would be not indicated in clinical care be allowed as part of a research study?

Generally, when a research study offers the prospect of direct benefit to participants, a greater level of risk is permitted than in studies that do not offer such a potential benefit. The possibility of direct, personal benefit justifies greater risk. However, the degree of risk must be appropriate. It is ethically problematic to justify substantial risks from an intervention carried out solely to answer the research question because some other part of the study offers a small prospect of direct benefit. For example, in Study 5.4 it would be unconvincing to argue that because the study drug might reduce heart attacks and mortality, the risks of repeat angiography were justified. Furthermore, it is problematic to justify such risks by collateral benefits, such as additional education or free care for other conditions. Thus, Study 5.4 illustrates the general question of how the risks and benefits of different components of a research project may be combined into a single assessment of whether the balance of risks and benefits is acceptable. Ethics commentators disagree on how best to address this question (14,15). The following sections offer a pragmatic approach.

ASSESS THE BENEFITS AND RISKS OF EACH STUDY INTERVENTION
Interventions That Offer the Prospect of Direct Benefit

Generally, a greater level of risk is allowed for interventions that offer the prospect of direct personal benefit compared to interventions carried out solely for research goals. For the former, the balance of benefits and risks should be comparable to the balance of benefits and risks in standard clinical care. In Study 5.4, the study drug should offer a balance of risks and benefits that is comparable to the balance for drugs used in standard clinical care for the condition. A broad perspective on benefits should be used; for example, the study drug might be somewhat less effective but much easier to administer or less expensive than a standard drug.

In Study 5.4, follow-up angiography offers a very small possibility of providing direct benefit to participants. It is conceivable that a participant might rapidly develop clinically silent critical stenosis of the left main coronary artery, an indication for revascularization. However, this possibility is so remote that in standard clinical practice it would not justify the risks of coronary angiography as a follow-up test after starting a lipid-lowering drug. It would be inconsistent to justify the risk of coronary angiography in a research setting on the basis of such unlikely potential direct benefit to the participant. Not every conceivable benefit to participants justifies an invasive procedure in a research study. If angiography can be justified in Study 5.4, it must be on the basis of the importance of the scientific knowledge gained by its use (compared to other means of assessing endpoints).

Interventions That do not Offer the Prospect of Direct Benefit

In Study 5.4, several study procedures are carried out primarily to answer the research questions in a rigorous manner, such as the follow-up exercise tolerance test and cardiac catheterization. For components of the study that are carried out solely for research purposes, the risks must be reasonable relative to the potential new knowledge to be gained, and must be minimized to an extent consistent with a valid research design (14). The cumulative effect of all such procedures needs to be taken into account. For example, repeat angiography poses a greater risk than a single angiogram.

Criteria that would justify invasive procedures done solely for research purposes include the following: the research question is important, the procedure is essential to answer the research question, alternative study designs that pose lower risks are not scientifically acceptable, the study design is sound, and experienced physicians are carrying out the procedure.

Just because a procedure is widely used in clinical care, for different indications, does not necessarily mean that it is acceptable to answer a research question by conducting a study that offers no countervailing benefits to the participant undergoing the procedures. Participants need to understand that the intervention has serious risks and is being done for research purposes, and that in this situation no direct benefit to them is expected.

STUDY 5.4   **(Continued).**

Several tests will be carried out primarily to answer the research questions. An exercise nuclear imaging study is noninvasive and has low risk when monitored carefully. Thus, its risks are acceptable to answer the research question.

Cardiac angiography is invasive and carries a small but definite risk of death (under 0.1%). The follow-up angiogram raises considerable concerns. Can another, noninvasive method of measuring the study endpoint be used? For instance, would CT angiography be sensitive and reliable enough to detect changes in the cross-sectional area of vessels? In another, similar trial, the risk of angiography was considered unacceptable, and instead Doppler blood flow in the carotid vessels was used as the primary study endpoint.

MINIMAL RISK

The concept of minimal risk plays a pivotal role in the federal regulations concerning human subjects research. The underlying idea is that minimal risk research requires less oversight than riskier research. The Common Rule relaxes oversight of minimal risk research in several ways:

- Minimal risk research projects may be eligible for *expedited IRB review*, rather than full IRB review.
- Informed *consent may be waived or modified* for certain types of minimal risk research.
- In some research that poses greater than minimal risk, vulnerable participants need to receive *more protection*. For example, some types of pediatric research that pose greater than minimal risk may only be approved by a national panel, not by a local IRB.

Although minimal risk is an intuitively appealing concept, it is hard to define precisely. According to the Common Rule:

Minimal risk *means that the probability and magnitude of harm or discomfort anticipated in the research are not greater in and of themselves than those ordinarily encountered in daily life or during the performance of routine physical or psychological examinations or tests.*

Several key terms in this definition are ambiguous. First, does "daily life" refer to healthy individuals or to persons who are eligible for the research study? If a study enrolls persons with a serious illness, they might regularly experience during their clinical care invasive procedures such as intravenous lines, bone marrow biopsy, or lumbar puncture. If minimal risk were defined in terms of individuals who are ill, research participants might receive less protection than healthy persons. However, this interpretation is ethically problematic because persons who already face greater risks in their lives need more protection, not less. Similarly, persons who are socioeconomically disadvantaged may face increased risks in their daily lives, such as violence. It would be ethically problematic to allow them to encounter greater risks in research simply because they are already disadvantaged. Thus, "minimal risks" should refer to the common risks that the general population faces, such as crossing the street, getting a blood test, or answering questions on the telephone (16). Furthermore, the concept of minimal risk involves a normative judgment: society must regard the risk as acceptable, rather than unfortunate or regrettable, as in the case of illness or poverty (17).

The second part of the definition of minimal risk also requires interpretation. "Routine physical examinations or tests" are generally interpreted by IRBs to include studies ordered for annual checkups, such as testing of blood samples obtained by venipuncture, electrocardiogram, or urine analysis. More invasive procedures should not be considered minimal risk, even if they are commonly carried out in patients with the condition being studied.

VULNERABLE PARTICIPANTS

Participants might be especially vulnerable in two ways. First, they might be unable to give free and informed consent, and thus might become research participants without their knowledge or permission. Second, they might be more susceptible to the risks of a specific project. For instance, they might be more likely to suffer adverse events, or the adverse events may be more severe. Vulnerable participants require additional protections, as in the following examples:

STUDY 5.3 and 5.4   **(Continued).**

In Study 5.3, the epidemiologic study of hepatitis C, commercial sex workers are at greater legal risk than other participants because they are engaging in illegal activities. Special care should be taken to protect the confidentiality of highly sensitive information, as we later discuss.

In Study 5.4, the study of a new cholesterol-lowering agent, some participants may be at greater risk for adverse effects of the study drug. For example, if the drug caused liver toxicity in preclinical studies, persons with preexisting liver disease or heavy alcohol intake might be at greater risk and should be excluded from the study.

Chapters 16–22 analyze how prisoners, children, and persons who lack decision-making capacity are vulnerable in research, and suggest what additional safeguards would be appropriate.

DIFFERENT ASSESSMENTS OF BENEFIT AND RISK

Participants and their advocates may weigh the risks and benefits of a study differently from investigators. In some studies, participants who are poor or members of disadvantaged minority groups may regard the risks as more serious than researchers (18).

STUDY 5.5   **Causes of asthma in children.**

Asthma is disproportionately common in inner-city areas that have low incomes, poor housing, and predominantly minority populations. To identify factors associated with asthma and asthma-related disability, researchers are planning a cross-sectional study in which they will collect dust samples from homes and test them for cockroach and dust mite antigens, and inspect the homes for mold. They will also administer questionnaires about respiratory symptoms, their impact on activities, and other triggers of asthma, such as cigarette smoke and pets.

Researchers characterized the physical risks of Study 5.5 as minimal because no invasive proce-dures would be carried out and no drugs would be administered. Community leaders and parents, however, might view the risks more broadly than medical risks. In Study 5.5, home visits entail an invasion of privacy because the researcher cannot help observing information not related to the re-search question. For instance, the researcher may notice that there are more people living in a rented unit than the lease permits. Someone in the household might be carrying out illegal activities, such as injection drug use. These observations might pose legal risks for parents of study participants or lead to recrimination from others in the household.

Furthermore, low-income, predominantly minority populations might object to being targeted for study. Community leaders might allege they are being treated as "guinea pigs," being studied while nothing is done about substandard housing conditions that are already known to cause or ex-acerbate asthma. They also might doubt that the community will benefit from the knowledge gained from the research, based on their experience with previous research projects. They might perceive that the researchers gain publications, grants, and promotions while the participants remain in substandard housing. They might want to know what the researchers will do to improve housing conditions.

Differences in expectations regarding risks and benefits should be explored during the research de-sign process. Researchers should discuss their protocol with community representatives and prospec-tive participants to ensure that they understand the community's concerns and try to address them.

OPTIMIZING THE BALANCE OF BENEFITS AND RISKS

Researchers should take steps to increase the benefits and reduce the risks to research participants. Investigators might use the following items as a checklist when designing a study.

INCREASING BENEFITS TO PARTICIPANTS

Increase Direct Benefits

If an intervention in a clinical trial proves to be effective, it could be provided to all participants who still qualify for it at the end of a clinical trial. In Phase I trials like Study 5.1, more rapid escalation of doses of a new cytotoxic agent or intrasubject dose escalation might make beneficial effects more likely. However, this strategy might also lead to greater toxicity because it is less likely to identify tox-icity that occurs at lower doses.

Increase Collateral Benefits

Researchers can educate participants and their communities about the condition being studied, and offer information about prevention and healthy lifestyles. They can also offer to refer participants for medical treatment that they need.

Provide Findings to Participants and the Community at the End of the Study

Offering to provide the overall results of the study to the participants at the conclusion of the study shows them respect, treats them as partners in research, increases their knowledge of the condition, and promotes community acceptance of the project (18,19). Several empirical studies have found that most participants want to be offered the aggregate findings (20). After an RCT, researchers need to be prepared for possible negative reactions from participants who were in the arm that was found to be inferior. Chapter 11 discusses the related issue of providing individual results from research tests to participants.

DECREASING RISKS TO PARTICIPANTS

Take Steps to Reduce Risks

Persons who are susceptible to adverse events can be identified by conducting screening evaluations and obtaining medical histories from their primary physician. In a Phase I clinical trial, researchers can start with a lower dose of the intervention or raise the dose more slowly. These precautions would be particularly important for studies involving a novel intervention with a radically different mechanism of action that has not previously been studied in humans (21,22). In some Phase I trials, there is a trade-off between safety and benefit: a lower dose may be safer, but may also be less likely to have a beneficial effect.

Monitor for Adverse Events

More frequent or more extensive follow-up evaluations may detect early signs of adverse events. Clinical trials should have formal procedures for monitoring interim data. Phase II/III clinical trials generally have an independent data and safety monitoring board (DSMB) (see Chapter 26).

Have a Plan for Responding to Adverse Events

When adverse events are identified, researchers must take steps to mitigate harm to patients. If an adverse event may be related to a study intervention, the intervention should be stopped. Furthermore, treatment for medical adverse events should be instituted—for example, by having the participant receive care in a clinic or emergency room.

Because serious adverse events may occur unexpectedly, the principal investigator or another senior investigator should be reachable at all times by pager or cell phone. Participants should be removed from the study if necessary to obtain care for a serious adverse event. In a blinded clinical trial, there must be provisions for unblinding if needed to guide a participant's clinical care (see Chapter 26).

Investigators should anticipate discovering that a participant is at risk for serious, imminent harm, such as domestic violence, child abuse, or elder abuse. Even though these conditions did not result from research interventions, investigators have a duty to try to prevent or ameliorate them (see Chapter 10).

Provide Free Care for Adverse Events

If participants require medical care for adverse medical events that are caused by the study agent, it seems fair that the study sponsor, not the participant, should pay for such care (23). Purchasing insurance for such a contingency would allow sponsors to spread the cost of such care. Having to present insurers information about the risks involved would provide an incentive for sponsors to analyze the risks and take steps to mitigate them. Such coverage would be particularly desirable in high-risk studies or first-in-human studies where the risks are uncertain. The state of California requires coverage of medical expenses for complications in another research context, donation of oocytes for stem cell research (24). To exclude coverage for long-term or indirect adverse events whose actuarial risk would be difficult to calculate, coverage is required only for "direct and proximate" complications.

Protect Confidentiality

Breaches of confidentiality may be a serious risk in many studies that involve stigmatizing conditions and sensitive data, such as Study 5.4. Chapter 7 discusses how researchers can strengthen confidentiality protections at each step of the research project (25). Basic safeguards include the following steps:

- *Choose a study name and location that do not stigmatize participants.* The name chosen for the study or the location of the study office should not identify participants as being in stigmatized, high-risk groups.
- *Train staff about why confidentiality is important and how to protect it.*
- *Work with coded or de-identified data, rather than identifiable data, whenever possible.*
- *Have good security precautions,* including locked offices and file cabinets, and password protection and encryption for electronic data. The code for linking data and identifiers should be stored separately from the data set.
- *Obtain a Certificate of Confidentiality* if the research topic or collected data are sensitive.

STUDY 5.5   (Continued).

To maximize the benefit/risk balance, researchers can educate participants and their parents about asthma and offer referrals to asthma specialists for children who have severe or poorly controlled disease. After publishing their research findings, they also can present the results to community groups, such as Parent-Teacher Associations and church groups. Furthermore, researchers can offer to testify at government hearings on housing. To minimize medical risks in this study, the researchers decided not to administer skin testing for sensitivity to dust mites and cockroaches. If a serious allergic reaction occurred in the home, it would be difficult to provide prompt medical attention.

DISCUSSING BENEFITS AND RISKS WITH PARTICIPANTS

Researchers should discuss the risks and benefits of research in ways that minimize participants' misconceptions.

Don't Use Misleading Terms to Explain Benefits

Consent forms in clinical trials often contain terms such as "experimental therapy" or "study treatment." The terms are oxymorons. "Treatment" and "therapy" imply that the experimental intervention is known to be safe and effective. However, the rationale for a clinical trial is that the safety and efficacy of the study drug are not known. Thus, these terms should be avoided.

Researchers sometimes tell participants in a clinical trial that they may or may not benefit from the study, or that personal benefit is not guaranteed. Such statements can be misleading (6). On the literal level, they are simply saying that something might or might not happen. However, participants may infer from the first statement that the chance of benefit is about 50/50, and from the second statement that although the probability of benefit is not certain, it is likely to be high. In Study 5.1, it is better to say, "The goal of this study is to find out what the side effects of the study intervention are and what dose might be used in future research studies. Although it is possible that your tumor may shrink or not grow, this is unlikely." In Study 5.5 (about the epidemiology of asthma), it is more accurate to say, "The goal of the research is to benefit future asthma patients. This study will not improve your child's clinical health." However, it is appropriate to say that some participants have a positive reaction to meeting with study staff and learning about their illness.

Explain the Clinical Significance of Possible Benefits

In Study 5.4, the Phase II trial of a cholesterol-lowering agent, it is possible that the participants in the active arm will receive a direct benefit. The investigators could say, "If you are in the group that receives the study agent, it is possible that the cholesterol deposits in your arteries may get smaller. It is also possible that you will be able to do more exercise." It is important to distinguish surrogate endpoints (improvements in cholesterol levels or angiogram) from clinical endpoints (exercise tolerance).

Group Risks by Likelihood and Severity

The National Cancer Institute (NCI) website suggests that adverse effects in a clinical trial be grouped in the consent form under the headings of "likely," "less likely," and "rare but serious." This grouping helps participants get a comprehensive overview of a complicated study.

Explain That the Outcomes of Research are Unknown

Even with promising preliminary results, the results of research cannot be predicted. The researcher should say, "We do not know whether the study agent will have good effects or not, and we are conducting this research to find out."

Address Common Misconceptions About Research

Because participants commonly believe that research will provide them with personalized care, it is important for researchers to clarify that this is not the case.

Several websites contain useful suggestions for discussing benefits and risks:

- NIH Guidance on Informed Consent for Gene Transfer Research at http://www4.od.nih.gov/oba/rac/ic/.
- National Cancer Institute at http://www.cancer.gov/clinicaltrials/understanding/simplification-of-informed-consent-docs/page3.
- The UCSF IRB at http://www.research.ucsf.edu/chr/Recruit/chrCFformats.asp.

TAKE HOME POINTS

1. The words researchers use in discussing the risks and benefits of research should be chosen to minimize participants' misconceptions. Researchers must be careful not to overstate the benefits of research. Participants tend to overestimate the benefits of research.
2. The risks of clinical research include medical risks, breaches of confidentiality, and psychosocial harm.
3. Vulnerable participants who are at greater risk for adverse events need to be protected.
4. Researchers should take steps to increase the benefits of a research study and decrease the risks.

ANNOTATED BIBLIOGRAPHY

Henderson GE, Churchill LR, Davis AM, et al. Clinical trials and medical care: defining the therapeutic misconception. *PLoS Med* 2007;4:e324.
    Analyzes "therapeutic misconception," showing how both conceptual articles and empirical studies use the term in different ways.
King NMP, Churchill LR. Assessing and comparing potential benefits and risks of harm. In: Emanuel EJ, Grady C, Crouch RA, et al, eds. *The Oxford Textbook of Clinical Research Ethics*. New York: Oxford University Press; 2008:514–526.
    Thoughtful conceptual review of risks and benefits.

REFERENCES

1. King NM, Henderson GE, Churchill LR, et al. Consent forms and the therapeutic misconception: the example of gene transfer research. *IRB* 2005;27:1–8.
2. Horstmann E, McCabe MS, Grochow L, et al. Risks and benefits of phase 1 oncology trials, 1991 through 2002. *N Engl J Med* 2005;352:895–904.
3. Joffe S, Miller FG. Rethinking risk-benefit assessment for phase I cancer trials. *J Clin Oncol* 2006;24:2987–2990.
4. King NMP, Churchill LR. Assessing and comparing potential benefits and risks of harm. In: Emanuel EJ, Grady C, Crouch RA, et al, eds. *The Oxford Textbook of Clinical Research Ethics*. New York: Oxford University Press; 2008:514–526.
5. Churchill LR, Nelson DK, Henderson GE, et al. Assessing benefits in clinical research: why diversity in benefit assessment can be risky. *IRB* 2003;25:1–8.
6. King NM. Defining and describing benefit appropriately in clinical trials. *J Law Med Ethics* 2000;28:332–343.
7. Marshall J, Martin T, Downie J, Malisza K. A comprehensive analysis of MRI research risks: in support of full disclosure. *Can J Neurol Sci* 2007;34:11–17.
8. Bosk CL. Obtaining voluntary consent for research in desperately ill patients. *Med Care* 2002;40:V64–V68.
9. Dresser R. *When Science Offers Salvation: Patient Advocacy and Research Ethics*. New York: Oxford University Press; 2001.
10. Appelbaum PS, Lidz CW. The therapeutic misconception. In: Emanuel EJ, Grady C, Crouch RA, et al, eds. *The Oxford Textbook of Clinical Research Ethics*. New York: Oxford University Press; 2008:633–644.
11. Lidz CW, Appelbaum PS. The therapeutic misconception: problems and solutions. *Med Care* 2002;40:V55–V63.
12. Henderson GE, Churchill LR, Davis AM, et al. Clinical trials and medical care: defining the therapeutic misconception. *PLoS Med* 2007;4:e324.
13. Steinbrook R. Protecting research subjects—the crisis at Johns Hopkins. *N Engl J Med* 2002;346:716–720.

14. Wendler D, Miller FG. Risk-benefit analysis and the net risks test. In: Emanuel EJ, Grady C, Crouch RA, et al, eds. *The Oxford Textbook of Clinical Research Ethics*. New York: Oxford University Press; 2008:503–513.
15. Weijer C, Miller PB. When are research risks reasonable in relation to anticipated benefits? *Nat Med* 2004;10: 570–573.
16. National Bioethics Advisory Commission. *Ethical and Policy Issues in Research Involving Human Participants*. Rockville, MD: National Bioethics Advisory Commission; 2001.
17. Wendler D, Belsky L, Thompson KM, et al. Quantifying the federal minimal risk standard: implications for pediatric research without a prospect of direct benefit. *JAMA* 2005;294:826–832.
18. Lo B, O'Connell ME, eds. *Ethical Considerations for Research on Housing-Related Health Hazards Involving Children*. Washington, DC: National Academies Press; 2005.
19. Partridge AH, Winer EP. Informing clinical trial participants about study results. *JAMA* 2002;288:363–5.
20. Partridge AH, Wong JS, Knudsen K, et al. Offering participants results of a clinical trial: sharing results of a negative study. *Lancet* 2005;365:963–964.
21. Wood AJ, Darbyshire J. Injury to research volunteers—the clinical-research nightmare. *N Engl J Med* 2006;354: 1869–1871.
22. Dowsing T, Kendall MJ. The Northwick Park tragedy—protecting healthy volunteers in future first-in-man trials. *J Clin Pharm Ther* 2007;32:203–207.
23. Steinbrook R. Compensation for injured research subjects. *N Engl J Med* 2006;354:1871–1873.
24. Lomax GP, Hall ZH, Lo B. Responsible oversight of human stem cell research: the California Institute for Regenerative Medicine's Medical and Ethical Standards. *PLoS Med* 2007;4:e114.
25. Panel on Institutional Review Boards, Surveys, and Social Sciences Research. *Protecting Participants and Facilitating Social and Behavioral Sciences Research*. Washington, DC: National Academies Press; 2003.

6

Informed Consent

Free and informed consent is a fundamental requirement of research with human participants. The Nazi "experiments" and the Tuskegee Study (see Chapter 1) caused outrage in
part because no valid consent was obtained. Carrying out research on persons without their
knowledge or permission violates their autonomy, liberty, and dignity. Consent also helps to protect
participants because people may decline to participate in research whose risks they consider unacceptable. Informed consent has several components:

- The researcher must disclose to the participant information about the research project that is
  pertinent to the decision to participate in the study (1). Such information should include the
  proposed procedures, their risks and benefits, and any alternatives.
- The participant must comprehend the disclosed information.
- The participant must have the capacity to make informed decisions.
- Consent must be free and voluntary.

The issue of consent continues to raise ethical dilemmas. First, research participants often
misunderstand the nature of clinical research and specific studies. In clinical care, patients' misunderstandings about their treatment are mitigated because physicians only recommend care that they
believe is in the patient's best interests. In contrast, research procedures primarily benefit society
through the generation of new knowledge; they generally are not intended to directly benefit participants. A common response to concerns that participants do not understand a study is to insert
additional material into the consent form. However, longer consent forms do not ensure that participants understand the study, and might even confuse participants.

A second question is whether there are circumstances in which consent is not required. For
example, much research with existing medical records or specimens poses no medical risks, and it
may be very difficult to contact participants to request consent. However, some participants may be
offended by certain uses of their data or biological materials.

A third issue is how research may be carried out with participants who are incapable of giving
consent, such as children or persons with severe dementia. These issues are addressed in Chapters 16
and 17. The following case illustrates some dilemmas regarding informed consent.

STUDY 6.1   Impact of air pollution on persons with asthma.

*A researcher is studying the impact of air pollution on pulmonary function. The hypothesis is
that levels of pollutants present in the air on a bad smog day might impair the lung function
of persons with asthma. If current levels of pollutants harm persons with chronic lung
disease, air quality standards may need to be tightened.*

*Under this protocol, persons with asthma will inhale in the laboratory particulate matter
equivalent to what is present in the air on a bad smog day. The participants' exercise tolerance*

STUDY 6.1   (Continued).

will be assessed through a treadmill test, which will be monitored by a physician. A subset of participants will also undergo bronchoscopic lavage to assess markers of lung inflammation after the exposure to pollutants. Participants will not take their usual asthma medications on the day they are studied. The consent form says, "One benefit of the study is information on whether your health may be adversely affected by air pollution. This information could influence decisions on whether to reside in a city with high levels of air pollution."

This study raises several questions regarding consent.

First, should participants be informed of rare but serious risks? For instance, bronchoscopy carries a very small risk of death.

Second, should participants be informed how the research procedures differ from standard clinical care? On bad smog days asthma patients are advised to stay indoors, take their medications, and not exercise.

Third, what claims may be made regarding the benefits of participating in such research?

In this chapter, we first describe what information researchers must disclose to participants. Second, we suggest how researchers can improve the consent process and participants' comprehension of essential information. Third, we analyze how consent may be compromised by undue influence and suggest how researchers can avoid undue inducements. Finally, we discuss situations in which consent is not required from research participants.

As discussed in Chapter 3, the Common Rule, which is the first part of the federal regulations for the protection of human research subjects, applies to virtually all research carried out in academic health centers and universities. Its main provisions concern IRB review (discussed in Chapter 4) and informed consent, which is discussed here. In addition to the Common Rule, the Health Insurance Portability and Accountability Act (HIPAA) Health Privacy regulations have provisions regarding informed consent that differ from those in the Common Rule, particularly regarding exceptions to the consent requirements.

THE INFORMED CONSENT PROCESS

WHAT INFORMATION MUST RESEARCHERS PROVIDE TO PARTICIPANTS?

Table 6.1 presents the information that the Common Rule requires researchers to provide participants, in language they can understand. If relevant to the study, additional information must also be provided, including any possibility of unforeseeable risks or financial costs to participants.

TABLE 6.1   Information Researchers Must Provide Participants

- The fact that the study involves research, and the purpose of the research.
- Research procedures, risks and discomforts, benefits, and alternatives. Experimental procedures must be identified as such.
- How confidentiality will be maintained.
- The fact that participation is voluntary and may be discontinued at any time.
- Whom to contact with questions about the study or the rights of participants.
- If the research involves more than minimal risk, what treatments and compensation are available if injury occurs.

The Common Rule generally requires that participants sign consent forms to document that informed consent has been obtained. The consent form needs to contain all of the above information. Alternatively, a short consent form may be used, which states that the required elements of informed consent have been presented orally. If a short form is used, there must be a witness to the oral presentation, and both the witness and the participant must sign it.

WHAT ARE SOME PROBLEMS WITH INFORMED CONSENT?

IRBs carefully review how information is disclosed in consent forms. Despite these efforts, many participants in research studies—perhaps the majority in some studies—have serious misunderstandings about important aspects of the research protocols (2–6).

Participants Often do not Understand the Purpose of the Research

Participants in Phase I cancer clinical trials usually expect that they will personally benefit from the trial, even after they are told that the primary purpose of Phase I trials is to test the safety and determine the dosage of an experimental agent (7). Furthermore, participants often do not understand how clinical trials differ from standard treatment. According to one study, 48% of participants in cancer clinical trials believed that all of the treatments and procedures in the clinical trial were standard therapy for their type of cancer (7). Thirty-eight percent believed that the clinical trial did not carry any additional risks or discomforts compared to standard treatments, while 29% believed that the treatment being studied was proven to be the best treatment for their type of cancer (7).

This failure to understand the differences between clinical research and ordinary clinical care has been termed "therapeutic misconception" (8,9). More specifically, participants might believe that the choice of interventions in the study will be based on their needs and interests or might overestimate the direct benefit they will receive from the study (10). This misunderstanding occurs in many kinds of research, not just cancer research (10). Some research participants cannot imagine physicians in a research study doing anything that is "not in their best interests" (4). A lively debate regarding the "therapeutic misconception" has been hampered because people define the term in different ways (9,11–13).

Participants Commonly Misunderstand Essential Features of the Research Design

Participants in clinical trials commonly do not understand that they may be in a control group rather than the intervention group, and that being in a clinical trial may restrict their therapeutic options (8). Randomization is also frequently misunderstood (14). In one study of leukemia clinical trials, researchers found that 50% of the parents did not understand randomization (14). However, a crucial difference between a randomized clinical trial and clinical care is that the intervention is determined by chance rather than by an individualized judgment of what is best for a particular patient.

IRBs Emphasize Consent Forms Rather Than Consent Discussions

Although IRBs spend considerable time reviewing and revising consent forms, significant problems still remain. Model consent forms posted on IRB websites are usually written above the 10th-grade reading level, which is the level that the IRBs themselves recommend (15). Many consent forms used in actual research projects are written at the reading level of a college graduate (4). In addition, revisions of consent forms by IRBs can actually reduce readability and thus fail to improve the consent process (16).

EMPIRICAL STUDIES ON IMPROVING COMPREHENSION

Misunderstandings are especially troubling in research studies that are controversial, complicated, highly innovative, or risky. Examples include some Phase I clinical trials and HIV prevention trials in resource-poor countries, where allegations of lack of consent have halted studies. How can investigators improve participants' comprehension of relevant information? Empirical studies provide some suggestions.

Spend More Time Talking With Participants

This intervention has the strongest empirical support and may be more effective than efforts to improve consent forms or develop multimedia presentations (17,18). Participants commonly report that discussions with research staff are more useful than consent forms (17). Additional measures to enhance discussions include giving the potential participant information to take home, and having a relative or friend present during the discussion. These interactions allow tailored discussions that address the needs and concerns of the individual participant.

Questions and Feedback

Participants can be tested on their understanding and given additional information on topics they do not understand (17). However, skeptics point out that if participants are asked the same questions after receiving more information, improved scores might indicate rote memorization rather than true understanding (18).

Simplify Consent Forms

Researchers might improve consent forms by making them shorter and more readable, using plain language with clearer formatting, and adding graphics (18,19). Specific suggestions include using familiar rather than technical terms, using shorter words and sentences, using bullet points to break up long explanations, and using readability checkers in word-processing programs (20). However, studies evaluating improved consent forms have not shown consistent improvements in understanding; the effects of these improvements might be attenuated because face-to-face discussions between the investigator and the participant also occur (18). Simplified consent forms must include all the information prescribed in federal regulations. Another option is a stepwise consent process in which participants are first given basic information about the research and then provided with more details only after they understand this key information.

Multimedia interventions, such as videotapes or CDs, do not consistently enhance participants' understanding of clinical trials, even though they may improve patients' comprehension in clinical care (18,21). It is possible that multimedia presentations do not add much to the information already required in consent forms or presented in discussions (18).

Use Multicomponent Interventions

Multiple interventions may be more effective than single interventions. In one project, researchers set the reading level of the consent form at the eighth grade, enhanced the visual display of consent documents, made an audiotape of the consent form for low-literacy participants, had educators independent of the research team discuss the project with participants, and provided opportunities for participants to ask questions (22). This intervention improved their understanding of key concepts about a hypothetical HIV vaccine trial.

In another multipronged innovation, the National Cancer Institute (NCI) developed a simplified informed consent form written at the eighth-grade level, using a question-and-answer format and graphics such as flow charts, diagrams, and calendars (23). In a cross-sectional study, participants in cancer trials who received the simplified NCI form, had a nurse present at the consent discussions, and had more time to deliberate had greater understanding about the research than control participants (7). These results highlight the idea that informed consent should be viewed as a process or an ongoing dialogue between researcher and participant, rather than as a legal document to be signed (24).

HOW CAN PARTICIPANTS' COMPREHENSION BE IMPROVED?

Although there is limited empirical evidence on how to improve comprehension, several rules of thumb might help researchers inform participants more effectively.

Design the Consent Process From the Participant's Point of View

People need to know information that will be pertinent to their decision to participate in the study or not. They want to know what will happen to them if they agree to participate in the study—for example, how often they will need to come in for visits, what procedures will be done, etc.

Use Simple Language That Laypeople can Understand

Avoid scientific and legal jargon. Keep sentences short. Use a sixth- to eighth-grade reading level. Many word-processing programs can check the reading levels of documents. Pretest consent forms on people who are not college graduates.

Disclose Serious but Rare Risks of the Research Procedures

In clinical care, patients must be informed of rare but serious risks. Research participants should receive at least as much information about risks when undergoing the same procedures. After healthy volunteers died as a result of research procedures (25,26), there was a public outcry because the participants had not been told that such a serious adverse event might occur.

Explain how the Research Procedures Differ From Standard Medical Care

Participants may mistakenly assume that the researcher's interventions are similar to what a doctor would do in clinical practice. Researchers should clarify what risks participants would face in the study that they would not face in ordinary clinical care.

Do not Overstate Benefits to Participants

A participant might benefit from knowing the results of common clinical tests obtained in the study. However, tests that are ordered without clinical indications have a low predictive value and uncertain clinical significance, and might lead to a cascade of additional tests.

Invite Questions

Researchers should ask participants if they have questions, instead of expecting them to take the initiative to ask.

Use Consent Form Templates Provided by the Local IRB

Local IRBs interpret the federal regulations for investigators at each institution. Most IRBs have sample consent forms and templates on their website, illustrating recommended language and format. Investigators should download and modify these templates as needed.

STUDY 6.1   **(Continued).**

Participants should be informed that death is a rare complication of bronchoscopy. Also, they should be reminded of standard medical advice to take prescribed medications during a smog alert and not to exercise. It seems disingenuous or even misleading to say that knowing one's response to inhaled pollutants is a benefit to the participant. To put the "benefit" in context, the participant needs to be told that comparable information could be obtained from observing symptoms or measuring peak flow during smoggy days.

HOW CAN THE ADEQUACY OF INFORMED CONSENT BE ASSESSED?

In high-risk, very innovative, or controversial studies, researchers will want to ensure that participants are truly informed. Some researchers simply ask participants, "Do you understand what I've told you?" However, participants may not admit that they do not understand or may not realize that they misunderstand.

A better approach is to administer to participants a questionnaire about the key features of the research study. If a participant does not understand an important point, the researcher can provide more information. Several international HIV prevention trials have used this approach to defend against allegations that consent was not informed (5,22,27–29). Participants in developing countries may be vulnerable because poor education, low health literacy, poverty, and limited access to medical care may compromise their ability to give informed and voluntary consent. Some researchers in these settings have used simple questionnaires to test whether participants understand key elements of the research. Community advisory groups can help identify issues that participants will have difficulty understanding, and help to develop more effective consent processes and materials (29). These trials provide proof of principle that informed consent is feasible under difficult circumstances. Participants in a randomized controlled trial should understand the following crucial items (27):

- Research is different from clinical care.
- The effectiveness of the research intervention is unknown.
- The research intervention has risks.
- The interventions are determined by chance and not by what a physician believes is best for the individual participant.

There may also be additional information specific to the trial that the participant should appreciate. For instance, participants in an HIV vaccine trial should understand that they are still at risk for HIV even if they receive the experimental vaccine, and that they should continue to use condoms. When retesting comprehension after providing more information, researchers should not ask the same questions they did previously, to ensure that correct answers are not the result of rote memorization (18).

VOLUNTARINESS AND UNDUE INFLUENCE

Ethically valid consent must be voluntary as well as informed. The following case illustrates common examples of undue influence.

STUDY 6.2

In the study of persons with asthma on a bad smog day, the investigators find it difficult to recruit participants. Several suggestions are made to increase enrollment:

- *Paying participants $3000 for the exercise test and bronchoscopy.*
- *Asking graduate students and staff in the pulmonary medicine division to participate in the study.*
- *Investigators personally asking their patients to participate in the study.*

A voluntary act is an act of free will or personal choice that must be "free from coercion and undue influence" (30). The Common Rule requires that investigators "minimize the possibility of coercion or undue influence." The IRB Guidebook explains that "offers that are too attractive may blind prospective subjects to the risks or impair their ability to exercise proper judgment" (31). Undue inducement or undue influence may be defined as "an offer of an excessive, unwarranted, inappropriate or improper reward or other overture in order to obtain compliance" (32).

Undue influence might occur when the researcher has power or authority over participants. Staff, students, and patients of the investigator might feel that if they do not participate in the research their employment, grades, or ongoing care may be compromised. For example, patients might fear that the physician will not be as interested in their care or that they might have difficulty getting timely appointments if they do not participate. Patients also might feel a sense of obligation to their treating physician.

Undue influence needs to be distinguished from coercion, which is the use of a threat of harm or punishment to influence behavior (2). For example, it would be coercive for a researcher to say that persons could no longer receive medical care at the clinic or hospital if they did not participate in a research project.

Very high payments to participants might be regarded as undue influences because they might induce persons to agree to inappropriately large risks. Emanuel et al (33) have argued that most concerns about undue influence are really concerns about excessive risk, problems with informed consent, and inadequate IRB deliberations. If these issues can be resolved, then a high payment level is not ethically problematical but rather a boon to the participants, particularly low-income persons. Moreover, if problems with risk and consent are not adequately addressed, reducing payments will not make the study ethically acceptable.

Concerns about undue influence should certainly heighten scrutiny about risk and consent; apparently excessive payments may be a warning of other problems with a study. However, undue influence *per se* is also problematic. Voluntary consent is an ethical requirement for human participants research even when the risks are acceptable and choices are informed.

STUDY 6.2   **(Continued).**

In Study 6.2, IRBs generally would not accept the proposed strategies to increase enroll-ment. First, the proposed level of payment is higher than what participants in other research studies are paid for similar procedures. IRBs typically allow payments of $500 to $700 for an invasive procedure such as bronchoscopy. Chapter 9 discusses payments to research partic-ipants in more detail. Second, people may not feel free to refuse a request to participate in research made by their boss, teacher, or treating physician.

WHICH PARTICIPANTS ARE VULNERABLE?

Some participants are vulnerable in the sense that they are "at greater risk for being used in ethically inappropriate ways in research" (27). They might have difficulty giving informed consent or making voluntary decisions, or they might be more susceptible to adverse events.

Federal regulations view vulnerability in terms of categories of research subjects, such as children, prisoners, and pregnant women. Subparts D, C, and B of the Common Rule respectively present special protections for these groups (see Chapters 17 and 21), which include limits on the level of risk permitted and heightened requirements for informed consent. Although the regulations also call attention to problems in research that involves "mentally disabled persons or economically or educationally disadvantaged persons," there are currently no special regulations for such participants.

This approach of analyzing categories of vulnerable participants is conceptually flawed for several reasons. First, the subparts fail to address many types of people who may be vulnerable, such as substance abusers or undocumented immigrants. Also, vulnerability depends on context; people who are vulnerable in one situation may not be vulnerable in others. For example, cancer patients may be vulnerable in Phase I trials because they mistakenly believe the purpose of the trial is to benefit them personally. However, they are not vulnerable with respect to a questionnaire study on out-of-pocket spending for care. Finally, a focus on vulnerable populations overlooks the variation among individuals within a group. An alternative approach identifies different reasons for vulnerability and suggests measures that might be taken to reduce each cause of vulnerability (27).

Vulnerability Because of Power Differences

As previously discussed, people may find it difficult to refuse requests by those who have power over them, such as control over their daily routine (34). Residents of nursing homes, military personnel, and prisoners may not appreciate the fact that they can decline to participate in research without fear of retaliation or jeopardy to other aspects of their everyday lives.

Cognitive or Communicative Impairments

Persons with impaired cognitive function may have difficulty understanding information about a study and deliberating about its risks and benefits. Chapter 16 discusses research with persons who have impaired decision-making capacity.

Social and Economic Disadvantages

Persons of low socioeconomic status may join a research study to obtain payment, a free physical examination, or screening tests, even though they would regard the risks as unacceptable if they had a higher income. Furthermore, poor education or low health literacy may lead to poor comprehension of information about the study or undue influence.

Whether or not a research participant might be susceptible to undue influence depends on both the nature of the influence and the vulnerability of the participants. Offers that most people could readily decline can strongly influence vulnerable persons.

STUDY 6.2   (Continued).

Some graduate students might be doubly susceptible to undue influence because of large educational debts as well as their dependent relationship with a teacher.

HOW CAN VOLUNTARINESS BE ENHANCED?

Reduce the Influence of More Powerful Persons

To avoid undue influence by the treating physician, patients might be invited to participate in a research study through flyers or posters rather than by a direct request from the physician. Alternatively, someone other than the treating physician, such as a research assistant, can discuss the research project with patients. The investigator should not know whether one of her patients decides to participate.

Frame Information About Payment to Minimize Undue Influence

To keep payment for participating in research in perspective, the researchers can describe it as payment per hour of time spent or per procedure completed on the study, rather than as a total payment, which might be considerable over the course of a long, complicated study. Also, payment should not be mentioned prominently in descriptions of the research, lest participants consider their participation primarily in terms of monetary gain. Chapter 9 discusses payments in more detail.

Check Whether Decisions are Voluntary

Investigators can ask participants whether their decision to enroll in the study was their own or whether they felt pressured by other people to join the study (35). The response can provide useful information if participants say that others influenced them. However, a negative response does not ensure that consent was voluntary, because people can be unconscious of strong influences on their behavior or hesitate to disclose them to others. Researchers can also ask community-based organizations or disease advocacy groups whether persons targeted for enrollment can make voluntary decisions about the study, and how to enhance their decision-making (6).

Monitor Refusal Rates

If a study involves significant risk, researchers should expect some eligible persons to decline to participate. An unexpectedly high enrollment rate should raise concerns about undue influence.

PARTICIPANTS WHO LACK DECISION-MAKING CAPACITY

When persons cannot provide informed consent, the Common Rule allows their "legally authorized representative" to give permission for them to participate in research. The regulations do not specify who may serve as the legally authorized representative; presumably, family members or health care proxies who under state law may make clinical decisions for such persons may also give permission for them to enter research studies.

In addition to surrogate permission, the participant also must give assent. For example, a person with dementia who refuses to have blood drawn for a research project should not be pressured into participating. In contrast, in clinical care family members may cajole or even pressure a patient who lacks decision-making capacity into having a blood test needed for clinical care, because the patient will benefit. Chapter 16 discusses in detail ethical issues concerning adults who lack decision-making capacity, including how to assess decision-making capacity. Chapter 17 discusses research with children.

FROM WHOM MUST CONSENT OR PERMISSION BE OBTAINED?

In some research projects, persons whom the researcher may not regard as research participants need to give permission for the study to proceed.

Participants With Whom the Investigator Does Not Interact

Some persons are research participants even though the investigator does not interact with them, as the following case illustrates:

STUDY 6.3	Questionnaire asking sensitive questions about family members.

A researcher carrying out a twin study is administering a questionnaire that asks about the health of the participant's parents and families. Some of the questions ask whether the father has a history of depression or abnormal genitalia. The father of an adult participant, who is living in the same household, sees a copy of the questionnaire and complains that his privacy has been violated and that he should have given consent for his daughter to participate in the research.

This father could be readily identified because he had the same last name and address as his daughter, even though the researchers did not know his name, Social Security number, or any other direct identifiers. His complaint to the federal Office for Human Research Protections led to the conclusion that IRBs need to determine whether family members in such studies should be considered research participants.

Under the Common Rule, participants include persons about whom the researcher collects identifiable private information, even though there is no personal interaction with them. However, in most circumstances, it is impossible to identify a person simply by knowing his relationship to a research participant (36). In Study 6.3, the requested information about the father is sensitive and potentially stigmatizing or embarrassing; therefore, the research cannot be considered minimal risk (36). Hence, as we will see later in the chapter, this study does not meet the requirements for waiver of consent.

Persons who Provide Access to Research Participants

Researchers may need to obtain permission for a project from persons who control access to participants but are not participants themselves. For example, to review records in a medical practice, the researcher needs to obtain the cooperation of the physician and office staff. For research in schools, the principal and teachers must agree to the study. To approach members of a village, religious congregation, or Native American tribe, the permission of the group leader is needed. Although such permission to approach participants is necessary, it does not replace the need for individual consent from the participants themselves.

THE HIPAA HEALTH PRIVACY RULE

The federal Health Privacy Rule generally requires that researchers obtain authorization from patients to use or disclose personally identifiable health information in research (37–39). These regulations are commonly known as HIPAA, which stands for Health Insurance Portability and Accountability Act. By definition, health information pertains to a person's health, health care, or payment for health care. These regulations apply to health information held by health care providers (such as hospitals and physicians) or health plans that transmit health information electronically. The Privacy Regulations do not apply to researchers who are not health care providers, who are employed by a health care provider, or who collect research information directly from participants and do not put it into medical records.

Research authorization forms must include certain core information, and such disclosures are in addition to what the Common Rule requires to be disclosed. Researchers must obtain authorization for each use of protected information for research. Research subjects may have the right to access health information and to obtain a record of disclosures of their protected health information. Many researchers regard these provisions as being burdensome without providing meaningful protection to participants.

HIPAA allows exceptions to authorization for research, as we discuss later in the chapter. These standards are stricter than the Common Rule because HIPAA enlarged the set of information that is considered identifiable. Chapter 7 discusses HIPAA in more detail.

EXCEPTIONS TO INFORMED CONSENT

Although informed consent is a fundamental requirement for research involving human participants, an exception may be made for many low-risk studies.

WHAT IS THE ETHICAL RATIONALE FOR EXCEPTIONS TO CONSENT?

Every patient has benefited from knowledge obtained from research that used existing records and specimens, such as Studies 6.4 and 6.5.

STUDY 6.4	Review of records of patients with hepatitis C.

After the discovery of the hepatitis C virus, a researcher studying its epidemiology proposes to review the records of patients diagnosed with hepatitis C at a clinic serving low-income and uninsured patients. At this clinic, patients with hepatitis are routinely asked about sexual orientation, number of sexual partners, injection drug use, and trading sex for money.

STUDY 6.5	Study using pathology samples.

A researcher has identified a possible new prognostic marker for breast cancer. He will use materials left over from biopsies of patients receiving care for breast cancer at a comprehensive cancer center. He will determine whether patients with localized breast cancer who have higher levels of the marker are more likely to be free of disease 15 years later.

Studies 6.4 and 6.5, which analyze existing data and specimens, address important research questions and would be impractical to carry out if informed consent were required from each participant. The risks of such research are very small. Confidentiality can be protected by appropriate safeguards. Few people would be offended that their data or materials are being used in such research. Every patient has benefited from knowledge obtained from research that used existing records and specimens. Fairness in the sense of reciprocity suggests that people who receive such benefits should be willing to participate in similar very low-risk research to benefit others. Empirical studies suggest that most people are willing to have their data and materials used for research (40). On the other hand, it is disrespectful to use a person's medical information for research without his or her knowledge or approval, particularly if the information is about sensitive topics, such as sexual activities.

Under the Common Rule and the HIPAA Privacy Rule, Study 6.4 and Study 6.5 are permitted without informed consent, subject to certain conditions. The value of the knowledge to be gained is considered sufficient to justify an exception to consent. Requiring individual authorization would greatly increase the cost and difficulty of such research, without adding significant protections.

Figure 6.1 provides a series of questions that investigators and IRBs may use to determine whether informed consent is required. These questions are based on the logical structure of the federal regulations. Investigators also need to understand how the Common Rule defines such terms such as "research," "identifiable," and "human subjects." Chapter 23 discusses these issues from a more pragmatic perspective, providing an algorithm for researchers to use to determine whether consent is needed in a specific project using existing data or specimens.

IS THE PROJECT RESEARCH?

The Common Rule defines research as "a systematic investigation . . . designed to develop or contribute to generalizable knowledge." Furthermore, the researcher must interact with participants—for example, to collect data through interviews or laboratory tests and to administer an intervention. IRBs often operationalize this definition by considering a project research if the researcher plans to disseminate the findings through publications or presentations at professional meetings. Chapter 2 discusses the definition of research in more detail and analyzes how research may be distinguished from innovative clinical care, public health practice, and most quality-improvement activities.

DOES THE RESEARCH INVOLVE HUMAN SUBJECTS?

Human subjects are living persons about whom the researcher obtains identifiable private information or with whom the researcher interacts or intervenes. If researchers obtain identifiable data or specimens, they are carrying out human subjects research, even if they do not interact with the subjects. Note that if the subjects are dead, identifiable private information may be used without consent. The federal Office for Human Research Protections (OHRP) has issued guidance to clarify the regulations regarding identifiable private information.

Does the Research use Identifiable Data and Specimens?

Data and specimens are *identifiable* if the identity of the participant is associated with the data or specimen, or can be readily ascertained by the investigator. In operational terms, identifiable data and specimens fall into two categories:

- Data and specimens contain an individual identifier. Researchers readily appreciate that a name, Social Security number, and medical record number can identify an individual. HIPAA defines identifiers much more broadly. In the computer era, individuals might be re-identified from such information as birth date and zip code, using existing databases such as reverse telephone directories, driver's license lists, and voting registries. HIPAA allows researchers to use or disclose health information without the person's authorization only if all 18 identifiers in Table 6.2 are absent.
- Data and specimens are coded (e.g., overt identifiers are replaced by 001, 002, etc.), and the investigators can obtain the link between the coded identifiers and the identities of the participants.

What Data and Specimens are not Identifiable?

In several situations, data and specimens are considered not identifiable. Thus, working with them does not fall under the definition of human subjects research and consent is not required.

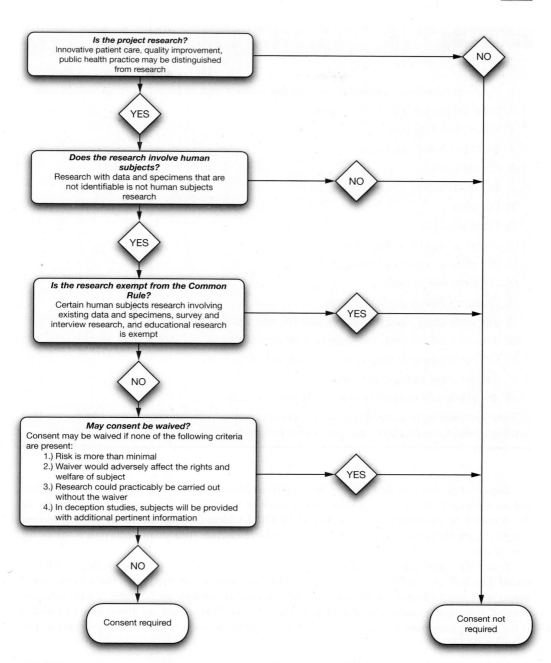

FIGURE 6.1. Questions to determine whether informed consent is not required.

TABLE 6.2	Personal Identifiers Defined by HIPAA

1. Names
2. Street address and all geographic units smaller than a state, except for the first three digits of a zip code
3. Social Security numbers
4. Medical record numbers
5. Health plan beneficiary numbers
6. Account numbers
7. Telephone numbers
8. Fax numbers
9. E-mail addresses
10. Internet protocol (IP) address numbers
11. Web universal resource locators (URLs)
12. Certificate/license numbers
13. Device identifiers and serial numbers
14. Vehicle identifiers and serial numbers, including license plate numbers
15. Biometric identifiers, including fingerprints and voice prints
16. Full-face photographic images and comparable images
17. All elements of dates except the year
18. Any other unique identifying number, characteristic, or code

These identifiers might allow individuals to be re-identified by computer experts using information in voting registries, reverse phone directories, lists of licensed drivers, etc.

Data and specimens include none of the 18 HIPAA identifiers. The data might have been collected anonymously (no identifying information was ever recorded). Alternatively, the data might be de-identified or anonymized by removing all 18 HIPAA identifiers. An electronic medical records system can readily generate a de-identified data set for researchers from identifiable data collected for clinical care.

Coded data and specimens if the investigators cannot decipher the code. According to OHRP, coded data and specimens are not identifiable if two conditions are met. First, the data and specimens were not collected for the current research project through an interaction with subjects. Second, investigators cannot readily identify the subjects. This second condition may be fulfilled if the investigators have no access to the key to decipher the code. This may be accomplished in several ways (41):

- The key may be destroyed before the study begins.
- The researchers and the holder of the key agree not to release it to the investigators.
- The repository or data management center has written policies and procedures that prohibit release of the key to investigators.
- There are other legal requirements that prohibit release of the code to the investigators.

The federal regulations allow release of the key to investigators if the subjects are deceased, because dead persons are not considered human subjects.

These provisions allow a repository or data center to keep identified specimens and data, and to release nonidentifiable coded materials and data to researchers without consent from the subjects.

The repository or data center may collect identifiable data prospectively for purposes other than the specific research project under construction. Examples include future information from medical records and tissue that will be donated to a repository in the future.

> **STUDY 6.4 and 6.5   (Continued).**
>
> *These studies can both be designed so that they do not involve human subjects. The investigators do not intervene with or interact with the individuals whose data they are studying; they merely obtain existing data and specimens. The clinic or the cancer center may give investigators coded data and specimens but promise never to release to the investigators the key linking codes to participant identities (the researcher can only recognize participants as 001, 002, etc.). Because some of the data in Study 6.4 are sensitive, researcher need to take rigorous precautions to avoid breaches of confidentiality, which could put participants in legal jeopardy.*

IS THE RESEARCH EXEMPT FROM THE COMMON RULE?

Even if the project is considered human subjects research, it still may qualify for an exemption from the Common Rule and therefore from requirements for informed consent. The main categories of exempt clinical research are as follows.

Publicly Available Data

If the research involves data that are publicly available, it is exempt from the Common Rule. The rationale is that there can be no harm to subjects from collecting and analyzing data that are publicly available and can be used for any purpose without consent and IRB review.

Research Involving Existing Data, Documents, Records, or Pathological or Diagnostic Specimens

As discussed previously, if research uses only existing data or specimens that are not identifiable, it is not considered human subjects research. Even if this is not the case, research may be exempt under two conditions. One situation is when the investigator records the information "in such a manner that subjects cannot be identified, directly or through identifiers linked to the subjects" (41). Researchers are permitted to look at identified medical records, but they may not record their data in a format that allows participants to be identified. However, under HIPAA, researchers need patient authorization to access identifiable personal health information, or else must obtain a waiver of permission from the IRB or Privacy Board.

Alternatively, such research is exempt if the data or specimens are publicly available, for example identifiable data from voting registries and telephone directories.

Surveys, Interviews, Educational Tests, or Observations of Public Behavior

Such research qualifies for exemption unless two conditions are met. First, the information must be recorded in a "manner [such] that subjects *can be identified*, directly or through identifiers linked to the subjects." This provision allows many questionnaire studies to be done without IRB review or formal consent, provided the responses are anonymous. Second, disclosure of subjects' responses beyond the research study would *place them at risk* for criminal or civil liability or damage their financial standing, employability, or reputation. Therefore, questionnaires on such sensitive issues such as drug addiction, sexual practices, depression, HIV risk behaviors, or illegal immigration are not exempt if the subjects can be identified.

Strictly speaking, this exemption does not apply if the questionnaire responses are anonymous but researchers can identify the participants, even though there would be no adverse consequences if the confidentiality of responses were disclosed. For example, researchers often want to know which persons have responded to a questionnaire so that they can send reminders to nonrespondents. This can be accomplished while still keeping the actual responses anonymous. For example, the questionnaire can be anonymous, but responders can return a separate card or envelope that is linked to their identity. However, this situation would qualify for expedited review, as discussed in a later section.

Research on Normal Educational Practices in Educational Settings

An example of research on normal educational practices in educational settings would be a study of how curriculum changes have affected test scores. Note that HIPAA does not apply to such research because it does not involve protected health information.

MAY CONSENT BE WAIVED OR MODIFIED?

Some human subjects research that does not qualify for an exemption from the Common Rule may be eligible for a waiver or modification of consent.

STUDY 6.6	Database study on outcomes in myocardial infarction.

A researcher is studying whether outcomes for myocardial infarction vary according to the number of cases the hospital and physician treat. The researcher plans to identify persons aged 65 and older who were hospitalized for a first myocardial infarction through a database of hospital discharge summaries, and to obtain additional information on these individuals from Medicare utilization records and death certificate records. To combine data from these different sources, the researcher will need to identify patients by name, birth date, address, and Social Security number. The researcher plans to study over 10,000 participants. It would be prohibitively expensive to obtain informed consent from so many persons.

In Study 6.6, the researcher needs identifiers attached to the data so that she can combine information from data sets held by different organizations; therefore, this project deals with identifiable private information and is human subjects research. Because participants can be readily identified, it does not qualify for an exemption. However, it may still qualify for a waiver of informed consent, as we discuss next.

Waiver of Consent Under the Common Rule

A waiver or modification of informed consent is permitted under the Common Rule if the following four criteria are satisfied:

1. The research involves no more than minimal risk to the subjects.
2. The waiver or alteration will not adversely affect the rights and welfare of the subjects.
3. The research could not practicably be carried out without the waiver or alteration.
4. Whenever appropriate, the subjects will be provided with additional pertinent information after participation.

In the first criterion, *minimal risk* means that "the probability and magnitude of harm or discomfort anticipated in the research are not greater . . . than those ordinarily encountered in daily life or during the performance of routine physical or psychological examinations or tests." Chapter 5 discusses the concept of minimal risk in more detail.

The second requirement recognizes that participants may be wronged even though they do not suffer physical or psychosocial harm. For example, it is disrespectful to use a person's biological materials for research they strongly object to, even if the materials are de-identified. This issue is discussed in more detail in the Appendix and Chapter 23.

The third criterion recognizes that a strict requirement of informed, explicit consent could preclude many important research studies, such as Study 6.6. Furthermore, unless a very high percentage of eligible participants agree to participate in a study, the findings might be biased. For example, persons who have poor functional status are less likely to return a consent form than healthier persons. However, the term "practicably" is ambiguous and not defined in the regulations. How much time, effort, and resources should be expended in trying to obtain individual informed consent? Ultimately, the researcher needs to explain her position to the IRB, and the IRB will answer that question.

The fourth criterion allows some research that involves deception, in the sense that explaining the purpose of the research would undermine the study. For example, a research project might ask how bystanders respond to a simulated call to assist someone who has collapsed in a parking lot. If the true nature of the study were explained to participants beforehand, they would alter their response to the simulated situation. After the completion of the research intervention, the researchers must explain to participants the purpose of the study and the nature of the deception.

Waiver of Consent Under HIPAA

HIPAA presents somewhat different criteria for waiving the requirements for patient authorization. As in Study 6.6, de-identification may remove some data that researchers need to answer important research questions. To study length of stay, for example, researchers need the full dates of hospital admission and discharge. Without full zip codes, researchers cannot use census-tract data to analyze how a health outcome varies by neighborhood demographics. To allow such research, HIPAA allows *limited data sets* to be used for research without patient authorization. Limited data sets may include zip codes and dates that include the month and day of the month, but not the other 16 specified identifiers. To use a limited data set, researchers must agree that they will use or disclose the information only for the specific purposes stated in the agreement, they will use appropriate safeguards to protect confidentiality, and they will not identify or contact the individuals. Researchers who violate a data use agreement are subject to criminal penalties.

Under the HIPAA Privacy Rule, researchers may obtain a waiver or alteration of the requirement for patient authorization to use or disclose protected health information for research purposes provided that:

1. The use or disclosure of the protected health information presents minimal risk to the privacy of individuals. There must be an adequate plan to protect health information identifiers, an adequate plan to destroy identifiers, and written assurances that the protected health information will not be reused or disclosed to others (except for other research permitted under the Privacy Rule or if required by law).

2. The research could not practicably be conducted without the waiver or alteration of authorization.

3. The research could not practicably be conducted without access to and use of the protected health information.

Waivers under the Privacy Rule may be granted either by an IRB or by an alternative review board called a Privacy Board. The requirements for membership and procedures for Privacy Boards are less detailed than the requirements for IRBs. Usually, requests for a waiver of consent qualify for expedited review rather than full review.

Several differences between HIPAA and the Common Rule regarding waiver of consent are noteworthy. HIPAA focuses only on privacy and confidentiality issues, with the implicit assumption that the unidentified information presents no violations of privacy. The Common Rule is broader, considering the "rights and welfare" of research participants. The distinction is important because, as discussed in the Appendix, some persons might strongly object to their information being used in certain types of research, even though identifiers have been removed.

STUDY 6.6 **(Continued).**

IRBs or Privacy Boards typically allow waivers of consent for research in this situation. The risk to privacy is minimal if adequate measures are taken to protect confidentiality. Because the researchers need identifiers to combine different data sets, de-identified data and limited data sets are not feasible. Thus, it would not be practicable to carry out the project without the waiver. To obtain a waiver, researchers will need to present a plan for destroying identifiers and protecting confidentiality.

DOES THE RESEARCH PROJECT QUALIFY FOR A WAIVER OF SIGNED CONSENT FORMS?

Even if consent is required, the IRB may waive the requirement for a signed consent form in two situations. In the first situation, the only record linking the subject and the research is the consent document and the principal risk is a breach of confidentiality. In the second, a consent form may be waived if the activity entails minimal risk and would not require written consent outside the research context. For example, telephone surveys may be carried out without written consent, just like public opinion polls and telemarketing surveys.

STUDY 6.4 **(Continued).**

A waiver of signed consent forms would be appropriate. The absence of a signed consent form would protect participants who are engaging in illegal activities, such as injection drug use or commercial sex work.

In some situations, informed consent procedures may be modified rather than waived, as in the following study.

STUDY 6.7 **Survey of high school students.**

Researchers plan to administer an anonymous questionnaire to high-school students about their diet, exercise, and weight. Students will be told about the nature of the questionnaire and that they may decline to participate. The questionnaire will be administered during assembly period. Students who do not participate can spend the time reading or doing homework.

The school district requires that research with students foster parental involvement with their children. To meet this requirement, the researchers propose to use "passive" permission from parents; that is, parents will be notified about the study through the school newsletter and a letter. Parents may refuse permission for their child to participate by returning a postcard, or calling or e-mailing the school. If they do not respond, the student will be permitted to participate if he or she so chooses.

So-called "passive consent" allows research to be carried out provided that the participant (or in this case, the parent) does not object. It contrasts with an "active" consent procedure in which people explicitly indicate their willingness to participate. Participation rates are higher with passive consent than with active consent because many people who are not opposed to having their children in the study may not make the effort to return a consent form. However, passive consent is a misnomer because there may be no consent at all. Passive consent is appropriate as an additional measure of respect for the participants or (as in Study 6.7) their parents, not as a replacement for consent.

> **STUDY 6.7   (Continued).**
>
> *Parental permission may be waived. Giving parents an opportunity to refuse respects their responsibility for their children and meets the school policy of fostering parental involvement.*

EXCEPTION FOR EMERGENCY RESEARCH

Federal regulations allow an exception to informed consent for certain emergency research, as Chapter 19 discusses in more detail.

PRACTICAL ASPECTS OF EXEMPTIONS AND WAIVERS

As we have discussed, the Common Rule does not require IRB review or informed consent in certain circumstances. However, most institutions do not allow researchers to decide for themselves that their study is not human subjects research. Investigators need to provide some information to an institutional official, who then determines whether the project is human subjects research. The rationale is that the IRB might identify psychosocial harms that researchers did not appreciate.

Does it make a practical difference whether a study is regarded as not human subjects research or as exempt from the Common Rule? The main consequence is likely to be the amount of information the investigator must provide the IRB. The forms for an exemption may require more information than the forms for research that does not involve human subjects.

In some situations, research projects need to undergo some level of IRB review beyond what is required by the Common Rule. A local IRB may enact policies that are stricter than the Common Rule. Furthermore, many medical journals require documentation demonstrating that the submitted research has received IRB approval or that IRB review was not needed. Therefore, before starting a study, a researcher might want to obtain documentation from the IRB that review and consent were not necessary, rather than later risk that a journal will decline to review the manuscript.

TAKE HOME POINTS

1. Federal regulations require that specific types of information about a research project be disclosed to participants.
2. Spending more time talking with participants improves the consent process.
3. Consent must be voluntary as well as informed.
4. Informed consent is not required for much survey research and research with existing data and specimens.

APPENDIX: CONSENT FOR RESEARCH WITH DE-IDENTIFIED SPECIMENS

Although researchers need to understand and comply with regulatory requirements, they must also appreciate that the regulations do not resolve some important ethical issues regarding consent. In certain situations, an investigator's ethical responsibilities regarding consent may go beyond her legal duties, as in the following project involving de-identified existing specimens.

> **STUDY 6.8   Derivation of stem cell lines from discarded oocytes.**
>
> *A researcher is deriving stem cell lines using somatic cell nuclear transfer. The researcher plans to obtain discarded oocytes (oocytes that failed to fertilize in vitro) from an infertility practice. The researcher plans to remove all identifying information from the specimens. Under the Common Rule, this project is not considered human subjects research, and therefore informed consent is not required.*

Stem cell research is controversial. Around one-third of Americans oppose embryonic stem cell research because they believe embryos have the moral status of persons. In one study (42), about 22% of infertility patients with frozen embryos reported that they intended to discard them rather than donate them for stem cell research. Furthermore, oocytes may have special significance compared to, for example, cancer tissue removed at surgery. Another study (43) reported that about 25% of women who provide oocytes to patients at infertility clinics would not want their oocytes to be used for research. Using a person's reproductive materials for purposes she would strongly object to violates the ethical principle of respect for persons. De-identifying the materials would not overcome her objections. Hence an IRB might decide not to exempt Study 6.7 from informed consent, even though no identifiable materials would be involved and thus, strictly speaking, it is not considered human subjects research. This example shows that cutting-edge research that is technically in compliance with the Common Rule may still be ethically problematic.

More generally, some persons might object if blood or tissue specimens left over from their clinical care were to be used in research projects they consider offensive (44–46). Anonymizing the specimens would not overcome their objections. Other examples of potentially offensive research using de-identified biological materials might include studies on contraception, ovulation, the genetic determinants of violence or criminal behavior, and research on human evolution. In such research, waiving requirements for informed consent would be disrespectful to persons who strongly object for deeply held moral reasons.

ANNOTATED BIBLIOGRAPHY

Flory J, Emanuel E. Interventions to improve research participants' understanding in informed consent for research: a systematic review. *JAMA* 2004;292:1593–1601.
    Critical review of empirical data on effectiveness of interventions designed to enhance informed consent.
Henderson GE, Churchill LR, Davis AM, et al. Clinical trials and medical care: defining the therapeutic misconception. *PLoS Med* 2007;4:e324.
    Analyzes the therapeutic misconception, showing how both conceptual articles and empirical studies use the term in different ways.
Jefford M, Moore R. Improvement of informed consent and the quality of consent documents. *Lancet Oncol* 2008; 9:485–493.
    Recent review on improving informed consent, with emphasis on using plain language in consent documents.
Nelson RM, Merz JF. Voluntariness of consent for research: an empirical and conceptual review. *Med Care* 2002;40: V69–V80.
    Analyzes how consent must be voluntary as well as informed.
Woodsong C, Karim QA. A model designed to enhance informed consent: experiences from the HIV prevention trials network. *Am J Public Health* 2005;95:412–419.
    Describes how a questionnaire can be used to assess whether low-literacy research participants in resource-poor countries have sufficient understanding of disclosed information about a research study to give informed consent.

REFERENCES

1. Berg JW, Lidz CW, Appelbaum PS. *Informed Consent: Legal Theory and Clinical Practice*, 2nd ed. New York: Oxford University Press; 2001.
2. Institute of Medicine. *Responsible Research: A Systems Approach to Protecting Research Participants*. Washington, DC: National Academies Press; 2003.
3. National Bioethics Advisory Commission. *Ethical and Policy Issues in Research Involving Human Participants*. Rockville, MD: National Bioethics Advisory Commission; 2001.
4. Advisory Committee on Human Radiation Experiments. *Final Report*. New York: Oxford University Press; 1998.
5. Wendler D, Emanuel EJ, Lie RK. The standard of care debate: can research in developing countries be both ethical and responsive to those countries' health needs? *Am J Public Health* 2004;94:923–928.
6. Lo B, O'Connell ME, editors. *Ethical Considerations for Research on Housing-Related Health Hazards Involving Children*. Washington, DC: National Academies Press; 2005.
7. Joffe S, Cook EF, Cleary PD, et al. Quality of informed consent in cancer clinical trials: a cross-sectional survey. *Lancet* 2001;358:1772–1777.
8. Lidz CW, Appelbaum PS. The therapeutic misconception: problems and solutions. *Med Care* 2002;40:V55–V63.

9. Henderson GE, Churchill LR, Davis AM, et al. Clinical trials and medical care: defining the therapeutic misconception. *PLoS Med* 2007;4:e324.

10. Appelbaum PS, Lidz CW. The therapeutic misconception. In: Emanuel EJ, Grady C, Crouch RA, et al, eds. *The Oxford Textbook of Clinical Research Ethics*. New York: Oxford University Press; 2008:633–644.

11. Kimmelman J. The therapeutic misconception at 25: treatment, research, and confusion. *Hastings Cent Rep* 2007;37:36–42.

12. Appelbaum PS, Lidz CW. Re-evaluating the therapeutic misconception: response to Miller and Joffe. *Kennedy Inst Ethics J* 2006;16:367–373.

13. Miller FG, Joffe S. Evaluating the therapeutic misconception. *Kennedy Inst Ethics J* 2006;16:353–366.

14. Kodish E, Eder M, Noll RB, et al. Communication of randomization in childhood leukemia trials. *JAMA* 2004;291:470–475.

15. Paasche-Orlow MK, Taylor HA, Brancati FL. Readability standards for informed-consent forms as compared with actual readability. *N Engl J Med* 2003;348:721–726.

16. Burman W, Breese P, Weis S, et al. The effects of local review on informed consent documents from a multicenter clinical trials consortium. *Control Clin Trials* 2003;24:245–255.

17. Flory J, Emanuel E. Interventions to improve research participants' understanding in informed consent for research: a systematic review. *JAMA* 2004;292:1593–1601.

18. Flory JH, Wendler D, Emanuel EJ. Empirical issues in informed consent for research. In: Emanuel EJ, Grady C, Crouch RA, et al, eds. *The Oxford Textbook of Clinical Research Ethics*. New York: Oxford University Press; 2008. 645–660.

19. Coyne CA, Xu R, Raich P, et al. Randomized, controlled trial of an easy-to-read informed consent statement for clinical trial participation: a study of the Eastern Cooperative Oncology Group. *J Clin Oncol* 2003;21:836–842.

20. Jefford M, Moore R. Improvement of informed consent and the quality of consent documents. *Lancet Oncol* 2008;9:485–493.

21. Agre P, Campbell FA, Goldman BD, et al. Improving informed consent: the medium is not the message. *IRB* 2003;Suppl 25:S11–S19.

22. Coletti AS, Heagerty P, Sheon AR, et al. Randomized, controlled evaluation of a prototype informed consent process for HIV vaccine efficacy trials. *J Acquir Immune Defic Syndr* 2003;32:161–169.

23. National Cancer Institute. Simplification of Informed Consent Documents. 2004. Available at: http://www.nci.nih.gov/clinicaltrials/understanding/simplification-of-informed-consent-docs/page2. Accessed November 28, 2008.

24. Federman DD, Hanna KE, Rodriguez LL, eds. Responsible Research: A Systems Approach to Protecting Research Participants. Washington, DC: National Academies Press; 2002.

25. Steinbrook R. Improving protection for research subjects. *N Engl J Med* 2002;346:1425–1430.

26. Steinbrook R. Protecting research subjects—the crisis at Johns Hopkins. *N Engl J Med* 2002;346:716–720.

27. National Bioethics Advisory Commission. *Ethical and Policy Issues in International Research*. Rockville, MD: National Bioethics Advisory Commission; 2001.

28. Fitzgerald DW, Marotte C, Verdier RI, et al. Comprehension during informed consent in a less-developed country. *Lancet* 2002;360:1301–1302.

29. Woodsong C, Karim QA. A model designed to enhance informed consent: experiences from the HIV prevention trials network. *Am J Public Health* 2005;95:412–419.

30. Nelson RM, Merz JF. Voluntariness of consent for research: an empirical and conceptual review. *Med Care* 2002;40:V69–V80.

31. Office for Human Research Protections. *IRB Guidebook*. 1993. Available at: http://www.hhs.gov/ohrp/irb/irb_chapter3.htm#e2. Accessed November 28, 2008.

32. National Commission for the Protection of Human Subjects of Biomedical and Behavioral Research. *The Belmont Report: Ethical Principles and Guidelines for the Protection of Human Subjects of Biomedical and Behavioral Research*. Washington, DC: U.S. Government Printing Office; 1979.

33. Emanuel EJ, Currie XE, Herman A. Undue inducement in clinical research in developing countries: is it a worry? *Lancet* 2005;366:336–340.

34. Goffman E. *Asylums: Essays on the Social Situation of Mental Patients and Other Inmates*. Garden City, NY: Anchor Books; 1961.

35. Pace C, Emanuel EJ, Chuenyam T, et al. The quality of informed consent in a clinical research study in Thailand. *IRB* 2005;27:9–17.

36. Botkin JR. Protecting the privacy of family members in survey and pedigree research. *JAMA* 2001;285:207–211.

37. Department of Health and Human Services. 45 CFR Parts 160 and 164. Standards for Privacy of Individually Identifiable Health Information. Available at: http://www.hhs.gov/ocr/hipaa/finalreg.html. Accessed December 2, 2008.

38. National Institutes of Health. Protecting Personal Health Information in Research: Understanding the HIPAA Privacy Rule. 2003. Available at: http://privacyruleandresearch.nih.gov/. Accessed July 28, 2008.

39. Gunn PP, Fremont AM, Bottrell M, et al. The Health Insurance Portability and Accountability Act Privacy Rule: a practical guide for researchers. *Med Care* 2004;42:321–327.

40. Wendler D. One-time general consent for research on biological samples. *BMJ* 2006;332:544–547.

41. Office for Human Research Protections. Guidance on research involving coded private information or biological specimens. 2008. Available at: http://www.hhs.gov/ohrp/humansubjects/guidance/cdebiol.htm. Accessed November 11, 2008.

42. Lyerly AD, Faden RR. Embryonic stem cells. Willingness to donate frozen embryos for stem cell research. *Science* 2007;317:46–47.

43. Kalfoglou AL, Geller G. A follow-up study with oocyte donors exploring their experiences, knowledge, and attitudes about the use of their oocytes and the outcome of the donation. *Fertil Steril* 2000;74:660–667.

44. National Bioethics Advisory Commission. *Research on Human Stored Biologic Materials.* Rockville, MD: National Bioethics Advisory Commission; 1999.

45. Nuffield Council on Bioethics. *Genetics and Human Behavior: the Ethical Concerns.* London: Nuffield Council on Bioethics; 2002.

46. Greely HT. The uneasy ethical and legal underpinnings of large-scale genomic biobanks. *Annu Rev Genomics Hum Genet* 2007;8:343–364.

CHAPTER 7

Confidentiality

WHY IS CONFIDENTIALITY IMPORTANT?

Confidentiality refers to protecting information obtained through the researcher-participant or doctor-patient relationship from inappropriate disclosure to third parties. Confidentiality is required by professional codes of conduct and by law. Furthermore, researchers promise confidentiality during the informed-consent process. Confidentiality is breached if researchers obtain or disclose personal information from medical records without authorization. The federal health privacy regulations (commonly known as HIPAA regulations) call attention to confidentiality problems associated with electronic medical records. Although electronic records facilitate clinical care and research, breaches of confidentiality can result from inadequate computer security or the re-identification of coded or de-identified data.

Confidentiality must be distinguished from the related concept of privacy. Privacy is violated if people are observed, touched, or intruded upon without their permission. In addition, privacy includes having control over information about oneself and about intimate relationships. Privacy is closely related to dignity, because most cultures regard certain sensitive information as embarrassing or even shameful (1).

In the context of research, "privacy pertains to the collection, storage, and use of personal information and addresses the question of who has access to personal information and under what conditions" (2). Specific privacy issues include whether specific types of information about an individual may be collected at all, and whether information collected for one purpose can be used for another purpose.

Privacy is violated if researchers contact individuals with whom they have no relationship, particularly if the research deals with a sensitive topic.

WHY ARE CONFIDENTIALITY AND PRIVACY IMPORTANT?

Research participants may suffer serious harm if their personal information is inappropriately divulged.

STUDY 7.1	Loss of Social Security numbers.

A researcher is conducting a survey of physicians to ask them about their experience with patients discontinuing medications because they cannot afford copayments. The investigators purchase a list of U.S. physicians from the American Medical Association's master file of physicians. A random sample of physicians will be selected and invited to participate in the survey. This list contains names, addresses, birth dates, Social Security numbers, medical license numbers, and identification numbers from the Bureau of Narcotics and Dangerous Drugs. The investigator downloads this list onto his laptop computer. This computer is stolen from his car.

In Study 7.1, the physicians whose names, Social Security numbers, and medical license numbers were lost do not know that the researcher had their personal information. As a result of this breach of confidentiality, these physicians might suffer inconvenience, identity theft, or economic harm. Thieves could open credit card accounts using the physicians' names and Social Security numbers. These physicians, who have not agreed to participate in research, would likely be upset that the investigator has obtained sensitive personal information about them. The researchers are ethically responsible for the loss of this personal information.

There are strong reasons for researchers to respect privacy and protect confidentiality. First, maintaining privacy and confidentiality shows respect to research subjects. Second, confidentiality may encourage people to participate in research. The loss of Social Security numbers in Study 7.1 may make people less willing to allow researchers access to identifiable information without express permission. Third, confidentiality prevents nonmedical harms, which might include:

- Psychological harm, such as shame or embarrassment.
- Social harm, such as disruption of relationships with friends or relatives, stigmatization, or discrimination.
- Economic harm, such as loss of employment or credit card fraud.
- Legal harm, such as prosecution for illegal behaviors such as illicit drug use or commercial sex work.

Research on certain topics is particularly likely to raise concerns about confidentiality, as in the following case.

STUDY 7.2	**Screening for domestic violence.**

A researcher wishes to evaluate the effectiveness of an intervention to increase screening for domestic violence in a primary care clinic. The interventions include posters and brochures in waiting rooms and examining rooms, reminder notices appearing as pop-up windows in the electronic medical record, and a brief online CME program for physicians on domestic violence. The outcome measure will be the percentage of cases in which domestic violence is mentioned as a problem in a clinic note. The researchers also plan to conduct a medical records review in 6 months of patients who are noted to have this problem to see whether follow-up is documented.

Study 7.2 illustrates the use of research information that is regarded as particularly private or sensitive. The psychosocial risks if confidentiality is breached might be particularly great. If the perpetrator of domestic violence knows that the victim has disclosed the situation, there may be increased violence. Other highly sensitive topics include:

- Illegal conduct
- Alcohol and substance abuse
- Sexually transmitted infections and HIV infection
- Sexual attitudes, behaviors, or preferences, and reproductive health
- Mental health and psychiatric illness

When carrying out research on these topics, researchers should give heightened attention to how they will protect the participants' privacy and confidentiality.

HOW IS CONFIDENTIALITY BREACHED?

Understanding how confidentiality can be breached enables researchers to take steps to protect it. Confidentiality protection is a chain that is only as strong as its weakest link.

SECURITY LAPSES

Unauthorized persons might obtain research records or databases if computer security is lax or the research staff is careless. In numerous highly publicized cases involving banks and insurers, laptop computers containing large databases with personal financial information were stolen or lost. Although most cases contained bank or payroll data rather than research data, people may be concerned that research records are also not secure. People may also be concerned that personal information they disclose to researchers might be passed on to employers or insurers without their permission.

STAFF MEMBERS KNOW PARTICIPANTS FROM OTHER CONTEXTS

Even without overt identifiers, research staff might be able to identify some participants from data about them. In some situations, physicians might be able to identify participants whose radiology images or pathology slides they have seen. Similarly, when persons have a rare disease or an unusual combination of clinical features, physicians and nurses might be able to ascertain or recall their identity. Furthermore, research staff may be able to identify participants from social contacts in the community or from previous clinical contacts.

RE-IDENTIFICATION OF DE-IDENTIFIED OR CODED DATA

Computer experts can identify some participants without knowing overt identifiers such as name, medical record number, address, or Social Security number. Through readily available databases such as voter registries, driver's license registries, and reverse telephone books, some individuals can be identified from their birth date, gender, and zip code. Because of this possibility of re-identification, HIPAA sets strict standards for de-identified data. According to these standards, de-identified data may not contain the 18 specified elements in Table 7.1.

TABLE 7.1	Personal Identifiers Defined by HIPAA

1. Names
2. Street address and all geographic units smaller than a state, except for the first three digits of a zip code
3. Social Security numbers
4. Medical record numbers
5. Health plan beneficiary numbers
6. Account numbers
7. Telephone numbers
8. Fax numbers
9. E-mail addresses
10. Internet protocol (IP) address numbers
11. Web universal resource locators (URLs)
12. Certificate/license numbers
13. Device identifiers and serial numbers
14. Vehicle identifiers and serial numbers, including license plate numbers
15. Biometric identifiers, including fingerprints and voice prints
16. Full-face photographic images and comparable images
17. All elements of dates except the year
18. Any other unique identifying number, characteristic, or code

IDENTIFICATION THROUGH GENOME SEQUENCING

As genome sequencing becomes cheaper, more research studies will carry out whole genome sequencing. Researchers working in publicly funded genome sequencing centers are required to make DNA sequences widely available to other researchers (3). However, individuals can be re-identified if a reference database exists that links DNA sequences with individual identities. The Department of Justice database has identifying genomic information on 4.7 million persons accused or convicted of various crimes. Thus research participants can be re-identified if someone with access to full genome sequencing data gains access to that database. As full genome sequencing data become widely shared, the possibility of re-identification may increase.

Although the risk of breaches may seem small, the consequences can be great for the participants whose confidentiality is violated. Moreover, if many participants in an electronic database can be identified, the scope of a breach would be large. Researchers have an obligation to take reasonable precautions against rare but serious adverse events.

THE HEALTH PRIVACY RULE

The U.S. Department of Health and Human Services (DHHS) issued federal regulations to protect the privacy of personal health information. These regulations are called the Privacy Rule or, more informally, HIPAA (after the Health Insurance Portability and Accountability Act that authorized them). HIPAA's provisions regarding research have been criticized as impeding valuable research while giving little additional protection to privacy (2).

BASIC PROVISIONS OF THE PRIVACY RULE

To Whom Does HIPAA Apply?

The Privacy Rule applies to *covered entities*, which are individuals or organizations that transmit health information electronically. Covered entities include health care providers (such as hospitals and physicians) and health plans (such as private health insurers, managed-care organizations, and public programs such as Medicaid, Medicare, and Veterans Affairs). The Privacy Rule does not protect individually identifiable health information held by an organization that is not a covered entity.

What Kind of Health Information is Covered?

The Privacy Rule protects all individually identifiable information related to a patient's health, health care, or payment for care that was created or received by a covered entity. This information is known as *protected health information* (PHI). Health information is identifiable if it includes any of the 18 specified identifiers in Table 7.1. These identifiers might allow individuals to be re-identified by computer experts using publicly available information in voting registries, reverse phone directories, lists of licensed drivers, etc. Information that includes none of these 18 identifiers is considered *de-identified* and may be used or disclosed without the individual's authorization. Information may also be considered de-identified if a qualified statistician determines that enough identifiers have been removed that the risk of identifying the individual is very small. However, this latter option is rarely used because the requirements are ambiguous.

Authorization to Use or Disclose Information

Covered entities must obtain specific written authorization from patients to use or disclose PHI, with certain broad exceptions (2,4–6). No patient authorization is needed to use or disclose protected information

- for treatment, payment, or clinical operations (which include quality improvement, quality assurance, and education);
- for legally required disclosures to public health officials, health oversight agencies, and courts; or

- for business associates, who are individuals or organizations that carry out for the covered entity functions or services that require the use or disclosure of PHI. A business associate must sign an agreement to use the information only for specific purposes and to safeguard information from misuse.

Privacy Safeguards

Providers generally must make reasonable efforts to use and disclose only the minimum identifiable information that is needed to accomplish their intended purpose. In addition, health care providers must take reasonable safeguards against prohibited or incidental use or disclosure of personal health information and maintain reasonable and appropriate administrative, technical, and physical safeguards to prevent violations of the privacy regulations.

Rights of Patients

Patients have the right to

- receive a notice of privacy practices from a health care provider or a health plan;
- inspect and copy their medical records and request that corrections be made; and
- obtain an accounting of disclosures (AOD) that the covered entity made of their PHI over the previous 6 years, including disclosures made for research purposes. The AOD must also include certain information related to each disclosure, including the date of the disclosure, the identity of the person who received the information, a description of the information disclosed, and the purpose of the disclosure. For research involving 50 or more participants, it suffices to provide a general list of all protocols for which a person's PHI might have been disclosed.

The Privacy Rule contains both civil and criminal penalties for violations. Because of these penalties, many covered entities have interpreted the regulations in a risk-adverse manner, often choosing not to participate in research projects rather than comply with the extensive administrative burdens needed to comply with the regulations.

USE OF PHI FOR RESEARCH

The federal Health Privacy Rule generally requires that researchers obtain authorization from patients to use or disclose identifiable health information in research (2,4–6).

Authorization for Research

Authorization for research use of protected health information (PHI) under the Privacy Rule differs from informed consent for research under the Common Rule. Under the Privacy Rule, each research project requires a separate authorization stating how and why the PHI will be used for research, and to whom it will be disclosed. In contrast, informed consent describes the potential risks and benefits of research, and how the confidentiality of the research records will be protected. The Privacy Rule permits, but does not require, review of authorization forms by an IRB or Privacy Board.

Use of PHI for Research Without Authorization

The Privacy Rule establishes a number of exceptions to authorization to use or disclose protected health information (PHI) for research (see Table 7.2).

De-identified information may be used in research without authorization from the persons whose data are studied. Research using nonidentifiable data and specimens requires neither consent under the Common Rule nor authorization under HIPAA. However, the criteria for de-identified data under HIPAA are more stringent than the criteria for information and specimens that are not identifiable under the Common Rule.

TABLE 7.2	Research That May be Carried out Without Patient Authorization

1. De-identified information
2. Waiver of authorization
3. Limited data set
4. Activities preparatory to research
5. Researchers not covered by the Privacy Rule
6. Hybrid entities
7. Business associates

Limited data set. Limited data sets may include zip codes and dates that include the month and day of the month, but not the other 16 specified identifiers. Such information is often needed to carry out certain types of research projects, for example, when the date of service must be known (see Chapter 23). To obtain a limited data set, researchers must sign a data use agreement promising that they will use or disclose the information only for the specific purposes stated in the agreement, they will use appropriate safeguards to protect confidentiality, and they will not identify or contact the individuals. Some health care organizations have been reluctant to sign data use agreements, creating barriers to potentially important research. Under the Common Rule, IRBs commonly allow such data sets to be used in research without consent from participants, provided the risk is minimal.

Waiver of authorization. Researchers may obtain a waiver or alteration of the requirement for patient authorization to use or disclose PHI for research purposes provided that:

1. The use or disclosure of the PHI presents minimal risk to the privacy of individuals. There must be an adequate plan to protect health information identifiers, an adequate plan to destroy identifiers, and written assurances that the PHI will not be inappropriately reused or disclosed to others.
2. The research cannot practicably be conducted without the waiver or alteration of authorization.
3. The research cannot practicably be conducted without access to and use of the PHI.

Waivers under the Privacy Rule may be granted either by an IRB or by an alternative review board called a Privacy Board. The requirements for membership and procedures for Privacy Boards are less detailed than those for IRBs.

Research institutions vary in how they interpret these HIPAA criteria for waiver, and often set such strict interpretations that even low-risk research cannot proceed. Some institutions interpret the term "impracticable" to mean "not at all possible," and require researchers to demonstrate that a study will fail without a waiver of authorization.

Activities preparatory to research. Covered entities may use or disclose PHI without obtaining authorization to plan research projects and identifying and recruiting participants, provided that the researcher will not remove PHI from the covered entity. According to the guidance from DHHS, only internal researchers (employees of the covered entity) may contact potential research subjects about enrolling in a study. External researchers must sign a business associate agreement or obtain a partial waiver of authorization from the IRB or Privacy Board to contact potential participants. This provision creates an artificial distinction between internal and external researchers. Furthermore, HIPAA provides less privacy protection than the Common Rule, which requires activities preparatory to research involving human subjects be approved by an IRB. This issue has lead to great confusion, and many institutions have been reluctant to release information to external researchers that is essential to carry out research.

Researchers not covered by the Privacy Rule. This includes individuals who are not health care providers or employed by a health care provider, collect research information directly from participants, and do not put it into medical records.

Hybrid entities. If a covered entity also performs functions unrelated to health care, it may designate itself a hybrid entity so that only its "health care components" are subject to the Privacy Rule. For example, if a university includes an academic medical center with a hospital, the entire university will be classified as a covered entity unless the university elects to be a hybrid entity by designating only the hospital as the health care component. Then only the hospital must comply with the Privacy Rule. Researchers within a hybrid entity are not subject to the Privacy Rule if they work outside the health care component, do not provide health care, and do not transmit health information electronically.

Business associates. Business associate agreements would allow the linking of PHI from various data sources to create a research data set. In practice, however, such agreements are used infrequently for this purpose because they are complicated and impractical to set up for individual research projects.

PROBLEMS WITH HIPAA
Differences Between the Privacy Rule and the Common Rule

The Privacy Rule and the Common Rule differ in several important ways (see Table 7.3). Overall, the Privacy Rule has been criticized for making it significantly more difficult to carry out research, particularly research with existing data and biological specimens (2). However, such research has great potential benefits for society (see Chapter 23). In addition, the Privacy Rule imposes such heavy

TABLE 7.3	Differences Between the Privacy Rule and the Common Rule
Under the Privacy Rule, research is more difficult.	
Privacy Rule	**Common Rule**
Definition of de-identified data is stricter.	
Authorization must be for specific project. Authorization for unspecified future research is not permitted.	IRB may approve consent for unspecified future research and must approve such research.
Under the Privacy Rule, administrative burdens are greater.	
Privacy Rule	**Common Rule**
Accounting of disclosure (AOD)	Not required.
Limited data sets require data use agreement.	Use of such data may be approved by IRB.
Criteria for waiver of authorization are interpreted very conservatively.	
Under the Privacy Rule, protections for participants are weaker.	
Privacy Rule	**Common Rule**
Hybrid entity may exclude some researchers from the Privacy Rule.	All research at covered institution or carried out by employees is generally subject to the Common Rule.
Privacy Board or IRB need not review research if subjects have authorized it.	IRB must review and approve such research.
In activities preparatory for research, internal researchers are not subject to to Privacy Board or IRB oversight.	IRB must review and approve all research activities, regardless of who is carrying them out.

administrative burdens on research institutions that many health care organizations have decided not to participate in important research projects. Finally, in several respects the Privacy Rule provides less protection to human subjects than the Common Rule. The next sections analyze several of the most serious barriers to research created by the Privacy Rule.

Future Research

The National Institutes of Health (NIH) encourages researchers conducting a study to obtain authorization to store data and biological materials and carry out future research with them. Under the Common Rule, it is permissible to obtain patient consent to store biological samples for future research, which will be overseen by an IRB. However, DHHS has determined that this requires a second authorization separate from the authorization to participate in the primary research project. According to DHHS, an authorization must be "study-specific," and authorizations for "unspecified future research" are overly broad and invalid. This interpretation sets up serious administrative barriers to secondary research using stored samples and existing data. Furthermore, the HIPAA Privacy Rule fails to provide strong protection to participants in secondary research because, unlike the Common Rule, it does not require IRB or Privacy Board review of research carried out with individual authorization.

Accounting for Disclosure (AOD)

Several advisory groups have sharply criticized the Privacy Rule's AOD requirements in the research context as a huge burden to providers and researchers that has led many covered entities to refuse to make PHI available to researchers (2).

Outcomes Research and Health Services Research

The Privacy Rule makes it difficult to carry out important projects in outcomes research and health services research. Such research is essential to understand the effectiveness and cost-effectiveness of medical therapies in actual clinical practice. The definition of de-identified data excludes data sets with the dates of service, which are often essential in such research. In addition, the requirements for obtaining a limited data set or a waiver of authorization, which are needed to combine data from two different sources, are administratively burdensome. Many health care organizations have decided not to participate in health services research, severely limiting the generalizability of findings and potentially introducing bias.

Recommendations

An Institute of Medicine consensus committee concluded that the HIPAA Privacy Rule does not protect privacy adequately and constrains important health research (2). The committee recommended a new approach to ensure privacy in health research that shifts the focus of privacy protections from individual authorization for research to enhanced security of personal information used for research. Furthermore, the protections should be required in all health research in the United States, not just research at institutions covered by HIPAA.

As an alternative to this comprehensive approach, the committee also proposed revisions to the current HIPAA Privacy Rule and the associated guidance from DHHS to eliminate some provisions of the HIPAA Privacy Rule that hinder research without providing meaningful privacy protections (2).

HOW SHOULD RESEARCHERS PROTECT CONFIDENTIALITY?

Researchers should anticipate problems with confidentiality and take steps to protect it.

WHAT ARE SOME BASIC STEPS TO PROTECT CONFIDENTIALITY?

Study Name and Site

The name chosen for the study or the location of the study office should not reveal sensitive conditions or stigmatize participants.

Staff Training

Staff members should receive training about why confidentiality is important and how to maintain it. For example, when leaving messages for patients, they should not mention the name of the study or the condition being studied. Staff members who input data, particularly identifiable data, need to be trained regarding confidentiality even if they do not interact with participants.

Use of Coded or De-identified Information

HIPAA requires researchers to use the "minimum necessary" identifiable data needed to achieve the research goals. Investigators should use coded or de-identified data and biological specimens whenever possible. In coded samples (sometimes called linked or identifiable samples), identifiers such as name, Social Security number, or medical record number are replaced with a code number such 001, 002, etc. The key linking the code numbers and the identities of participants should be secure, as discussed in the next section.

Data Security

File cabinets and offices should be locked. Electronic safeguards to protect sensitive identifiable data should include password protection and encryption. Such data should not be downloaded onto laptops, which are commonly lost or stolen. The code for linking data and identifiers, as well as headers for data fields, should be stored separately from the data set.

> **STUDY 7.1**   **(Continued).**
>
> *The investigators should have considered whether they needed to obtain or retain Social Security numbers and medical license numbers. If such personal information was necessary, it should have been password-protected and encrypted, and it should not have been placed on a laptop.*

WHAT ARE SOME SPECIAL STEPS TO PROTECT CONFIDENTIALITY?

In certain circumstances, researchers should take additional steps to protect confidentiality because the data they are collecting is particularly sensitive or the risks of a breach of confidentiality would be particularly great.

Certificates of Confidentiality

Certificates of Confidentiality allow the investigator to withhold the names or identifying characteristics of research participants in the event of a subpoena or court order. Certificates of Confidentiality are particularly helpful if the research project involves highly sensitive information (7,8). Investigators can obtain a Certificate of Confidentiality from the NIH and should do so at the onset of sensitive studies. The research need not be federally funded. The NIH Certificate of Confidentiality Kiosk website can be accessed at http://grants.nih.gov/grants/policy/coc/.

Certificates of Confidentiality have limitations that should be kept in mind. They do not apply to audits by funding agencies or the Food and Drug Administration. Nor do these certificates prevent the researcher from disclosing information to comply with state reporting laws, such as domestic violence in Study 7.2. Furthermore, certificates do not prevent investigators from releasing de-identified data in accordance with a court order.

Promises not to Re-identify Participants

HIPAA requires researchers to promise not to try to re-identify or contact participants when they obtain a "limited data set," which may contain dates and zip codes, unless they have explicit authorization to do so from the patients whose data are used. It would be prudent for all investigators using de-identified data or specimens to promise not to try to re-identify participants as a condition of obtaining the data or approval from the IRB.

Publication of Identifiable Data

In most research reports, only aggregate data are presented. However, in some research publications or presentations, distinctive clinical data, photos, videos, radiology images, or pathology slides may be presented. Even if explicit identifiers such as name are withheld, health care workers who cared for a patient might infer the identity of individual participants from distinctive clinical characteristics (9).

Researchers should take steps to reduce the risk of such breaches of confidentiality. First, some details that might identify participants can be omitted from presentations and publications. For example, it is usually not necessary to report exact dates or specific locations. In a photo, if the face is not shown or the eyes are obscured, it is less likely that the subject will be readily identified. Second, researchers should obtain explicit permission to publish or present information that is so unique that participants can be identified. Some other suggestions for altering data are problematic. For example, some have suggested modifying a family pedigree to protect the identity of a family or individual (10). However, such modifications might be scientifically misleading and therefore ethically problematic.

WHAT SHOULD RESEACHERS DO IF CONFIDENTIALITY IS BREACHED?

If a breach of confidentiality occurs, the investigator should first try to minimize harm to participants. Institutional officials should be notified immediately of a breach of security, and police should be called if data or computers are stolen or lost. Participants should be notified so that they can take steps to mitigate risks. It is appropriate for researchers to apologize for breaches of confidentiality.

STUDY 7.1   **(Continued).**

The researcher should promptly notify persons on the list so that they can notify their banks and credit card institutions and check their credit scores to see if anyone is trying to open accounts in their name. The institution should pay for persons on the list to monitor their credit ratings for a reasonable period of time. Because the researchers are clearly at fault, there is little to be gained by not being forthright about the breach and apologizing for it. Compensation for harm should be offered by risk management.

As with any error, health care professionals should use the episode as an opportunity for quality improvement. These researchers need to upgrade their confidentiality and security protections. In addition, the IRB may clarify security practices they expect researchers to have in place when using identifiable data. Furthermore, the IRB may want to researchers to justify why they need identifying information in their data set (e.g., in Study 7.1 the physician's Social Security and medical license numbers). Researchers should be required to delete unnecessary identifiers from their files, in keeping with the spirit and letter of HIPAA.

MAY RESEARCHERS OVERRIDE CONFIDENTIALITY?

Researchers may be required by law to override confidentiality if they identify conditions such as child abuse, domestic violence, elderly abuse, certain infectious diseases, and serious threats of violence by psychiatric patients.

These exceptions to confidentiality are ethically justified as a last resort to prevent serious and imminent risks to participants or third parties. The rationale is similar to the rationale for overriding confidentiality in clinical medicine and public health (11–13):

- The potential harm to identifiable persons is of serious magnitude and high likelihood.
- Overriding confidentiality will allow steps to be taken to prevent harm.
- There is no less invasive alternative to overriding confidentiality to warn or protect those at risk.

Harms resulting from overriding confidentiality are minimized and acceptable. Disclosure should be limited to information essential for the intended purpose. Persons should receive the information only if they have a need to know. The greater the number of these criteria that apply in a specific situation, the stronger will be the ethical reasons for an overriding confidentiality.

If confidentiality needs to be overridden in a particular case, researchers should minimize harms by informing the person that the case will be reported and, whenever possible, obtaining their assent. These discussions may identify additional steps that could reduce harms. In cases of domestic violence or elder abuse, such reports might lead to retaliation against the victim. If this is the case, it would be prudent to set up plans for moving the person to a safe place or having a friend or family member move in temporarily.

When planning a research project, researchers should anticipate what kinds of sensitive information participants might disclose that would require confidentiality to be overridden. During informed-consent discussions, researchers need to inform prospective participants of readily foreseeable situations in which confidentiality might be overridden.

STUDY 7.2   (Continued).

Most states require physicians to report domestic violence. States vary regarding who has a duty to report or permission to report. A Ph.D. sociologist or a research assistant who is not a licensed health care worker may not be required to report, but may be legally protected if they make a good faith report. However, the principal investigator may have responsibility for reporting any cases discovered by the project. Investigators need to consult with the institutional legal services department to determine what their legal obligation is. Reporting raises ethical issues because the victim may suffer retaliation when the perpetrator learns that the case has been reported. Thus, reporting should be coordinated with measures to protect the victim, such as obtaining space at a shelter. Reports can usually be made with the help of the domestic violence response team at the hospital, who are familiar with procedures and resources.

OTHER CONFIDENTIALITY ISSUES IN RESEARCH

Researchers may face confidentiality issues that do not arise in clinical practice. They should anticipate such situations and consider how to respond to them.

CONFIDENTIALITY DURING PEER REVIEW

During the peer review of a grant or article, researchers obtain information that other scientists expect to be kept confidential. The author could be harmed if other researchers learned of her ideas and took advantage of them in their own work. Hence, confidentiality is a condition of serving as a reviewer. Reviewers should not disseminate the author's ideas to others or incorporate them into their own work.

RESPONDING TO SUBPOENAS FOR RESEARCH DATA

Researchers may receive a subpoena for their research data. Such requests are often disconcerting and time-consuming for investigators. In some cases, raw data or data from unpublished studies have been subpoenaed (14). Researchers should realize that there are legal measures they can take to quash or modify a subpoena. Consulting with institutional legal counsel is an essential first step. Investigators should try to protect identifiable information and seek to provide de-identified information. In some studies, there may be other legal obligations. For instance, in some clinical trials the sponsor owns the data. Anticipation and prevention are useful. Researchers who anticipate that their data will be sensitive and of interest to litigants or police officials should obtain a Certificate of Confidentiality before the study begins, to protect their data from subpoena.

TAKE HOME POINTS

1. Researchers should take reasonable precautions to protect confidentiality, including using coded data whenever possible and keeping identifiable data secure.
2. In exceptional circumstances, researchers may override confidentiality to avert serious and imminent harms.

ANNOTATED BIBLIOGRAPHY

Gostin LO, Nass S. *Beyond the HIPAA Privacy Rule: Enhancing Privacy, Improving Health Through Research.* Washington, DC: National Academies Press; 2009.
    Consensus report on the impact of the federal health privacy (HIPAA) regulations. Contains a conceptual overview of privacy and confidentiality. Can be accessed through http://www.nap.edu/.

REFERENCES

1. National Bioethics Advisory Commission. *Ethical and Policy Issues in Research Involving Human Participants.* Rockville, MD: National Bioethics Advisory Commission; 2001.
2. Gostin LO, Nass S. *Beyond the HIPAA Privacy Rule: Enhancing Privacy, Improving Health Through Research.* Washington, DC: National Academies Press; 2009.
3. National Research Council. *Reaping the Benefits of Genomic and Proteonomic Research: Intellectual Property Rights, Innovation, and Public Health.* Washington, DC: National Academies Press; 2005.
4. Department of Health and Human Services. 45 CFR Parts 160 and 164. Standards for Privacy of Individually Identifiable Health Information. Available at: http://www.hhs.gov/ocr/hipaa/finalreg.html. Accessed December 2, 2008.
5. National Institutes of Health. *Protecting Personal Health Information in Research: Understanding the HIPAA Privacy Rule.* 2003. Available at: http://privacyruleandresearch.nih.gov/. Accessed July 28, 2008.
6. Gunn PP, Fremont AM, Bottrell M, et al. The Health Insurance Portability and Accountability Act Privacy Rule: a practical guide for researchers. *Med Care* 2004;42:321–327.
7. Wolf LE, Zandecki J. Sleeping better at night: investigators' experiences with certificates of confidentiality. *IRB* 2006;28:1–7.
8. Wolf LE, Zandecki J, Lo B. The certificate of confidentiality application: a view from the NIH institutes. *IRB* 2004;26:14–18.
9. Hecht FM, Wolf LE, Lo B. Lessons from an HIV transmission pair. *J Infect Dis* 2007;195:1239–1241.
10. Botkin JR. Protecting the privacy of family members in survey and pedigree research. *JAMA* 2001;285:207–211.
11. Gostin LO. *Public Health Law: Power, Duty, Restraint.* Berkeley: University of California Press; 2000:85–109.
12. Lo B. *Resolving Ethical Dilemmas: A Guide for Clinicians,* 3rd ed. Philadelphia: Lippincott Williams & Wilkins; 2005:36–44.
13. Beauchamp TL, Childress JF. *Principles of Biomedical Ethics,* 5th ed. New York: Oxford University Press; 2001: 303–312.
14. Racette BA, Bradley A, Wrisberg CA, et al. The impact of litigation on neurologic research. *Neurology* 2006; 67:2124–2128.

The Researcher-Participant Relationship

CHAPTER 8

Identification and Recruitment of Participants

To carry out clinical research, investigators need to identify and contact eligible participants. There is often an ethical tension between enrolling participants efficiently and respecting them as persons. Often the most feasible procedures to identify and contact participants would intrude on their privacy and confidentiality. Different approaches for contacting potential participants balance these conflicting goals in different ways.

STUDY 8.1

A researcher is studying access to screening mammography in women with breast cancer. The researchers are particularly interested in studying women with poor access to care to identify barriers to screening. The study will involve a 30-minute questionnaire administered by phone within 6 months of diagnosis.

The researchers identify potential participants through the state cancer registry. In this state, physicians and hospitals must report patients with breast cancer to the registry. State law allows researchers to access information in the registry for IRB-approved studies without individual consent. Health care providers are requested to give cancer patients information about the registry and its importance for epidemiological tracking and research studies.

The researchers send eligible women a letter explaining the study. Women may opt out of further contact with the researchers. The researchers provide a toll-free number and a self-addressed envelope for patients to decline further contact. Women who do not opt out will be telephoned by the researchers and invited to participate in the study.

One of the first women telephoned is angry at being contacted. "How did you get my name and number? What happened to my privacy? Who else knows that I have cancer? I don't want everyone in town to know."

Contacting people to invite them to participate in research might raise ethical concerns, even though there is no physical risk. First, people may consider it an invasion of their privacy to be contacted by researchers they do not know and have not authorized to communicate with them. Second, patients may regard it as a breach of confidentiality if their personal medical information is given to researchers, even though state law and federal regulations permit it. In Study 8.1, even if cancer patients must be reported to the state registry, some women may not have been told about the cancer registry and its use in research, or they may not remember being told. In recent years, state cancer registries have become increasingly sensitive to such privacy and confidentiality concerns and less willing to allow researchers to contact eligible subjects directly (1). Because of heightened sensitivity to privacy and confidentiality, researchers need to think carefully about ethical issues when identifying and contacting eligible participants.

HOW MAY ELIGIBLE PARTICIPANTS BE IDENTIFIED?

Various approaches for identifying participants present different trade-offs. Generally, procedures that efficiently identify eligible participants involve some infringement on privacy and confidentiality. In some approaches, the identification of eligible participants and contact with them are separate steps, while in other approaches they occur simultaneously.

RESEARCHERS IDENTIFY PARTICIPANTS USING MEDICAL RECORDS

Often the most efficient way for a researcher to identify participants with a specific disease or condition being studied is through electronic medical records. However, as Study 8.1 illustrates, patients may believe their privacy and confidentiality have been violated if researchers obtain personal medical information about them without their approval. These violations of confidentiality need to be weighed against the benefits of research. Without such use of medical records, it would be prohibitively difficult to identify eligible participants for many studies. Under HIPAA, researchers are permitted to use medical records to identify eligible participants without their explicit authorization (see Chapter 7).

INTERMEDIARIES WHO KNOW ELIGIBLE PARTICIPANTS IDENTIFY THEM

Privacy and confidentiality are respected if treating physicians and their office staff invite patients to participate in a research study. Hence IRBs commonly require researchers to involve treating physicians in the recruitment process. For instance, the researcher and treating physician may cosign a letter to suitable patients.

Another example of recruitment through intermediaries is "snowball sampling" (also called respondent-driven sampling), in which participants already enrolled in a study ask other eligible persons to contact the researcher. Such recruitment does not involve personal health information protected by HIPAA. This approach is useful for contacting populations that are stigmatized or perform illegal activities, such as injection drug use and commercial sex work. However, there are ethical concerns about undue influence or coercion if the intermediary receives a financial incentive to refer eligible participants.

ELIGIBLE PARTICIPANTS IDENTIFY THEMSELVES TO RESEARCHERS

Invitations at the Site of Care

A hospital or clinic may set up a procedure for patients to indicate that they are willing to be contacted for research. Because researchers only contact patients who have given permission to be contacted, there are no violations of privacy. The clinic may not require patients to allow researchers to contact them as a condition of care, which would be coercive. However, this approach has practical disadvantages. The clinic or hospital must fund staff to ask patients for permission to be contacted and to keep records of who is willing to be contacted. Furthermore, if only a small percentage of eligible patients agree to be contacted, samples might be biased.

Advertising

Researchers may recruit through advertisements in the media, on the Internet, in public places, or in clinical sites. Persons interested in a project can then contact researchers. There are no concerns about privacy and confidentiality because participants take the initiative to make contact. However, the yield of this approach may be low.

Advertising for research differs from commercial advertising in several important ways. The goal of commercial advertising is to stimulate consumers to buy a product even if they really do not need it or want it. Indeed, advertising may try to stimulate impulse buying, in which consumers do not weigh the benefits and costs of the product. Commercial advertisers have no obligation to provide complete and balanced information about their product. Although they may not give false information, they may exaggerate the benefits and need not mention the disadvantages. In contrast, researchers have an ethical obligation to explain the risks of research and to obtain informed consent. The decision to enroll or not in a research project should not be made on impulse. Thus, advertisements should not make misleading claims about the benefits of the study. Moreover, payments for participation should not be the first or most prominent item in the ad. The IRB must approve all advertisements and recruitment materials.

RESEARCHERS RECRUIT PARTICIPANTS WITHOUT KNOWING PERSONAL INFORMATION ABOUT THEM

Researchers may not know any personal information about the participants they recruit.

STUDY 8.2

A researcher is conducting a population-based study to determine the prevalence of obesity in the community and its relationship to diet, exercise, proximity to parks and recreation centers, and density of fast food restaurants in the zip code. The researchers want to enroll a population-based sample so that their results will accurately describe the public health burden of obesity. The researchers plan to contact participants directly, through door-to-door interviews. The sampling strategy will take into account multifamily buildings and apartments.

Random-digit telephone calls and door-to door canvassing are commonly used in survey research. Although the privacy of the participants is invaded, medical confidentiality is maintained because the researcher does not know their medical condition before contacting them. Moreover, the researcher need never know their name or identity. However, this is an inefficient way to recruit participants, particularly when the eligibility criteria are narrow.

Another way to recruit participants without knowing personal information about them is to approach them at a specific site of care. For example, a researcher might wish to study all patients receiving care in a cardiology practice or a walk-in clinic.

HOW MAY ELIGIBLE PARTICIPANTS BE CONTACTED?

After researchers identify eligible participants, they must next determine how to contact them to invite them to participate in the study. When contacting eligible participants, researchers need to explain how they were identified.

RESEARCHERS CONTACT ELIGIBLE PARTICIPANTS

As previously discussed, because of increasing concerns about confidentiality and privacy, many IRBs do not allow researchers to contact patients with whom they have no existing relationship (1). Although an IRB might allow researchers to identify eligible participants from hospital records without obtaining their permission, it might require researchers to contact them only through the treating physician or clinic director.

USE OF INTERMEDIARIES TO CONTACT PATIENTS

One option is for treating physicians or their staff to personally approach patients about the study and invite them to participate. However, this approach may raise other problems. Busy clinicians may have little time to discuss a research project or may forget to do so. Thus, few participants may be recruited. In addition, there is a potential for undue influence because patients may find it difficult to decline requests from their treating physician and office staff, on whom they depend for care. Another approach is for the treating physician or director of the clinic to cosign with the researcher a letter to eligible participants explaining the study and stating that the research team will contact them. Alternatively, the clinic receptionist or nurse may ask permission for the researcher to speak with patients.

HOW SHOULD FIRST CONTACT BE MADE?

Participants may view certain means of contact as a greater violation of their privacy. A letter from a researcher describing a study may be regarded as less intrusive than a telephone call because it does not require a response or interaction. Hence it is respectful for the first contact to be a letter to eligible participants to briefly describe the study and to inform them about how additional contact will occur and offer a means to prevent it.

AFTER INITIAL CONTACT, WHAT SHOULD BE DONE?

Opt-in Strategy

After sending a letter to eligible participants, researchers should make additional contact only with those who return a postcard or make a telephone call giving permission to be contacted about the study. Having participants give permission for further contact maximizes their privacy and confidentiality, and is preferable when the study concerns a sensitive condition. However, recruitment rates may be much lower than they would be with an opt-out strategy (2). Moreover, persons who take the initiative to contact researchers may not be representative of the target population of the study in clinically important ways (2,3). Thus an opt-in strategy may lead to bias and lack of generalizability (1,3).

Opt-out Strategy

Researchers can send eligible participants an introductory letter saying that they will call about the study, unless the person makes a phone call or returns a postcard refusing contact. The participant therefore has the burden of taking steps to avoid further contact. The rationale is that the vast majority of persons who do not reply are willing to be contacted (2,4). Compared to an opt-in strategy, this approach usually leads to higher participation rates and thus more rapid completion of the research.

STUDY 8.1 **(Continued).**

In Study 8.1, researchers have legal permission to contact eligible participants directly. However, to reassure participants about privacy and confidentiality, it is prudent to have a physician who has a relationship with the patient cosign with the researcher a letter informing patients about the study. For example, the director of cancer programs at the hospital where the woman was treated could cosign the letter.

Recontact nonresponders. Under an opt-out strategy, researchers usually want to try again to contact prospective participants whom they are unable to reach but who have not refused contact. Such persistence increases response rates and therefore enhances the generalizability of the research findings. However, some people who do not want to be contacted again may fail to return a postcard or telephone call indicating this. They may consider it an invasion of privacy if researchers continue to try to reach them. They may also feel upset that they have to do something to keep from being bothered. Thus researchers should set limits on the number of attempts to contact nonresponders.

Oversight of research staff. Research staff who contact participants or respond to participants' inquiries need appropriate training and supervision. The principal investigator must develop scripts for these discussions and obtain IRB approval for them. Front-line staff should practice role-playing and observing several conversations with participants before holding interviews themselves. Senior investigators should conduct an ongoing review of interviews with front-line staff.

STUDY 8.1   (Continued).

In Study 8.1, research staff need to respond with empathy to participants' concerns about privacy and confidentiality, reassure them that only authorized researchers have access to their diagnosis, and explain how the cancer registry works.

ELIGIBLE PARTICIPANTS CONTACT RESEARCHERS

If persons interested in the research project contact the investigators, there are no concerns about confidentiality and privacy. For example, people may respond to an advertisement about the study.

INCENTIVES FOR ENROLLING PARTICIPANTS

To enroll the target number of participants, investigators and sponsors may consider giving physicians incentives or paying them to refer patients. It is appropriate to compensate physicians a reasonable amount for the actual time spent in identifying patients who are eligible for a study, discussing the project with them, and making the referral. However, in some studies, referral fees may be much greater than the actual expenses of going through records and contacting a research coordinator. Such large financial arrangements may raise serious ethical concerns regarding conflicts of interest and undue influence. For example, such large incentives might lead physicians to underplay the risks of the study or exaggerate the benefits. Researchers need to describe to the IRB any incentives and referral fees used, and be able to justify the amount.

RECRUITING VULNERABLE POPULATIONS

If low-income minority persons are targeted as research participants, either explicitly in the eligibility criteria or de facto as a result of demographics and epidemiology, they may object that they are being treated as "guinea pigs" and question why the study is not being done with more affluent, Caucasian populations. Furthermore, they might be skeptical that the community will benefit from the knowledge gained. Thus researchers need to explain to community leaders, potential participants, and the IRB why these disadvantaged persons are being targeted. For example, the disease may be more common or more severe or have worse outcomes in that population.

TAKE HOME POINTS

1. There is often an ethical tension between enrolling participants efficiently and respecting their confidentiality and privacy.
2. Researchers need to consider a range of options for identifying and contacting eligible participants, and be able to provide reasons for selecting a particular option.

REFERENCES

1. Beskow LM, Sandler RS, Weinberger M. Research recruitment through US central cancer registries: balancing privacy and scientific issues. *Am J Public Health* 2006;96:1920–1926.
2. Armstrong D, Kline-Rogers E, Jani SM, et al. Potential impact of the HIPAA privacy rule on data collection in a registry of patients with acute coronary syndrome. *Arch Intern Med* 2005;165:1125–1129.
3. Tu JV, Willison DJ, Silver FL, et al. Impracticability of informed consent in the registry of the Canadian Stroke Network. *N Engl J Med* 2004;350:1414–1421.
4. Littenberg B, MacLean CD. Passive consent for clinical research in the age of HIPAA. *J Gen Intern Med* 2006; 21:207–211.

9

Payment to Research Participants

Payments may be necessary to recruit and retain participants in a research project; however, the reasons for paying participants and the amount paid may raise ethical concerns. Too low a payment may be considered taking advantage of volunteers, while too high a payment may be regarded as an undue influence. Although there are often no clear-cut answers regarding payment, researchers need to consider the pertinent ethical issues and be ready to justify their approach to payment.

The term "compensation" is often used to refer to compensation for research-related injuries. To avoid confusion in this chapter, we use the term "payment" when referring to payments that are given to participants, whether or not an injury occurs.

STUDY 9.1   **Children's Environmental Exposure Research Study (CHEERS).**

The Environmental Protection Agency (EPA) proposed a prospective cohort study of children's household exposure to pesticides (such as bug spray) and other chemicals. Over the course of 2 years, the study would follow 60 young children whose parents routinely sprayed pesticides. Participants would be recruited from a Florida area with a high prevalence of insects and high pesticide use. Parents would use pesticides as if the study were not being conducted. Findings from the study would help set standards for safe home use of pesticides.

Data would be collected every 6 months. To collect urine samples, parents would save and label diapers, and have the child subject wear a one-piece outfit with socks attached. To document what the children ate, parents would prepare and submit a duplicate of everything that the child subject ate and drank during a 24-hour period. To record the child's activities, parents would keep a diary of the child's activities during a 5-day period and videotape the child's behavior. Parents would also record what pesticides they used in the home. During these 6-monthly follow-ups, researchers would visit homes to take swabs of floors and other surfaces and pick up samples collected by parents.

Families participating in the study would receive about $1000 in payment over 2 years plus a video camera. Some critics charged that the researchers were paying parents to expose their children to pesticides. In their view, the payment would induce low-income families to enroll their children in inappropriately risky research. Critics also objected that the researchers would not warn parents of the risks of pesticides or check that they were storing and using pesticides safely. Other critics believed that pesticides damage the environment and public health, and that the study results would be used to increase permitted levels of pesticides.

Parents were asked to do many tasks over a 2-year period. The payment rate was $20 to $40 per day of active participation, and this amount was defended as being consistent with hourly rates that research participants receive in other research that requires considerably less effort.

The EPA accepted an additional $2 million funding from the chemical industry to measure levels of common household chemicals, such as flame retardants and ingredients in plastic products, as well as pesticides. Critics charged that this funding from the chemical industry compromised the EPA's independence.

Study 9.1 shows how concerns about payment often are intertwined with concerns about excessive risk, lack of consent, and conflicts of interest (1,2). It also illustrates that for a long and complicated study, even if payment for each activity is modest, the total payment may be regarded as an undue inducement.

Risk. The researchers regarded the CHEERS study as a natural-history study that presented no risks beyond those that the children were already facing in their everyday lives. Parents were asked to do what they would ordinarily do with regard to pesticide use, diet, and activities. The gathering of data, although time-consuming and inconvenient, posed no physical risks to the children or parents. Critics, however, charged that the study and the study payments encouraged parents to use and, in their view, overuse pesticides. Some critics in effect accused the researchers of paying parents to use their children as guinea pigs. Critics also objected that researchers were not checking to see whether parents were using pesticides in dangerous ways. In their view, failure to call attention to inappropriate pesticide use condoned and even encouraged it. As discussed in Chapter 24, in observational studies researchers may sometimes observe a level of risk that they did not cause but is so great that they should intervene. Deciding whether and how to intervene is particularly challenging because the goal of protecting participants may conflict with the goal of answering the research question in a valid manner. Nonetheless, researchers have a fundamental ethical obligation to protect subjects from unacceptable risks.

In Study 9.1, researchers could have reduced the risks and thereby decreased concerns about undue influence by:

- Educating parents about the risks, proper storage, and application of pesticides, and ensuring that they understood the disclosed information.
- Checking to see that parents were following the recommended storage and application procedures.
- Warning parents if excessively high levels of pesticides were found in the collected samples. (However, advocates of the study responded that for most pesticides, no standards for dangerous levels existed. Indeed, the purpose of the study was to provide evidence on which standards might be based.)

Lack of consent. It is ethically problematic to carry out risky research with young children who have not consented to the risks and inconvenience of the research. Furthermore, Study 9.1 provides no prospect of direct benefit to participating children. As discussed in Chapter 17, federal research regulations provide special protections to children participating in research.

Conflict of interest. Some critics charged that the financial support from the chemical industry compromised the integrity of the study and introduced bias into the study design. Assurances by the EPA that the chemical industry had no input into the design of the study other than to include measurements of chemical levels failed to persuade critics.

STUDY 9.1   **(Continued).**

Because of heated public criticism, Study 9.1 was canceled. However, without information on how the use of pesticides in the home is associated with levels of the pesticides in children, evidence-based standards for home pesticide use cannot be developed.

WHAT ARE REASONS FOR PAYING PARTICIPANTS?

Researchers need to distinguish the different reasons for paying participants.

TO REIMBURSE FOR OUT-OF-POCKET EXPENSES

Reimbursing actual expenses for parking, bus fare, or child care presents no ethical problems because it ensures that participants will have no net financial gain or loss from participating in the research. Such reimbursement may be particularly important for poor people to reduce barriers to participating in research.

TO REIMBURSE LOST WAGES

Paying for actual lost wages is consistent with the idea that research participants should not lose money by taking part in research. Reimbursing their lost wages provides them the income they would have received if they had spent time at work rather than in the research project. However, reimbursement for lost wages raises concerns about equity, as we later discuss.

TO PAY PEOPLE FOR THEIR TIME AND EFFORT

Payments that recognize the time spent and the inconvenience of participating in research may be justified as a matter of reciprocity and respect. People should not have to make excessive sacrifices to participate in a time-consuming activity that is designed to advance scientific knowledge rather than benefit themselves directly. Moreover, without some payment for participating in research projects that require considerable time, the burden on poor persons might be prohibitive.

TO EXPRESS APPRECIATION FOR PARTICIPATION

Tokens of appreciation, such as $25 in cash or gift certificates, are often provided as a thank you and a manifestation of respect for participants.

TO INCREASE ENROLLMENT

Studies suggest that financial incentives increase people's willingness to participate in research. Economic models of behavior suggest that incentives are required to overcome opportunity costs, distrust, and inertia (3). Payment may be a particularly strong incentive when people hesitate to enter studies that involve considerable inconvenience, discomfort, or risk.

WHAT MODELS OF PAYMENT ARE CONSIDERED?

Different conceptual models of payment lead to different payment practices and raise distinct ethical concerns (4).

A *reimbursement* model prevents participants from losing money if they participate in research. There are no ethical objections to reimbursing reasonable out-of-pocket expenses, such as travel, parking, or child care. However, lavish expenses, such as staying in a luxury hotel, are difficult to justify because they may be an undue inducement.

In a *wage-payment* model, participants receive compensation for their time and inconvenience. The justification is that it would be unfair to ask participants to donate large amounts of time, particularly in a long or complicated study. However, as discussed below, choosing the level of wages to pay presents challenges.

In a *market* model, payments are set by supply and demand. Payments would be increased until the research had achieved the target enrollment in the study. Supporters of this model point out that in the workplace employers pay higher wages to fill riskier jobs. This practice is accepted on the grounds that individuals are in the best position to judge whether it is worthwhile to assume risks in exchange for higher wages.

An *appreciation* model, in which participants receive token gifts, raises no concerns about undue influence. However, when poor communities are the target population for a study, some participants may feel that receiving only token acknowledgment belittles their time and contribution. These concerns might better be addressed, not by increasing payment, but by other measures, such as increasing collateral benefits (e.g., education on related health topics), sharing the results of the study with the participants after the study is completed, and collaborating with community advocacy groups to improve the condition that was studied.

WHAT ARE ETHICAL CONCERNS ABOUT PAYING PARTICIPANTS?

UNDUE INFLUENCE

Payments that are too high may distort participants' perceptions of the balance of risks and benefit, or lead them to disregard or downplay the risks, to not consider their decision carefully, or to enroll in the study against their better judgment. Concerns about undue influence are greatest if the research involves high risk or the participants are poorly educated, have few financial resources, and have few other options.

Emanuel et al. (5) have argued that most concerns about undue influence are really problems about excessive risk, inadequate informed consent, and weak IRB oversight. If these problems can be addressed, a high payment level would not be an ethical problem, but rather a boon or "good deal" for the participants. Furthermore, unless problems with risk and consent are adequately resolved, reducing payments will not make the study ethically acceptable.

Certainly, concerns about undue influence should heighten scrutiny about risk and consent. Very high payments under a market model may be a warning that the risks are unacceptable and need to be reduced. However, even if the risks are acceptable and consent is informed, voluntariness is an independent ethical requirement in research. It may be difficult to address concerns about voluntariness. In the clinical context of organ donation from living donors, in-depth interviews with prospective donors are conducted to determine whether they felt free to decline. Simple, valid measures of voluntariness need to be developed for research settings.

Empirical studies suggest that there is indeed a level of payment that might impair potential participants' ability to think critically about the risks and benefits of a research study (6). One study suggested that the levels of payment commonly offered in research studies do not distort participants' views of the benefits and risks of a study (7). However, these studies were limited because few respondents had low incomes or poor education, and because they addressed a hypothetical situation, not an actual research project that posed serious or unknown risks. The issue of whether certain payments are an undue influence may be difficult for IRBs to determine without input from people whose socioeconomic backgrounds are similar to those of the participants.

Undue influence is a particular concern if payment for a long study is made only if the subjects complete the entire study. In contrast, if payments are prorated and made after the completion of each phase of the study, participants could decide to withdraw from the study without forgoing all payment.

FAIRNESS

The issue of fairness, in several senses of the term, raises important ethical concerns regarding payments to research participants.

Similar Payments for the Same Research Procedures

The level of payment must be chosen carefully. Payment that is trivial for well-off participants may be substantial for economically disadvantaged participants and might be considered an undue influence (8). To reduce concerns about undue inducement, usually the rate is similar to wages for unskilled labor.

The amount of payment made to different participants may also raise concerns regarding fairness. The idea of equal pay for equal work seems fair. All participants undergo the same research procedures and spend similar time in the study. However, this principle may conflict with the idea that people should neither gain nor lose financially by participating in research, which forms the basis for only reimbursing out-of-pocket expenses. However, payment for actual lost wages means that participants with higher wages will receive more money than persons with lower wages. Participants who receive a fixed salary or are self-employed or unemployed would not be able to demonstrate an actual loss of earnings, and therefore are not reimbursed. Consequently, participants receive different amounts of money depending on their employment status, even though they all spend the same amount of time and effort on the research project. It also seems unfair to pay economically disadvantaged participants less than more affluent participants if they all spend the same time and undergo the same research procedures.

The needs of participants are also relevant. In a multisite study, the cost of living may vary markedly among different sites. The payment needed to obtain sufficient enrollment in a region with a high cost of living may be significantly greater than what is needed in a low-cost area. These different conceptions of fairness may lead to different conclusions regarding payment. It may be considered unfair if participants in one area get markedly higher payments than participants from another area. On the other hand, if the same payment level is used for each area, the amount for those in the lower-cost area might be considered an undue inducement.

Not Taking Unfair Advantage of Participants

Although low payments may address concerns about undue influence, they may also raise criticisms that researchers are taking unfair advantage of participants who might spend many hours in research or undergo inconvenient or risky procedures for the benefit of others. If the research participants are poor or members of minority groups who have suffered discrimination in other ways, the study may be criticized as exploitation.

Equitable Selection of Participants

An additional concern about low payments to research participants is that most participants may have low incomes and few other options. Few wealthy individuals will participate in research unless they are strongly motivated by altruism and are willing to accept the opportunity costs of forgoing other activities. If the participants in a project are predominantly from lower socioeconomic groups, the guidelines for equitable selection of research subjects may be violated.

Payments in research projects involving children raise additional concerns, which are discussed in Chapter 17.

WHAT PAYMENTS DO IRBs ALLOW?

PAYMENT LEVELS

IRB policies vary considerably in what payments to research participants are allowed. A 1997 study found considerable variation in IRB payment policies (9). A few IRBs allowed hourly payments ranging from $4 to $10 per hour ($5 to $13 in 2007 dollars). A few other IRBs allowed a flat rate of between $25 and $125 per visit or day ($32 to $158 in 2007 dollars). Several allowed higher payments for procedures. Most IRBs would not allow participants to be paid only if they completed the study. However, completion bonuses to encourage completion of the study were permitted.

Actual payments to research participants also vary considerably (10). In a 2005 study, the median amount paid to healthy subjects was $100 ($104 in 2007 dollars). Generally the payment was not broken down by procedure. When a per-hour amount was specified, it varied from $10 to $250 per visit, with a median of $20 ($21 in 2007 dollars). In multisite studies, the payment at different sites for the same procedure varied. The median difference between sites was $120 (with a mean difference of $228).

The University of California San Francisco IRB suggests that the upper limit for lengthy or repeated research visits should be the average hourly wage in the area, which was $15 to $20 an hour in 2007. A payment of $100 for invasive procedures such as bronchoscopy is acceptable, but payments of $200 to $300 trigger concerns about undue influence.

Under federal regulations, IRBs may not consider payment a benefit when evaluating the benefits and risk of a research project. Thus, studies that have an unacceptable balance of benefit and risk may not be made acceptable by paying participants more money.

LOTTERY TICKETS

Some researchers may propose to offer lottery tickets rather than cash payments to participants. They may offer tickets for a state lottery or give participants a chance to win something purchased by the investigators, such as a gift certificate. Lottery tickets are particularly useful when the researcher has a small budget and cannot afford to give each participant a payment.

Critics have objected to lottery tickets on several grounds (11). Only one participant gets paid, which may be considered unfair because all participants experienced the same inconvenience and risk. Lottery tickets may undermine informed consent. Because people overestimate their chances of winning, lottery tickets may be undue inducement. Furthermore, participants may not be told the number of people who have a chance of winning the prize.

However, others reject these objections because all participants have an equal chance of winning the lottery prize. Moreover, people are familiar with lotteries and can be told the number of participants in the study. Offering a chance to win a lottery is particularly appropriate if the only risk of participation is time and inconvenience, and there is no physical or psychosocial risk.

PRACTICAL CONSIDERATIONS

Practical considerations about the method of payment may be important. Many research institutions prefer that payments to participants be made by check, and that participants' Social Security numbers be recorded to facilitate financial audits and reduce concerns about financial misconduct. However, these practices may inconvenience certain participants or put them at risk. For example, low-income participants may need to pay high fees to cash a check, and some participants may not have a Social Security number. Furthermore, in a study of a stigmatizing or illegal condition, the identity of participants might be ascertained using the Social Security number. In these situations, participants are commonly paid in cash. As another practical matter, payments may be provided as gift certificates for clothing or food rather than as cash because of concerns that cash payments might make researchers complicit in supporting addictive behaviors, such as alcohol or substance abuse.

No bright line separates acceptable payments from unacceptable ones. A consensus Institute of Medicine panel (12) noted that:

> *A mix of . . . circumstances may determine when a particular type or level of payment crosses the line. What is excessive in one situation may not be in another, and reasonable people may sometimes differ in their judgments.*

In light of differing perspectives regarding acceptable payment and undue influence, community representatives can help determine whether levels of payment are appropriate. They can help researchers understand how payments might influence potential participants' decisions in the context of a particular study and study population. Such advice can help avoid payments that may constitute undue influence as well as those that discourage enrollment or are regarded as exploitative.

TAKE HOME POINTS

1. Researchers need to anticipate potential criticisms about payment.
2. Researchers should be prepared to explain how they chose the level and method of payment and how they decided that this amount was neither too high nor too low.

ANNOTATED BIBLIOGRAPHY

Grady C. Payment of clinical research subjects. *J Clin Invest* 2005;115:1681–1687.
  Conceptual analysis of the rationales for paying research subjects, and how different rationales lead to different levels of payment.

REFERENCES

1. Stokstad E. Toxicology. EPA criticized for study of child pesticide exposure. *Science* 2004;306:961.
2. Lo B, O'Connell ME, eds. *Ethical Considerations for Research on Housing-Related Health Hazards Involving Children*. Washington, DC: National Academies Press; 2005.
3. Dunn LB, Gordon NE. Improving informed consent and enhancing recruitment for research by understanding economic behavior. *JAMA* 2005;293:609–612.
4. Grady C. Payment of clinical research subjects. *J Clin Invest* 2005;115:1681–1687.
5. Emanuel EJ, Currie XE, Herman A. Undue inducement in clinical research in developing countries: is it a worry? *Lancet* 2005;366:336–340.
6. Casarett D, Karlawish J, Asch DA. Paying hypertension research subjects. *J Gen Intern Med* 2002;17:650–652.
7. Halpern SD, Karlawish JH, Casarett D, et al. Empirical assessment of whether moderate payments are undue or unjust inducements for participation in clinical trials. *Arch Intern Med* 2004;164:801–803.
8. Wendler D, Rackoff JE, Emanuel EJ, et al. The ethics of paying for children's participation in research. *J Pediatr* 2002;141:166–171.
9. Dickert N, Emanuel E, Grady C. Paying research subjects: an analysis of current policies. *Ann Intern Med* 2002;136:368–373.
10. Grady C, Dickert N, Jawetz T, et al. An analysis of U.S. practices of paying research participants. *Contemp Clin Trials* 2005;26:365–375.
11. Brown JS, Schonfeld TL, Gordon BG. "You may have already won." An examination of the use of lottery payments in research. *IRB* 2006;28:12–16.
12. Field MJ, Behrman RE. *Ethical Conduct of Clinical Research Involving Children*. Washington, DC: National Academies Press; 2004.

Responsibility for Incidental Risks

I n the course of their research, investigators may become aware of risks that participants already face, whether or not they participate in the research. Researchers might learn of such risks incidentally through what they hear or see, even though the investigators do not ask about them explicitly and they are not related to the topics of the study. Such risks should be distinguished from risks that result from research procedures, which investigators are obligated to minimize and respond to. In addition, such incidental risks should be distinguished from incidental findings on research tests, as discussed in Chapter 11. When investigators personally observe or hear that a participant is at risk, they often may feel a greater sense of responsibility than when they detect an incidental finding on a test. What obligations do researchers have to respond to incidental risks that are not caused by their research interventions?

STUDY 10.1	Elder abuse in a research participant.

Researchers are carrying out a longitudinal study of risk factors for progression of renal failure in persons with mild renal impairment. As part of the interview, participants are asked about their psychosocial functioning. When answering questions about psychosocial issues, an elderly participant begins to get tearful. "I don't know if I can go on like this. My daughter yells at me all the time. She takes my Social Security check and doesn't give me any money for expenses. If I don't do what she says, she shakes me. It's humiliating, but what can I do? I don't want to be put in a nursing home." Later at a research team meeting, one of the physicians on the research team says, "This is not clinical practice, where a doctor has to address all of the patient's problems. Our project is only concerned with renal function. She needs to tell her treating physician about this awful situation."

DO RESEARCHERS HAVE RESPONSIBILITY FOR RISKS THEY DO NOT CAUSE?

In Study 10.1, the elder abuse did not result from the researchers' actions, and the protocol did not even ask about it. The researchers learned about it incidentally while carrying out their interviews. Should researchers respond to such information or simply consider it outside the scope of their work? In their professional training, physicians are trained to help persons in need—for example, by providing treatment for medical problems they identify. The researcher-participant relationship has different goals than the doctor-patient relationship. Nonetheless, there are good reasons for researchers to respond to some risks that participants incidentally disclose to them (1).

First, researchers often are in a special position to prevent harm because they have expertise or a unique opportunity to intervene. No one else with similar expertise may know about the risk. If researchers do not act, an opportunity to prevent serious harm may be lost. Nonmaleficence—preventing harm—is morally commendable and should be encouraged. The more serious and likely the risk, and the less able participants are to act on their own behalf or obtain help from others, the greater the researcher's ethical obligation to try to prevent harm. In Study 10.1, researchers could not assume that the treating physician had identified and responded to the possibility of elder abuse.

Second, researchers also have a special relationship with participants (2). They invite participants to talk with them and disclose information, often information that treating physicians have not asked about. Having elicited information to achieve their research goals, investigators have some reciprocal obligation to respond to serious risks the participants disclose. Otherwise, researchers might be viewed as using participants simply as a means to achieve their research goals. The more serious and likely the risk and the more direct, frequent, and prolonged the researcher-participant relationship, the stronger the researcher's ethical responsibility (3). For example, researchers' obligations would be stronger in a longitudinal study in which they have cultivated an ongoing relationship with participants. Moreover, participants might expect researchers to act upon information they receive, just as they expect a physician in clinical care to respond to information they provide.

HOW SHOULD RESEARCHERS RESPOND TO INCIDENTAL RISKS?

Table 10.1 summarizes how researchers should respond to risks they identify incidentally during a study.

ANTICIPATE SERIOUS RISKS

When planning a research project, the investigators should anticipate serious risks participants are likely to reveal, including:

- elder abuse
- child abuse or neglect
- domestic violence
- severe psychiatric illness, such as major depression or suicidality
- threats of violence by a person against third parties

EVALUATE THE LEVEL OF RISK

Investigators should balance the level of harm that can be averted against the burdens and risks of intervening, including the harms of overriding confidentiality (3). Intervention by researchers to prevent harm is more warranted when the benefit from intervening is greater than the risk of intervening. The following specific criteria justify intervention:

- The harm to the participant or a third party is serious and highly likely.
- The intervention is effective at averting harm.
- There is no less invasive alternative for protecting those at risk.
- The risks and burdens of intervening are minimized and acceptable.

The strongest warrant for intervening is when risks are serious and imminent.

TABLE 10.1	How to Respond to Incidental Risks
Anticipate serious risks.	
Evaluate the level of risk.	
Carry out legal duties regarding serious, imminent risks.	
Develop a plan for responding to other incidental risks.	
Inform participants if confidentiality might be overridden.	

CARRY OUT LEGAL DUTIES REGARDING SERIOUS, IMMINENT RISKS

Most states have legal requirements for health care workers to override confidentiality to prevent certain serious and imminent risks (see Chapter 7). Elder abuse reporting laws vary from state to state, but generally physicians and other "designated reporters" have an obligation to report elder abuse, and certain other persons may report it. Nurses and clinical psychologists may be designated reporters, as well as persons working under the supervision of a designated reporter. Persons making reports in good faith receive legal protections. The reporter does not need definitive proof of abuse, but simply enough evidence to warrant having elder protective services investigate the case further. State laws also differ in their definitions of abuse and neglect, protections for reporters, and time frames for submitting a report.

States generally also require that child abuse and domestic violence be reported. Researchers need to understand and obey applicable state reporting laws. It is prudent to consult with legal counsel for the research institution or with protective services agencies regarding reporting requirements. Health care institutions commonly have interdisciplinary teams to respond to cases of elder abuse, child abuse, and domestic violence, and researchers can ask them to handle the case.

DEVELOP A PLAN FOR RESPONDING TO OTHER INCIDENTAL RISKS

Even if there are no legal obligations to do so, researchers have an ethical obligation to try to prevent or mitigate imminent and serious risks. For instance, although there is no legal requirement to intervene when a participant is suicidal, there are strong ethical reasons to do so. Researchers should do what is reasonable under the circumstances.

If the risks are not imminent and serious, researchers have less responsibility to prevent or mitigate harm. Again, researchers should do what is reasonable under the circumstances. Generally, a discussion with the participant on how to mitigate the risk will suffice. The researcher may also refer the participants to appropriate community resources.

> ### STUDY 10.1   (Continued).
>
> *In the longitudinal study of renal failure, a 58-year-old man tells researchers that because he has been laid off from work, he no longer has health insurance and cannot afford medications for high blood pressure and Type II diabetes. One researcher declares, "We can't help him get his medicines—we would be intervening, and then it wouldn't be a natural history study any longer!" A colleague responds, "We can't just stand by without trying to help him, when we know how important those medicines are for his health."*
>
> *Researchers in a prospective cohort study can anticipate that some participants will lose their health insurance and access to medications. To mitigate predictable harms, the investigators should have a plan to provide referrals to community organizations that can help them obtain affordable or free medications. Although such referrals will have an impact on the study endpoints, the humanitarian response to help someone in medical need should take priority. With respect to research design, the researchers can include lack of insurance and level of blood pressure as potential risk factors for renal failure.*

The protocol should specify plans for responding to serious risks that participants are likely to disclose incidentally, rather than having front-line staff respond to them on an ad hoc basis. Furthermore, researchers should be available by pager or cell phone to back up staff if unanticipated or highly complicated situations arise.

INFORM PARTICIPANTS IF CONFIDENTIALITY MIGHT BE OVERRIDDEN

During the consent process, investigators need to explain that they might learn about serious and imminent risks to participants that will require them to override confidentiality. Researchers should specify these foreseeable situations, such as legally mandated reporting of elder abuse (as in Study 10.1) or domestic violence. Potential participants need such information to make an informed decision about whether to participate in a study.

TAKE HOME POINTS

1. Researchers need to anticipate learning about risks that participants face whether or not they participate in the study.
2. Researchers have an ethical obligation, and in many situations a legal duty, to intervene to prevent serious and imminent risks.

ANNOTATED BIBLIOGRAPHY

Lo B, O'Connell ME, eds. *Ethical Considerations for Research on Housing-Related Health Hazards Involving Children.* Washington, DC: National Academies Press; 2005.
   Analysis of how to respond to incidental observations when carrying out research in participants' homes.

REFERENCES

1. Lo B, O'Connell ME, eds. *Ethical Considerations for Research on Housing-Related Health Hazards Involving Children.* Washington, DC: National Academies Press; 2005.
2. Miller FG, Mello MM, Joffe S. Incidental findings in human subjects research: what do investigators owe research participants? *J Law Med Ethics* 2008;36:271–279.
3. Wolf SM, Lawrenz FP, Nelson CA, et al. Managing incidental findings in human subjects research: analysis and recommendations. *J Law Med Ethics* 2008;36:219–248.

11

Offering Results of Research Tests to Participants

During clinical research, investigators commonly carry out clinical tests, such as laboratory tests, x-ray imaging, and other imaging studies to answer the research questions. Many of these tests are used in clinical care, and their validity and clinical interpretation are established. Other tests carried out in the study might be innovative tests that are being developed as part of the research project. In this book, we term these latter tests "research tests."

This chapter analyzes whether research participants should be provided individual results of tests carried out as part of a research study. We distinguish results from tests that are available in clinical practice, results of research tests developed as part of the study, and incidental findings that are unrelated to the purpose of the test. Investigators need to balance the benefits, risks, and burdens of providing test results in various situations.

CONSIDERATIONS IN GIVING TEST RESULTS TO PARTICIPANTS

The following case illustrates the types of tests that participants may undergo in a research study.

STUDY 11.1   **Research tests for hepatitis C.**

After the hepatitis C virus was characterized, researchers proposed a prospective cohort study of incidence and risk factors. Persons at high risk for blood-borne infections, such as injection drug users and persons with multiple sexual partners, will be eligible for this study. Participants will be evaluated every 6 months. Blood samples will be collected for liver function tests, viral hepatitis serologies, and HIV testing. One of the tests is a new test for detecting hepatitis C infection that researchers hope will be more sensitive in early infection than the standard test for anti-HCV antibodies. The research team wonders whether they should provide the results of the new hepatitis C test to the participants.

Some of the tests used in Study 11.1 are commonly used in clinical practice, such as tests for liver function, hepatitis B, and antibodies to hepatitis C. One of the aims of the study is to determine the accuracy of the new hepatitis C test, particularly in early infection. When deciding whether to offer test results to participants in a research study, investigators need to take into account the characteristics of the test and arguments for and against providing the results.

VALIDITY AND SIGNIFICANCE OF TESTS

Analytic validity indicates how well a test measures the property or characteristic it was intended to measure (1). In Study 11.1, the new hepatitis C test should give the same result if it is repeated on a different day or by a different technician. Analytic validity includes assay development, laboratory proficiency, and quality control (2). If analytic validity has not been established, the test results will be unreliable and impossible to interpret.

Under the federal Clinical Laboratory Improvement Act (CLIA), test results that are provided to patients must be carried out in laboratories that comply with specified quality control standards. Virtually no research laboratories meet these standards. Thus, research tests using innovative methods generally would need to be repeated in a CLIA-certified laboratory. However, specialized research tests often cannot be performed in regular clinical laboratories. To date, the federal government has not enforced these CLIA requirements on so-called "home brew" tests, which are developed by a laboratory and used only by that laboratory. However, the FDA has announced its intention to regulate home brew tests that apply an algorithm to data from in vitro assays to generate patient-specific results, and to require evidence of analytic and clinical validity. The research hepatitis C test in Study 11.1 would be covered by these draft regulations. This proposed oversight would also cover tests to identify genes and the proteins they encode. If adopted, this policy would limit the research test results that research participants may receive.

Clinical validity refers to whether the test correctly identifies the presence or absence of a disease (in Study 11.1, the presence of hepatitis C). The sensitivity and specificity of the investigational hepatitis test must be confirmed in a second, independent study population.

Clinical significance is established if the test results would change recommendations for medical care. Persons found to have hepatitis C should be advised regarding what follow-up is recommended, how to avoid infecting others, and what follow-up care should be obtained.

The *personal significance* of test results to a participant is broader than clinical significance. Participants might regard uncertain information as useful even if their medical care would not change. For instance, they might be more motivated to change their lifestyle or plans regarding employment, education, marriage, or reproduction.

STUDY 11.1 **(Continued).**

Liver function tests and standard hepatitis serologies have well-established analytic and clinical validity and clinical significance. If the results of these clinical tests are abnormal, the participant will need clinical follow-up, including repeat liver function tests over time, a more detailed history to identify other causes of liver disease, and advice on avoiding the transmission of viral hepatitis to others.

With regard to the research hepatitis C test, the analytic validity may have already been established by previous research. However, the clinical validity has not yet been established; in fact, that is a goal of the research project. Nonetheless, the research test might have clinical significance. Because transmission of hepatitis C to others is a serious issue, participants who test positive on the research test but negative on the standard clinical test for hepatitis C might want to take precautions to prevent transmission to others, just as if they were known to be infected.

WHAT ARE SOME REASONS TO PROVIDE TEST RESULTS?

To Show Respect for Participants

Some writers contend that research participants have a right to have access to information about their health even if the clinical significance of that information is unknown or unclear (3). Empirical studies suggest that most participants want to know their own results, and do not suffer psychosocial distress from learning them (4). Moreover, participants report that they want to receive results even though there might be adverse psychological consequences. Some participants may simply want to know as much information about their health as possible, even if its interpretation is uncertain. Furthermore, participants may expect researchers to notify them of abnormal test results, and might assume that if they are not notified, the results are normal.

To Benefit Participants

Patients might benefit from learning of a previously undiagnosed medical condition or susceptibility to a condition. Researchers who have test results may be in a unique position to benefit participants or to prevent harm to them or to others, with relatively minor inconvenience and effort to themselves. The level of benefit will depend on the nature of the condition and test result. In some situations, after learning a result, a participant might be able to obtain effective treatment or preventive measures for a serious condition. For other conditions, however, there may be no proven preventive measures or therapies. Nevertheless, even if knowing the test results would not change the participant's medical management, the results might have personal significance. The benefit of offering test results is greatest if the condition is serious or life-threatening, the validity of the test is established, and effective therapies or preventive measures are available.

To Reciprocate for Contributions Participants Make to Research

Offering individual test results may also be justified on the grounds of reciprocity and justice. Participants give permission to researchers to obtain personal health information. Therefore, in exchange for helping researchers carry out the study, research participants should have access to information about themselves that the researchers have found. The more the participants have contributed to the research project in terms of time, inconvenience, or risk, the greater claim they have on the researcher to reciprocate by providing them benefits (2).

WHAT ARE SOME CONCERNS ABOUT PROVIDING RESULTS?

Compared with clinical tests, the benefits of disclosing the results of research tests may be less and the risks greater.

Test Results May not be Valid

Participants may be harmed by receiving information whose analytic validity has not been established (5). Such information is so unreliable that it should not be used as the basis of medical or personal decisions.

Even if analytic validity has been established, both false-positive and false-negative test results may occur. If there are no clinical indications for a test, the pretest probability and therefore the positive predictive value may be low. Positive test results may be falsely positive, leading to a cascade of additional tests.

Participants May Suffer Clinical and Psychosocial Risks

Positive results may require confirmation or further testing to clarify their clinical significance. Participants may need to have invasive tests, which have medical risks. If positive test results are confirmed, participants may suffer adverse psychosocial consequences, such as depression, anxiety, or stigmatization.

Some Participants do not Want to Know Results

For some conditions, participants may not want to know the results of individual tests. When a test for the gene for Huntington disease was developed, many participants in the research did not want to know their individual results because they did not want to live with the knowledge that they would develop this progressively debilitating, untreatable disease. Similarly, in research studies that led to the development of BRCA1 and BRCA2 testing for hereditary breast cancer, some participants did want to learn their individual test results.

The balance of benefits and risks in providing results will vary according to the clinical situation. In subsequent sections, we analyze the balance of benefits and risks in several situations: aggregate study results, clinical tests, research tests, and incidental findings on research tests.

SHOULD PARTICIPANTS BE OFFERED AGGREGATE STUDY RESULTS?

There are good reasons for researchers to provide participants with the overall results of a research study, such as by offering to send them a copy of publications or press releases accompanying those articles. By doing so, the researcher shows respect for participants as partners in the research, rather than regarding them merely as sources of data. Moreover, if participants learn the study results through the media or the Internet, they may feel slighted. In cancer clinical trials, most participants have positive feelings about being offered the overall results, even if they are negative (6). Furthermore, such information might benefit participants by educating them. In some situations the results may have clinical implications, such as when they suggest that a change in medication might be beneficial for a certain category of patients. In addition, providing study results enables researchers to reciprocate for the participants' contributions to the research study.

The risks of providing aggregate study results are small and can be minimized. Aggregate results may have personal implications for individual participants (7). Some participants might infer that they are at increased risk for poor outcomes and become anxious. In a clinical trial, participants might become discouraged to learn that the intervention proved ineffective or that they were in the control rather than the intervention group. However, these risks can be minimized if participants are offered the choice of whether or not to receive the results, the risks and benefits of the information are explained, and investigators answer questions or provide counseling if needed.

In general, the benefits of providing aggregate study results outweigh the risks, and participants should be offered the overall results of the study.

SHOULD INDIVIDUAL RESULTS FROM CLINICAL TESTS BE OFFERED?

There are strong reasons for researchers to offer to participants and their primary physicians the results of tests carried out during the study that are available in ordinary clinical care. The results may benefit the participant or avert harm. For example, the research participant might learn about a serious medical problem that has not been previously diagnosed. Because they perform clinical tests on participants, researchers have a unique opportunity to avert or ameliorate adverse medical outcomes. The risk of disclosing results is small and acceptable. The validity and clinical significance of tests available in routine care are established. Physicians are used to addressing the issues of false-positive or false-negative test results and the psychosocial impact of receiving such results. Although most participants want to know their individual test results, some may not. Their informed refusal should be respected, just as refusal to be tested in a clinical setting or to learn the results of testing should be respected. Thus researchers should offer results of clinical tests to participants, but generally may not insist that the participants receive them. If participants will be required to receive test results (for example, HIV test results in federally funded research), this should be disclosed during the informed consent process.

For results that require urgent or emergency attention, the investigators should have a plan for notifying participants in a timely manner. Participants should be encouraged to allow the results to be sent directly to their personal physician as well as to themselves.

SHOULD INDIVIDUAL RESULTS FROM RESEARCH TESTS BE OFFERED?

The researcher needs to decide whether to offer individual results from research tests to participants, and to provide the IRB with the reasons for that decision. The issue of results from genomic sequencing presents additional ethical issues and is discussed in Chapter 27.

WEIGH THE BENEFITS, RISKS, AND BURDENS OF DISCLOSURE

When designing a study, investigators should carefully consider whether to offer individual results from research tests. The benefits of disclosing individual research test results need to be balanced against the risks and burdens. Factors that should be considered include the validity and clinical significance of the tests, the seriousness of the condition, and CLIA regulations.

If analytical validity has not been established, results should not be offered to participants because the information is so unreliable that no inferences are warranted.

If clinical validity has not been established, even if analytic validity has been shown, the presumption should be not to disclose the results because researchers will not be able to say whether an abnormal test result means that the patient has the condition being studied. However, there may be exceptions in which this presumption is overridden. In Study 11.1, preventing harm to third parties justified offering to disclose uncertain information.

In another possible exception, participants, advocacy groups, or community groups may want access to results of research tests, even though their analytic and clinical validity has not been established. In some cases, it may be difficult to enroll participants without offering them the results of research tests. In such situations, researchers need to negotiate with advocacy and community groups. Some ethics experts go even further, advocating that researchers should routinely offer participants choices about receiving results of experimental tests (8), because only the individual participant can determine what value to place on knowing uncertain information.

If clinical significance has not been established, even though analytic and clinical validity have been established, the crucial issue is whether participants are likely to find personal significance in knowing their results. Because participants and researchers may place a different value on learning test results, it is helpful for investigators to consult with disease organizations and patient advocacy groups to understand their perspective on obtaining research test results and to explain to them the limitations of the tests.

If clinical significance has been established, there are compelling reasons to offer results to participants. In this situation, abnormal results would change clinical management, and participants would benefit from receiving results.

OBTAIN INFORMED CONSENT FOR RECEIVING RESEARCH TEST RESULTS

Because people vary in their preferences for information, receiving results of research tests should be optional rather than mandatory. If participants are offered the opportunity to receive research test results, they should have the option to decline them. Because participants may change their minds over the course of a longitudinal study, participants who indicate at the onset of a study that they wish to receive individual results should be asked before the results are provided, to confirm that they still wish to receive them (9).

Investigators need to anticipate that some participants may have a "therapeutic misconception" that the research tests are like clinical tests, with established validity and significance. Investigators should discuss explicitly during the consent process the limitations of the research tests, their own professional background if it is not in clinical medicine, and their plans for disclosing incidental findings.

If results of research tests will not be provided, researchers should be prepared to explain why this is the case. If results of research tests will be offered, participants should know when and how they will be available. If some tests are batched and run only at the end of the study, patients should understand this so that they will not have unrealistic expectations about when they will receive their results.

MAXIMIZE THE BENEFITS AND MINIMIZE THE HARMS OF OFFERING RESULTS

If possible, participants should get a confirmatory test in a CLIA-approved laboratory. Researchers should help participants understand the results by providing interpretation and counseling and explaining the limitations of research tests (9). Clinical decisions generally should not be based solely on research tests. Investigators need to be prepared to respond to questions and to emotional reactions to "bad news." Participants should be encouraged to have their results sent to their treating physicians, who can help put the results in clinical context. Often this will require educating the physicians about the research tests. Because research tests by definition are innovative, researchers must anticipate that both the participants and the treating physicians will not appreciate the limitations of the results.

INVOLVE THE IRB

Researchers must obtain approval from the IRB for any plans to disclose the results of research tests to participants. Furthermore, subsequent research may establish clinical validity, providing strong reasons to notify participants. In these situations, the researcher should not change plans about disclosure unilaterally, but should submit a plan to the IRB for approval.

STUDY 11.1   (Continued).

The individual results from the research test for hepatitis C provide fewer benefits than the clinical tests. The analytic validity is uncertain. Clinical validity cannot be determined until after the study is completed. The optimal cutoff point for abnormal tests cannot be determined until all the data are collected and analyzed. Furthermore, the specificity and sensitivity calculated from this study need to be confirmed in a separate independent population.

In addition, the clinical significance of the test is unknown. Should people who are found to be positive on the newer test before they are found to be positive on the standard clinical test be regarded as having early hepatitis C infection? Are they contagious? Does any intervention during this "window" period modify the subsequent course of the illness? Some individuals will have indeterminate results because they repeatedly test positive on the new test but have normal results on the conventional hepatitis C test. Should these people be considered to have hepatitis C? These important questions can only be answered through additional research. Nonetheless, from a public health perspective, the most prudent approach would be for persons who are positive on the more sensitive test to regard themselves as infected and take measures to prevent transmitting a blood-borne infection to others, such as by not donating blood for transfusions, sharing injection drug paraphernalia, or engaging in unprotected sexual intercourse.

The risks of disclosing individual results from research tests are significant. Persons who test positive might suffer psychosocial harm. They might be stigmatized by sexual partners if they disclose that they have an early infection. However, if they know they have an abnormal result on this research test but do not disclose it, they may suffer recriminations if the partner is infected during this window period. Overall, the balance of benefits and risks in terms of offering results to participants in Study 11.1 is a close call.

It would be permissible for researchers to offer the results to individuals, provided that steps are taken to educate and counsel those who have abnormal or indeterminate results, who should obtain additional follow-up testing.

SHOULD INCIDENTAL FINDINGS BE OFFERED TO PARTICIPANTS?

When investigators carry out research tests, they may discover abnormalities that are unrelated to the research question the test was intended to answer; these are called incidental findings. For example, on a radiology imaging study, researchers may note abnormalities outside the anatomical area of research interest. In genome testing, mutations may be noted at locations that are not in the region being studied. The term "incidental" derives from Latin terms meaning to fall upon or happen onto. The modern dictionary definition refers to something in fortuitous conjunction with something else of which it forms no essential part.

STUDY 11.2   **Incidental findings on a radiology study.**

A researcher is studying which areas of the brain are involved when people are shown images of favorite foods and tables of the food's nutritional contents. The hypothesis is that different functional areas of the brain are involved in obese and nonobese participants. As part of the study, participants undergo a functional magnetic resonance imaging (MRI) study and an anatomical MRI study of the brain. When researchers review these tests at the end of the study, they find a number of incidental findings, including mild cortical atrophy, scattered demyelinating plaques, and mass lesions in the brain.

The anatomical MRI study did not use contrast, used lower intensity than clinical MRI studies, and acquired only T1-weighted images. Thus the images were less sensitive than those obtained in MRI studies for clinical purposes. The images were read by the study team, a psychologist, and a basic neuroscience researcher. The researchers question whether they should inform participants of these abnormal findings.

CONCERNS ABOUT NOTIFYING PARTICIPANTS OF INCIDENTAL FINDINGS

Study 11.2 illustrates how disclosing incidental findings generally provides fewer benefits than disclosing the results of research or clinical tests. Furthermore, the risks may be greater.

Benefits of Offering Participants Incidental Findings

Some incidental findings may alert the participant to a previously undiagnosed serious condition for which early treatment would be beneficial. For example, an asymptomatic participant might be found to have a high-risk aneurysm that should be treated before it causes an intracerebral bleed.

Risks of Offering Participants Incidental Findings

Test results may not be valid. In Study 11.2, the analytic and clinical validity of the MRI research images is not well established. Their resolution and ability to identify very small lesions of research images is lower than that of clinical-quality studies. The researchers have not had formal training in reading MRI scans. Hence their interpretations are likely less reliable than interpretations by board-certified radiologists.

Positive results may be false positives. The prevalence of incidental findings on research-quality MRI scans is around 20% (10–12). The prevalence varies according to the imaging technique used, the experience of the reader, and participant characteristics, with older persons having more incidental findings. In one series, about 2% of the incidental findings required urgent referral for follow-up studies and care, and a larger percentage called for routine referral. The majority of incidental findings were of uncertain clinical significance, including unidentified bright objects, mild cortical atrophy, and small demyelinating plaques (13). The prevalence of potentially clinically serious conditions, such as tumors and aneurysms, has been reported to be between 0.2% and 3.4% (10–12). The appropriate management of such serious findings may be controversial; for example, although small, asymptomatic aneurysms have a very small risk of rupture, the consequences would be severe.

Negative results may be false negatives. Research-quality MRI cannot detect very small lesions. Also, researchers who are not board certified in radiology might miss subtle findings. Thus participants may receive false reassurance if they are told that they have no abnormalities.

Participants may suffer clinical and psychosocial risks. Incidental findings may require confirmation or further testing to clarify their clinical significance. In Study 11.2, participants would need a clinical-quality MRI of the brain with contrast. If a finding is confirmed, they might need additional tests, such as angiography, which entails medical risks such as renal toxicity and procedure complications. While awaiting the results of additional testing, participants may suffer adverse psychosocial consequences, such as depression, anxiety, or stigmatization.

Some participants do not want to know results. When a test for the gene for Huntington disease was developed, many participants in the research did not want to receive their individual results. Although the clinical significance was clear, they did not want to live with the knowledge that they would develop an untreatable, progressively debilitating disease. Similarly, in research studies that led to the development of BRCA1 and BRCA2 testing for hereditary breast cancer, some participants did want to learn their individual test results (14,15).

Burdens of Offering Participants Incidental Findings

Offering participants incidental findings on research tests may be burdensome for researchers. As in Study 11.2, researchers who notice incidental findings may not be trained in radiology or clinical medicine. Such investigators would need to consult with an appropriate clinical specialist to interpret the incidental findings.

A related issue is how much time and effort researchers should spend to look for incidental findings that are outside their areas of research interest. Some radiologists have recommended that all research brain MRI scans should have the same quality as clinical MRI scans and be read by board-certified radiologists (16). However, the resources required for investigators to follow this suggestion would be substantial, potentially adding significantly to the cost and time of a study or exceeding the available funding. In addition, ethics and policy experts have warned against expecting researchers to carry out the same responsibilities as clinicians who order a similar test on a patient (17). One risk is that participants will have a "therapeutic misconception" that they will receive direct clinical benefit from the research project. Another risk is that researchers who become highly involved in providing clinical information to participants will compromise their ability to carry out their research objectives. Therefore, it is necessary to set limits on the actions researchers must take regarding incidental findings (17).

RECOMMENDATIONS REGARDING INCIDENTAL FINDINGS

The researchers need to state in the protocol whether participants will be offered incidental findings, and justify that decision, as well as the procedures used to notify participants, to the IRB.

Use Reasonable Care in Identifying Incidental Findings

Generally speaking, researchers should do what a reasonable researcher with similar expertise would be expected to do under the circumstances. They should not be required to do what a treating physician would do when ordering a similar test in clinical practice for a patient. The researcher's primary goal is to obtain rigorous scientific knowledge, whereas the clinician's goal is to act in the best interest of the individual patient. Although the roles of researcher and clinician are similar, they should be distinguished. A clinician ordering an MRI scan should order the test at a facility that generates high-quality images, and the studies should be interpreted by board-certified radiologists. However, a researcher should not be expected to review all aspects of an MRI scan. A researcher who is not trained as a neuroradiologist should not be expected to have the expertise in reading and interpreting scans that a board-certified researcher would, assuming of course that such expertise is not needed to adequately carry out the research project. Incidental findings are by definition incidental to the research, and not part of the fundamental responsibility of the researcher. However, a researcher should be expected to notice abnormalities that are so obvious that even a nonspecialist could reasonably be expected to identify them. Hence, researchers would be expected to identify gross abnormalities such as large mass lesions causing asymmetry.

When investigators do identify an incidental finding, they should do what is reasonable under the circumstances: consult with a neuroradiologist about the clinical significance of the findings. Concerns about confidentiality can be addressed by showing the neuroradiologist de-identified images.

Disclosure to Participants Should Depend on the Balance of Benefits and Risks

At one extreme, the strongest argument for offering participants incidental findings is that the abnormality signifies a serious condition for which early treatment or prevention is effective. In this situation, the participant should be informed unless he has indicated he does not want to be told about findings.

At the other extreme, the weakest argument for disclosure occurs when the finding is not clinically important, and if it were observed in a clinical study, the patient would not be notified or would be told only that it is a minor abnormality that does not require follow-up.

In most cases, the findings will fall between these extremes. The clinical significance will be uncertain, and the treatments will usually be risky or of unproven effectiveness. Researchers should offer to disclose results only if knowing the results offers a clear net benefit to the participant (18).

A helpful rule of thumb is that the obligation of a researcher to disclose incidental findings should not be greater than the obligation of a treating physician to disclose the same findings on tests ordered for clinical purposes. After all, the treating physician has an ethical duty to act in the patient's best interests, whereas the researcher has no such obligation to participants. Thus, if a clinician would not disclose an incidental finding on a clinical-quality MRI scan (except perhaps to mention that it is present but does not require follow-up), it would be inconsistent to expect an investigator to provide more information if it were noted on a research-quality scan.

Disclosure of Incidental Findings Should be Discussed During the Informed Consent Process

Participants' expectations about disclosure of incidental findings should be consistent with the researchers' plans. Investigators need to anticipate that some participants may have a therapeutic misconception, and may believe that in return for participating in the study they will get a free clinical-quality brain scan. Thus, researchers should discuss explicitly during the consent process the limitations of the research tests, their own professional background if it is not in clinical medicine, and their plans for disclosing incidental findings. In Study 11.2, it would be accurate to say that participants should not expect any direct benefit, even though in exceptional cases an incidental finding could be noted that would have clinical expectations.

TAKE HOME POINTS

1. When researchers consider offering research participants their individual test results, they need to take into account the benefits, risks, and burdens of knowing those results.
2. Researchers should offer to disclose incidental findings on research tests only if there is a clear net benefit to the participant.

ANNOTATED BIBLIOGRAPHY

Miller FG, Mello MM, Joffe S. Incidental findings in human subjects research: what do investigators owe research participants? *J Law Med Ethics* 2008;36:271–279.
    Lucid conceptual analysis of responsibility for incidental findings.
Shalowitz DI, Miller FG. Communicating the results of clinical research to participants: attitudes, practices, and future directions. *PLoS Med* 2008;5:e91.
    Review of empirical studies on attitudes and consequences of receiving research results.
Wolf SM, Lawrenz FP, Nelson CA, et al. Managing incidental findings in human subjects research: analysis and recommendations. *J Law Med Ethics* 2008;36:219–248.
    Summary of consensus conference on incidental findings.

REFERENCES

1. Secretary's Advisory Committee. Enhancing the oversight of genetic tests: recommendations of the SACGT (2000). Available at: http://www4.od.nih.gov/oba/sacgt/gtdocuments.html. Accessed November 16, 2007.
2. Ravitsky V, Wilfond BS. Disclosing individual genetic results to research participants. *Am J Bioeth* 2006;6:8–17.
3. Shalowitz DI, Miller FG. Disclosing individual results of clinical research: implications of respect for participants. *JAMA* 2005;294:737–740.
4. Shalowitz DI, Miller FG. Communicating the results of clinical research to participants: attitudes, practices, and future directions. *PLoS Med* 2008;5:e91.
5. National Bioethics Advisory Commission. *Research on Human Stored Biologic Materials.* Rockville, MD: National Bioethics Advisory Commission; 1999.
6. Partridge AH, Wong JS, Knudsen K, et al. Offering participants results of a clinical trial: sharing results of a negative study. *Lancet* 2005;365:963–964.
7. Miller FA, Christensen R, Giacomini M, et al. Duty to disclose what? Querying the putative obligation to return research results to participants. *J Med Ethics* 2008;34:210–213.
8. Rothstein MA. Expanding the ethical analysis of biobanks. *J Law Med Ethics* 2005;33:89–101.
9. Renegar G, Webster CJ, Stuerzebecher S, et al. Returning genetic research results to individuals: points-to-consider. *Bioethics* 2006;20:24–36.
10. Illes J, Chin VN. Bridging philosophical and practical implications of incidental findings in brain research. *J Law Med Ethics* 2008;36:298–304.
11. Katzman GL, Dagher AP, Patronas NJ. Incidental findings on brain magnetic resonance imaging from 1000 asymptomatic volunteers. *JAMA* 1999;282:36–39.
12. Vernooij MW, Ikram MA, Tanghe HL, et al. Incidental findings on brain MRI in the general population. *N Engl J Med* 2007;357:1821–1828.
13. Royal JM, Peterson BS. The risks and benefits of searching for incidental findings in MRI research scans. *J Law Med Ethics* 2008;36:305–314.
14. Biesecker BB, Ishibe N, Hadley DW, et al. Psychosocial factors predicting BRCA1/BRCA2 testing decisions in members of hereditary breast and ovarian cancer families. *Am J Med Genet* 2000;93:257–263.
15. Foster C, Evans DG, Eeles R, et al. Non-uptake of predictive genetic testing for BRCA1/2 among relatives of known carriers: attributes, cancer worry, and barriers to testing in a multicenter clinical cohort. *Genet Test* 2004;8:23–29.
16. Mamourian A. Incidental findings on research functional MR images: should we look? *AJNR Am J Neuroradiol* 2004;25:520–522.
17. Miller FG, Mello MM, Joffe S. Incidental findings in human subjects research: what do investigators owe research participants? *J Law Med Ethics* 2008;36:271–279.
18. Wolf SM, Lawrenz FP, Nelson CA, et al. Managing incidental findings in human subjects research: analysis and recommendations. *J Law Med Ethics* 2008;36:219–248.

Responsible Conduct of Research

CHAPTER 12

Research Misconduct

In several recent scandals, researchers have committed egregious acts of scientific misconduct, including fabrication and falsification of data, to obtain desired results. In light of these episodes, scientists need to acknowledge the possibility of serious scientific misconduct, understand the definition of scientific misconduct, and respond vigorously and fairly to allegations of misconduct. Clinical research increasingly requires collaboration and interdisciplinary teams. Collaborations depend on trust because it is impossible for an investigator to monitor or be expert in all aspects of a project.

IS RESEARCH MISCONDUCT A SERIOUS PROBLEM?

RESEARCH MISCONDUCT BY A TRAINEE

STUDY 12.1	Cardiology research.

John Darsee, a fellow at a leading research cardiology department in the United States, published over 100 papers (1). Most of the papers were co-authored with senior scientists, including an eminent professor who was chief of the cardiology department and chairman of medicine at his hospital. Darsee falsified tracings in full view of colleagues in the laboratory, labeling data that had been collected over a few hours to appear as if they had been obtained over a few weeks.

Darsee's supervisor initially believed that he had cracked under the pressure to publish. An investigation by his mentor, who examined Darsee's notebooks, concluded that this falsification was an isolated incident. Darsee's co-workers were not notified.

Subsequently in a multicenter trial in which Darsee was an investigator, data from that one site differed markedly from data from other sites. The university appointed a committee to conduct a review. The committee did not conduct an independent investigation, but supported the findings of the internal investigation.

An investigation convened by the National Institutes of Health (NIH) reanalyzed data from five papers Darsee had written in collaboration with his mentor and found "extensive irregularities." The panel questioned whether there had been sufficient direct supervision of the research group. The university also was criticized for not reporting the incident to the NIH, which funded Darsee's training, or to co-authors of his papers.

Subsequently most of his papers, some of which involved research with human subjects, were found to contain serious inconsistencies in data and statistical analysis. Many of the participants and some co-authors simply did not exist. In retrospect, one of his collaborators acknowledged that the data were "too good, too neat, too perfect to be believed" (1).

This scandal forced scientists and research institutions to recognize that egregious misconduct may occur despite academic supervision and peer review. This episode occurred at a leading academic health center and the falsified work was published in prestigious scientific journals. The university's response to the incident was inadequate. Because of this and other cases of serious misconduct, the NIH established a definition of misconduct and procedures for responding to allegations of misconduct, as detailed further below.

This episode also revealed problems with authorship of scientific publications. Darsee did not notify some persons that they were listed as co-authors, and others who accepted co-authorship admitted that they did not review the drafts of the manuscript carefully. Thus some co-authors accepted credit for authorship although they did no significant work on the project, and later disclaimed responsibility for the errors. In response to this and similar incidents, journals clarified what responsibilities authors are expected to carry out, as discussed in Chapter 13.

This case also raised questions about appropriate supervision of a research group. If a mentor or supervisor fails to carry out rigorous review of raw data and preliminary analyses, fabrication and falsification may be more difficult to discourage and detect.

WHAT IS RESEARCH MISCONDUCT?

Research misconduct is defined by the federal Department of Health and Human Services (DHHS) as (2):

- *Fabrication*: "making up data or results and recording or reporting them."
- *Falsification*: "manipulating research materials, equipment, or processes, or changing or omitting data or results such that the research is not accurately represented in the research record." In short, investigators may not change the data to obtain the results they want to see.
- *Plagiarism*: "the appropriation of another person's ideas, processes, results, or words without giving appropriate credit."

The actions must be a "significant departure from accepted practices" in the scientific field. Research misconduct may occur when writing a research proposal, carrying out research, reviewing research or a proposal, or presenting results of research. The website of the Office of Research Integrity (ORI) provides detailed information at http://ori.dhhs.gov/.

The federal definition of research misconduct is narrow and excludes a number of ethically blameworthy actions. According to this definition, the misconduct must be intentional; carelessness, sloppiness, laziness, and poor scientific methods do not constitute research misconduct. Furthermore, the federal definition of research misconduct excludes unintentional, "honest" errors and differences of opinion or interpretation. This definition also excludes other unethical behaviors, such as violations of informed consent, financial mismanagement, poor mentoring, discrimination, and sexual harassment. Research institutions should have other procedures for addressing such misbehavior.

WHY IS RESEARCH MISCONDUCT ETHICALLY PROBLEMATIC?

Invalid data compromise scientific knowledge and the evidence base for clinical medicine. If investigators fabricate or falsify their data or findings, readers of scientific journals cannot trust their conclusions. Other scientists will waste resources and time trying to build on invalid results. Research participants may be subjected to risks without any valid knowledge being gained. If clinicians base their patient-care decisions on invalid findings, patients may be harmed.

Research misconduct is unfair, resulting in unmerited rewards for those who cheat. Publishing a larger number of papers can give a researcher prestige, jobs, promotions, and grants. As a result of such scandals, some universities now give more weight to the quality of publications than to the quantity.

Research misconduct weakens public support for biomedical research. The federal government, through the NIH, is the largest funder of investigator-initiated research. In contrast to research sponsored by pharmaceutical and biotechnology companies, the NIH sponsors basic and methodological studies that are not directed toward marketable products.

A powerful congressman warned that scandals would undermine the public's willingness to fund research, noting that "[e]very time a researcher takes taxpayer money and publishes fabricated, falsified, or plagiarized findings, the taxpayer has in effect been swindled. Furthermore, given our budget deficit, there is never enough money to go around" (3). Thus, although serious research misconduct may be rare, it causes serious damage to the entire research enterprise. To ensure Congress that research funded by NIH grants and training programs meets high ethical standards, NIH grantees and trainees must receive training about research ethics.

RESEARCH MISCONDUCT IN A MULTIDISCIPLINARY PROJECT

In the Darsee case, misconduct was detected when the perpetrator falsified data in full view of his colleagues. In the current era of large multidisciplinary projects and digital images, another scandal showed how difficult it can be to detect research misconduct.

STUDY 12.2   **Stem cell lines using somatic cell nuclear transfer (SCNT).**

In February 2004, a research team led by Professor Woo Suk Hwang in South Korea published a paper claiming they had derived the first human stem cell line using SCNT. In May 2005, the researchers published a second paper showing that they had made their techniques much more efficient and had derived 11 different human stem cell lines using SCNT. In August 2005, the team reported that they had successfully cloned a dog, Snuppy.

Acting on a tip from a junior member of the research team, a South Korean news reporter investigated allegations that data had been falsified and that members of the research team had contributed oocytes. The television station that broke the story was harshly criticized for being unpatriotic and unethical. The reporters had used hidden cameras to record interviews and overstated what they knew to induce interviewees to speak out. After the identity of the whistleblower was leaked, he had to resign from his position.

In December 2005, anonymous postings on the Internet showed that photographs of the cloned line were identical to photographs of an earlier stem cell line. Subsequent postings demonstrated that other key data in the articles were also falsified. Investigations by Seoul National University concluded that there was no evidence that the Hwang team had produced any SCNT stem cell lines. All the data and images in the 2005 paper were from two previously derived embryonic stem cell lines.

The investigation also determined that Hwang had lied about how the oocytes had been obtained. The publications claimed that 427 oocytes were used and no donors were paid. However, at least 2221 oocytes from 119 donors were used, and 66 of 119 donors received compensation. A graduate student and technicians were asked to donate eggs, contrary to previous denials. Donors were not properly informed of the risks. Furthermore, at one hospital, two out of 79 oocyte donors required hospitalization for serious ovarian hyperstimulation syndrome. The report also found that institutional review boards failed to provide appropriate oversight. A separate government investigation found that $2.6 million in funds the laboratory received could not be accounted for.

The senior (last) author on the 2005 paper was a U.S. scientist named Gerald Schatten. He did not participate in the actual research but revised the manuscript, negotiated with the editors of the journal in which it was published, and participated in interviews after publication. Upon learning of problems with oocyte donation, he cut ties with the Hwang group. An investigation found no evidence that he falsified anything or was aware of any misconduct. However, the investigators criticized his "concerted and deliberate effort . . . to further distance himself from Dr. Hwang and their joint publications," which was "in sharp contrast to the full participation of Dr. Schatten in the media spotlight following publication of the paper" (4). Furthermore, the panel declared, "We have no reason to doubt [his] statement to

STUDY 12.2 **(Continued).**

us that his major contribution . . . was a suggestion that a professional photographer be engaged so that Snuppy would appear with greater visual appeal." It is less clear that this contribution fully justifies co-authorship." The panel also criticized Schatten's consultation fee of $40,000, which it characterized as "far above normal honoraria for consultation."

The original publication of a human stem cell line derived using SCNT was hailed as a breakthrough. Supporters of stem cell research cited this work as evidence that NIH funding restrictions on embryonic stem cell research were putting U.S. scientists at a disadvantage. Many investigators tried to form collaborative relationships with the Hwang team.

Study 12.2 dramatizes how science depends on trust and how fragile that trust is. After this scandal, some opponents of stem cell research attacked the entire field of embryonic stem cell research as being unethical and irresponsible. Other persons, while not opposing all stem cell research, questioned whether research in this sensitive, rapidly moving field was under appropriate ethical oversight. As research becomes increasingly interdisciplinary, it is becoming apparent that most scientists lack the expertise to personally review all primary data from collaborators. They must trust that others have done their part of the collaboration carefully and with integrity. In Study 12.2, for example, one collaborating researcher carried out a series of tests to determine whether the putative stem cells had markers and properties characteristic of stem cells. When he performed tests in his laboratory on materials sent by the lead author, he could not verify that the cells were derived as claimed.

As was the case in Study 12.2, junior researchers and staff in a laboratory may be the first to suspect or observe scientific misconduct. The case illustrates that research institutions need to encourage whistleblowers to come forward, to take allegations of research misconduct seriously, and to investigate them promptly.

In that study, the peer review process failed to detect evidence of fabrication. Neither the reviewers nor the editors realized before publication that the figures had been manipulated and altered. Computer multimedia programs readily allow digital images to be manipulated, and journal editors concede that the peer review process is no guarantee against scientific misconduct.

The co-authors of that study also failed to prevent research misconduct. It is not clear which author took responsibility for retrieving the oocytes or producing the images in the published article. After the scandal was exposed, the last author of the paper disclaimed responsibility. Furthermore, he had not made substantial intellectual contributions to the manuscript. As discussed in Chapter 13, his contributions did not justify authorship.

In that study, the oocyte donors suffered serious physical harm. The incidence of serious ovarian hyperstimulation syndrome was much higher than that in high-quality clinical in vitro fertilization programs.

RESEARCH MISCONDUCT IN PATIENT-ORIENTED RESEARCH

Although many cases of research misconduct involve laboratory research, some cases have important implications for patient care and clinical trials.

STUDY 12.3 **Nonsteroidal anti-inflamatory drugs (NSAIDS) and risk of oral cancer.**

A researcher published a series of papers on oral cancer showing that aneuploidy (abnormal numbers of chromosomes) in noncancerous mouth lesions strongly predicted the development of oral cancer. A second study, based on analysis of medical records, claimed that long-term use of NSAIDs reduced the risks of oral cancer. Based on these data, the NCI approved a $9 million trial to prevent oral cancer using the NSAID celecoxib.

An astute reader noted that the researcher claimed to have analyzed archived health records that were not yet available to researchers. The reader was the director of this archive. She alerted the journal editors, who notified the hospital where the investigator worked. An investigation found that all of the data had been fabricated. Of the 908 study subjects, 205 had the same birthday, a coincidence that is unlikely in the extreme. The scientist also cited a grant that he had applied for but failed to get. An earlier paper was also found to be fabricated. One image in that paper was simply a magnified version of another image. These articles had all been published in top-tier medical journals (5,6).

This case is troubling because it demonstrates that fabrication and fraud can occur with research involving large data sets containing clinical records. Although lying about research results is always wrong, it is particularly harmful when it may result in risk to participants in research trials or future patients. If the planned prevention trial had taken place, the participants in the trial would have been at risk for medical complications from the study celecoxib (including gastrointestinal bleeding and heart attacks), with no scientifically founded expectation of contributing new knowledge or experiencing personal benefit through cancer prevention. Furthermore, the resources needed for the clinical trial would have been wasted and other meritorious research would not have been funded.

WITHHOLDING NEGATIVE RESULTS

In several recent pivotal clinical trials, investigators withheld data on negative outcomes or failed to report negative results for several years after the conclusion of the trial (see Table 1.1). Intentionally omitting clinically significant negative data to make the results from the study drug more favorable can result in bias in favor of the study drug. Failing to report negative outcomes in clinical trials is also ethically problematic because the participants in a study may be exposed to risks without any scientific knowledge being gained.

Negative studies should be submitted for abstract presentations at professional meetings and for publication as manuscripts. It may be difficult to publish negative results because of publication bias; however, findings can be presented on the sponsor's website.

PREVALENCE OF MISCONDUCT

Surveys of NIH-funded researchers have provided some indication of the prevalence of research misconduct. In a 2005 survey, respondents were asked whether they personally had engaged in specific unethical behaviors during the past 3 years (7). Their responses are summarized below:

	% Yes
Failed to present data that contradict one's previous research.	6.0%
Unauthorized use of confidential information in one's own research.	1.7%
Used another's ideas without attribution or credit.	1.4%
Ignored major aspects of human subjects requirements.	0.3%
Falsified data.	0.3%

Mid-career scientists who had recently received their first NIH R01 award were more likely to engage in these behaviors than trainees.

A 2006 survey asked respondents whether they had personally observed suspected research misconduct in their own department during the past 3 years (8); 4.4% said they had observed fabrication or falsification, and 2.7% had observed plagiarism. More than one-third of the cases were not reported to anyone.

ALLEGATIONS OF RESEARCH MISCONDUCT

HOW CAN RESEARCH MISCONDUCT BE IDENTIFIED?

Because research misconduct is difficult to detect, investigators need to be sensitive to possible warning signs, such as:

- Progress in the study is much faster than expected.
- Enrollment at one site of a study is far greater than at other sites.

- The data are too good to be true; for example, the effect may be much greater than anticipated or the variation among participants may be much less than expected.
- There are inconsistencies in the data; for example, the data at one site differ strikingly from data at other sites.

These warning signs are sensitive for research misconduct but not specific. There may be other explanations for the situation. It is the researcher's responsibility to explore the situation, rather than simply rejoice that the research is going better than expected. Other warning signs should raise even greater suspicions of misconduct:

- Data cannot be validated or replicated.
- Reviewers note that the wording in a new manuscript or grant looks very familiar.

HOW SHOULD INSTITUTIONS RESPOND TO ALLEGED RESEARCH MISCONDUCT?

When an allegation of misconduct is raised, the institution where the research occurred needs to take it seriously and look into it further. It is a mistake to dismiss at the onset allegations of misconduct as implausible or as personality clashes. Under NIH requirements, each institution must appoint a research integrity officer, who may speak confidentially about the situation with a whistleblower (technically called the complainant) before a formal compliant is made. An allegation must be sufficiently specific so that pertinent evidence can be gathered.

When allegations involve federally funded research projects or trainees, the institution must carry out a two-step response.

An *inquiry* is an initial review to determine whether the allegations have enough merit to warrant a full investigation. The goal is not to decide whether misconduct occurred. The person or committee conducting the inquiry must interview the complainant, the accused scientist (technically called the respondent), and key witnesses, as well as perform an initial review of evidence. A full review of all evidence is not required. A final report on the inquiry must be prepared and the respondent must have the opportunity to comment on it.

An *investigation* is a more extensive and formal process to determine whether research misconduct occurred. There must be additional procedural safeguards. The respondent must receive written notification of all allegations so that he can respond to them. All testimony before the investigational body must be recorded or transcribed, and the persons interviewed must have the opportunity to review and correct their testimony. The respondent must have an opportunity to comment on the draft of the investigation report and to review the evidence on which the report is based.

Throughout an inquiry and investigation, the research institution must ensure a fair process and protect the rights of both the complainant and the respondent. Specifically, the institution must:

- Protect the complainant, witnesses, and committee members from retaliation. Many complainants have reported adverse consequences, including loss of position, promotion, or salary increases.
- Protect or restore the reputation of those accused of research misconduct who are found innocent.
- Ensure that persons carrying out misconduct proceedings have no conflict of interest with the complainant, respondent, or witnesses.
- Protect confidentiality. The identity of the complainant and respondent should be disclosed only to those who have a need to know, for example, those carrying out an inquiry or investigation.

These procedures are designed to ensure a fair, thorough, and timely judgment regarding the allegations. Ad hoc or informal investigations can sometimes result in incomplete or unfair findings.

An investigation is expected to begin within 30 days after the inquiry concludes that an investigation is warranted, and it should generally be concluded within 120 days. An institution may have a process for respondents to appeal judgments of research misconduct, but is not required to have one. The institution may impose penalties if misconduct is judged to have occurred.

When an institution initiates an investigation, it must make a report to the Office of Research Integrity (ORI). The ORI has the power to review misconduct proceedings carried out by the institution, make a final determination of misconduct, recommend that DHHS conduct an inquiry or investigation, or propose penalties. A respondent may contest an ORI judgment of misconduct and any penalties through a hearing before an administrative law judge.

WHAT ARE THE CONSEQUENCES OF RESEARCH MISCONDUCT?

The federal government may suspend a grant or other federal funding, or debar a person from receiving future federal funding. The research institution may suspend or terminate employment. In addition, there may also be civil or criminal penalties.

HOW CAN RESEARCH MISCONDUCT BE PREVENTED?

Several measures can help prevent misconduct, as well as improve the quality of research data.

Education of investigators and staff. In some early cases of alleged research misconduct, scientists claimed that they did not know that fabrication, falsification, and plagiarism were wrong. In response, the NIH now requires courses in research ethics for investigators, key personnel, and trainees who receive its grants.

Data audits ensure that the protocol is followed and that the data are valid (9–11). Audits of a sample of on-site research records improve the quality of research data and encourage compliance with requirements for informed consent and IRB approval. On rare occasions, audits may also detect improper conduct.

In research that involves contact and interventions with participants, it is worthwhile to recontact a sample of participants for quality assurance purposes. Such interviews can verify that participants met eligibility criteria, the consent process was appropriate, and the research procedures were carried out as planned. Audits discourage fabrication of data, and because data audits enhance the quality of research data, their costs can justifiably be included in grants. The FDA also conducts audits of data submitted to it.

Close involvement of the principal investigator in all aspects of project. The principal investigator sets the tone for the entire project. Regular reviews of primary data, preliminary analyses, and internal data audits establish the importance of data integrity (12).

TAKE HOME POINTS

1. Research misconduct is defined as intentional fabrication, falsification, or plagiarism. Such misconduct undermines the integrity of research findings and public trust in research.
2. Because research misconduct is difficult to detect, investigators need to be sensitive to possible warning signs, including data that are much better than expected.
3. When allegations of research misconduct are raised, the research institution should institute an inquiry, followed by a full investigation if warranted. The rights of both the whistleblower and the accused must be protected.

ANNOTATED BIBLIOGRAPHY

Martinson BC, Anderson MS, de Vries R. Scientists behaving badly. *Nature* 2005;435:737.
Titus SL, Wells JA, Rhoades LJ. Repairing research integrity. *Nature* 2008;453:980–982.
    Two surveys of NIH-funded researchers on the prevalence of research misconduct.

REFERENCES

1. Culliton B. Coping with fraud: the Darsee case. *Science* 1983;220:31–35.
2. Department of Health and Human Services. 42 CFR Parts 50 and 93. Public Health Services Policies on Research Misconduct; Final Rule. 2005. Available at: http://ori.hhs.gov/policies/. Accessed December 5, 2008.
3. Dingell JD. Shattuck lecture—misconduct in medical research. *N Engl J Med* 1993;328:1610–1615.
4. Holden C. Korean stem cell scandal. Schatten: Pitt panel finds 'misbehavior' but not misconduct. *Science* 2006; 311:928.
5. Marris E. Doctor admits Lancet study is fiction. *Nature* 2006;439:248–249.
6. Couzin J, Schirber M. Scientific misconduct. Fraud upends oral cancer field, casting doubt on prevention trial. *Science* 2006;311:448–449.
7. Martinson BC, Anderson MS, de Vries R. Scientists behaving badly. *Nature* 2005;435:737.
8. Titus SL, Wells JA, Rhoades LJ. Repairing research integrity. *Nature* 2008;453:980–982.
9. Weiss RB, Vogelzang NJ, Peterson BA, et al. A successful system of scientific data audits for clinical trials. A report from the Cancer and Leukemia Group B. *JAMA* 1993;270:459–464.
10. Shapiro MF, Charrow RP. The role of data audits in detecting scientific misconduct. Results of the FDA program. *JAMA* 1989;261:2505–2511.
11. Shamoo AE, Resnik DB. *Responsible Conduct of Research*. New York: Oxford University Press; 2003:110–112.
12. Wright DE, Titus SL, Cornelison JB. Mentoring and research misconduct: an analysis of research mentoring in closed ORI cases. *Sci Eng Ethics* 2008;14:323–336.

Authorship and Its Responsibilities

Is there any researcher who has not looked up his or her own articles using a computerized literature search, such as PubMed? Authorship provides recognition for research achievements. Investigators naturally feel pride in seeing their name on a published article. However, authorship commonly causes ethical problems and disagreements among collaborators on a research project. In a 1996 survey, 38% of postdoctoral fellows reported being an author on a paper where one co-author didn't deserve to be an author (1), 37% had been asked to make someone an author who did not deserve it, and 20% had been omitted as an author even though they deserved authorship. Authorship disputes are particular stressful for fellows and young faculty members, who need publications to launch their careers and cannot alienate more senior researchers upon whom they depend for recommendations and mentoring. This chapter analyzes the criteria investigators must meet to merit authorship, common problems regarding authorship, and suggestions for resolving disputes over authorship.

WHAT IS THE PURPOSE OF AUTHORSHIP?

Authorship brings a researcher recognition and prestige. The expectation of seeing one's name in print is an incentive to work hard on research projects. In addition to subjective rewards, authorship leads to tangible benefits such as job offers, promotions, and grants.

Authorship also promotes accountability because authors are held responsible for the validity of the data and conclusions. This accountability discourages fabrication, fraud, and plagiarism. From a societal point of view, holding authors accountable is the quid pro quo for the recognition they receive.

WHAT ARE THE CRITERIA FOR AUTHORSHIP?

To earn authorship, a researcher should have made substantial intellectual contributions to a project. Major medical journals require that every author meet three criteria for authorship (Table 13.1).

Some journals also require authors to specify what contributions each author made or to specify which author was responsible for each phase of the study (e.g., design, data acquisition, data analysis, drafting the manuscript, and revising the manuscript).

Some activities that historically qualified someone to be an author are no longer sufficient. Merely providing funding, office space, or equipment for a project, collecting data, or supervising the research group, while essential, do not warrant authorship. Such assistance is not a substantial intellectual contribution and does not allow a person to vouch for the data and conclusions. Such contributions can and should be recognized by a generous acknowledgment.

Researchers often want to include research assistants or students as authors. This is praiseworthy and may be justified if the person fulfills the criteria for authorship. For example, in addition to

TABLE 13.1	Criteria for Authorship

Authors must:

1. Make substantial contributions to the conception and design of the project, data acquisition, or data analysis and interpretation.
2. Draft the article or revise it critically for intellectual content.
3. Approve the final manuscript.

helping with data analysis, the research assistant or student could draft part of the Methods section of the paper and help revise the paper.

If the research is to be carried out by a large, multisite group, a few individuals should be designated as a writing committee to take responsibility for the manuscript. These individuals should meet all the criteria for authorship.

Some journals now require that one or more authors serve as "guarantors" who take responsibility for the entire project from its inception to publication. This requirement serves to enhance accountability.

Details about recommendations by the International Committee of Medical Journal Editors regarding authorship can be accessed at http://www.icmje.org/#author.

WHAT ARE SOME COMMON PROBLEMS WITH AUTHORSHIP?

Problems with authorship are common and fall into several major categories:

TOO MANY AUTHORS

Many papers have authors who do not meet the criteria for authorship. About one-fifth to one-quarter of papers in major medical journals list "honorary" authors who made no substantial intellectual contribution to the project (2,3). These colleagues may have provided subjects, materials, or laboratory and technical assistance, or collected data (3). Most honorary authors have neither drafted nor revised the article.

TOO FEW AUTHORS

Articles may have too few authors as well as too many authors. A 1998 study (2) reported that 13% of articles in major biomedical journals had "ghost" authors—people who met the criteria for authorship but were not listed as authors. None of the ghost authors were even acknowledged in the papers. Typically, ghost authors work for for-profit companies, such as drug manufacturers or medical education and communication companies under contract with drug manufacturers. They draft the article for a university-based researcher who serves as the lead author. These academic authors may lend an aura of objectivity to the article. There are numerous ethical problems with this practice (4). It is misleading and dishonest, and it violates the guideline of giving credit where it is deserved. Furthermore, ghost authorship may mask conflicts of interest (5). Finally, the material in ghostwritten articles may be biased in favor of the company's product (4,6,7).

Because of concerns about bias in articles by ghost authors, many journals are now requiring that all persons who had input into the writing of a manuscript must either be listed as an author or acknowledged (8). Furthermore, all persons named as authors or acknowledged must complete a financial disclosure.

PUBLICATION OF ARTICLES THAT SHOULD NOT BE PUBLISHED

Some articles are published even though they should not be. Articles that contain plagiarized, fabricated, or falsified data should not be published, and should be retracted if they already have been published. Duplicate articles also should not be published because they waste space in journals and are misleading. Patients who are reported in duplicated articles may be counted more than once in systematic reviews, leading to biased conclusions, which usually favor the interventions studied.

A study of primary articles included in systemic reviews found that 8% of articles were duplicates (9). In the majority of cases there were no cross-references to the other articles, which made the duplication difficult to detect. Such duplication results in a misleading impression of the effectiveness of therapies. Several types of duplication occurred, including publishing the identical sample and outcomes, publishing part of a previous article, and combining several previous articles. Other studies have also documented that duplicate publication occurs (10).

FAILURE TO PUBLISH ARTICLES THAT SHOULD BE PUBLISHED

In several highly publicized cases, research sponsors discouraged scientists from publishing articles with "negative" findings (see Chapter 1, Table 1.1). The following case illustrates the ethical issues (11):

STUDY 13.1   **Pressure not to publish negative results.**

In 1996, a randomized controlled trial (RCT) was conducted to evaluate an immunologic modifier in HIV-infected persons. The study intervention was intended to boost the immune system's ability to better control HIV replication. The study intervention was inactivated HIV stripped of envelope proteins. The study agent plus antiretroviral therapy was compared with placebo plus antiretroviral therapy. The study endpoint was survival without HIV progression.

At the second interim data analysis, the data and safety monitoring board (DSMB) recommended that the study be terminated. There was no difference between the intervention and control groups with regard to the primary endpoint, and continuation of the study was highly unlikely to show a significant difference between the arms. Furthermore, the intervention group also failed to achieve prespecified benefits in HIV titers or CD4 counts.

The study sponsor did not provide the study leadership with a complete and final data set, despite multiple requests. The study leadership finally decided to publish an article based on the information available to the DSMB, which included 95% of the endpoints that would have been available in the final data set.

The sponsor threatened the principal investigator with a lawsuit if he submitted the article. The principal investigator had to spend considerable time with legal counsel. He was also concerned that he would be unable to obtain future industry funding for his research.

The editor of the journal that published the study commented, "The integrity of the research process rests on a sound study design and the disclosure of all pertinent results, whether positive or negative, based on analysis of all necessary data" (12).

Major medical journals have now established requirements for publishing industry-sponsored research. At least one author should have full responsibility for conducting the clinical trial, access to all study data, and control over publication, including data detrimental to the product (13). In addition, the manuscript must describe the role of the study sponsor in all phases of the study. Some major journals also require that someone independent of the for-profit sponsor carry out biostatistical analysis. Pertinent financial relationships for all authors must be disclosed. Finally, all clinical trials must be registered at the onset in an acceptable public clinical trials registry (14). The registry ensures that other researchers and clinicians are aware of trials that subsequently are not published.

Restrictions by corporate sponsors on publishing negative results have also led to changes in research agreements between universities and research sponsors. Currently, many universities insist that contractual agreements provide the principal investigator all data and control over publication. These conditions should be required for all sponsors, not just industrial sponsors.

WHAT IS THE APPROPRIATE ORDER OF AUTHORS?

Traditionally, the order of authorship has reflected the contributions individuals make to a project and therefore the recognition they should receive. However, because research is increasingly becoming a team effort, with fewer single-authored articles, authorship disputes may become more common.

The first author has primary responsibility for the paper and receives the most recognition. The last author is traditionally the senior author. The second author is regarded as having major responsibility, but middle authors are viewed as making less important contributions. Investigators should appreciate that for papers with more than six authors, according to the standard citation format, authors are not listed by name after the third one, and instead are merely referred to as "et al."

Unfortunately, these conventions about the order of authors are not clear in practice. First, conventions may vary from field to field. Furthermore, academic leaders, such as deans and journal editors, do not agree on the significance of the order of authors. One study concluded that department chairs had "little idea of the roles of any author" (15). However, respondents did agree that the corresponding author deserved more recognition than what his position in the list of authors would ordinarily merit (15).

Because of these inconsistencies regarding the order of authors, as well as concerns about scientific misconduct, many journals now require that the manuscript specify the contributions of each author. In addition to clarifying each author's contribution, this requirement ensures that one author will vouch for each component of the study.

HOW CAN DISPUTES OVER AUTHORSHIP BE RESOLVED?

Disagreements over authorship are common and can be stressful for younger investigators who are understandably concerned about establishing their credentials. Several types of disagreements can occur.

UNWARRANTED REQUEST TO BE AN AUTHOR

STUDY 13.2   **Request to add an author.**

After carrying out a research study, a postdoctoral fellow asks her division chief to comment on a draft of the manuscript. He returns it with a few comments, which are helpful, and asks to be added as an author. He previously made some suggestions at works-in-progress seminars and on the abstract submitted for presentation at a meeting. However, he did not participate in the design of the study or the data analysis.

Such a request places the researcher in a dilemma. Strictly speaking, the chief does not meet the criteria for authorship. However, a junior researcher is dependent on a division chief for recommendations, promotions, and other assistance. One response might be surprise, delay, and consultation; the researcher might say, "I'm flattered that you want to be included. I'd like a chance to discuss your request with the other authors" (16). It is appropriate to ask the other authors to help inform the person making the request that he does not meet the requirements for authorship. Alternatively, the junior investigator can fall back on the journal's requirements. She could say, "I'm afraid that the journal insists that all authors must sign a fairly stringent list of requirements. I feel very awkward asking you to sign a statement that isn't true. Instead, I would like your permission to give you a generous acknowledgment" (16).

If the person making the request is willing to sign the statement, the junior scientist needs to be realistic. It is not worth jeopardizing a career over this issue, particularly if in that field the division chief or lab head traditionally is the senior author.

Colleagues who provided some assistance to a research project but do not meet the requirements for authorship may request to be listed as authors. Often a response such as, "I'm sorry, but the manuscript is already written and the author list is set" (16), together with a promise to acknowledge their contributions, will suffice.

In some countries, it is the custom for the head of a department or clinic to be the last author on every paper, regardless of the actual contributions. This is considered respectful and perhaps also a quid pro quo for allowing access to patients. Without such honorific authorship, the research would not be carried out. An absolute condemnation of this practice would preclude important research to understand and ameliorate important health problems in the host country. Taking everything into account, honorific authorship may be the lesser of several evils.

Sometimes a colleague who fully deserves authorship will request to be given a higher place on the authorship list, perhaps because he is up for promotion and wants to strengthen his curriculum vitae. One approach is to say, "I can understand your desire to be first author, given your upcoming tenure decision. But I'm sure you'd agree that this has been my project from the beginning and you can understand that being first author is important to me also" (16).

FAILURE TO DO THE WORK AGREED UPON

A colleague on a project may not carry out the work he agreed to do. For instance, the first author may not produce a draft of the manuscript, perhaps because he has taken a new position or moved to another university. Alternatively, the person who agreed to perform the data analysis may fail to do so. Colleagues may make creative excuses for not carrying out their tasks, such as (17):

- It's in the pipeline.
- It's next in the pipeline.
- I'm reanalyzing the data.
- The data are on a Windows-incompatible computer.
- I can't find the right statistical test to prove it worked.

One approach to such delays is to indicate that you are willing to take over those tasks, with a corresponding change in the order of authors. You could say, "I know you're incredibly busy. I'm willing to take over as first author and write a draft. If I haven't heard from you in 3 weeks, I'll assume you're too busy to be first author, and I'll take over that role." It is also prudent to discuss the situation with the other authors on the paper, particularly the senior author, and get their approval for the proposed new arrangement.

SUGGESTIONS FOR AUTHORSHIP DISPUTES

Consult Colleagues

Talking with colleagues can provide emotional support during a difficult period and may also provide good suggestions on what to do. The senior author on the project or your mentor may be willing to intervene on your behalf.

Rehearse

Because responding to such requests is difficult, it is worthwhile to practice what words you might say. The phrases suggested above may help you find words that work for you. It is important to say clearly what you need to say without causing the other author to lose face, making him your enemy, or destroying your relationship with your other colleagues. The goal is to be firm yet diplomatic.

Be Your Own Advocate

If you are not willing to advocate for yourself, it is less likely that others will do so. At a minimum, researchers who feel that they are being treated unfairly need to be willing to talk with a mentor or another senior person.

Be Realistic

In authorship disputes, a keen sense of fairness may need to be tempered with pragmatism. A young investigator is dependent on more senior persons for recommendations and career assistance. It may not be worth it to alienate a powerful person, be labeled a troublemaker, or put your career at risk. Although it is unfair to receive less recognition than one deserves, it may be better to be second or third author than for the paper to not be published at all.

PREVENTING AUTHORSHIP DISPUTES

Because authorship disputes can become bitter, it is important to try to prevent them and address them when they become apparent, rather than hope things will work out by themselves (they generally do not). It is a good idea to clarify authorship at the beginning of a project. Sometimes friends will decide to do a joint project without specifying who will take the lead and be first author, and what each person will contribute. Although it may seem inconsistent with friendship to make these expectations explicit, it is usually better in the long run to agree in writing at the onset of the project about roles, expectations, and deadlines. If there are signs that the authorship arrangements are not working, it is better to address the problems directly when they arise than to delay addressing them and hope things will work out. Bringing up concerns early can prevent future problems by clarifying expectations and setting realistic deadlines.

SHARING OF RESEARCH MATERIALS AND DATA

> **STUDY 13.3** **Request for data.**
>
> *After a manuscript is published from a survey of 1000 patients, the corresponding author receives requests for information and data. One request is for the questions in a subscale. Another request is for the entire data set. The senior investigator wants to protect the interests of a new postdoctoral fellow, who is planning to carry out a secondary analysis of the data.*

Sharing of methods, findings, and research materials is considered a fundamental norm in scientific research (18). It expedites scientific progress by allowing researchers to build on the discoveries of others. Such sharing is similar to reciprocal altruism—an investigator shares her own data and findings with the expectation that others will share their information with her. The corresponding or senior author has the responsibility to respond to requests.

However, this expectation is frequently violated in practice. In a recent survey, just over one-half of graduate students and postdoctoral fellows said that their research had been delayed by another scientist's refusal to share information or data (19); 27% of trainees in the life sciences said that they had requested but been denied information, data, or materials associated with published research; and 6% reported that they had personally denied other scientists' requests for information related to their own published research. Trainees from highly competitive labs and those who had received industry support were more likely to be denied access.

In a 2002 survey of faculty-level genetics researchers, 47% of the respondents said they had been denied a request for information, data, or materials during the past 3 years (20), and 12% said that they had denied another researcher's request for data concerning published results during that time period. The reasons given included the effort to produce the materials or information, and the need to protect publication opportunities for themselves or junior colleagues.

Different types of sharing need to be distinguished. There is little warrant for refusing to share methods used to derive published results; indeed, without such information readers cannot interpret the paper and other scientists cannot build on those methods. Similarly, the sharing of genomic sequence data is now expected as a condition of receiving NIH funding, so that others can make use of this information when searching for other associations between alleles and other clinical conditions.

Under some circumstances, it is understandable that scientists will hesitate to share data and materials. As in Study 13.3, a researcher may fear that a competitor from a larger or better-funded research group will "scoop" additional studies that are planned. In other cases, a researcher may refuse to share data or materials with a group that has refused to share its own data in the past.

Sharing limited biological specimens, such as blood or tissue, is more complicated than sharing methods or data because these biological materials are scarce resources that should not be wasted. It seems reasonable to have some priority system for sharing materials, and to give priority to requests for scientifically meritorious and significant projects.

The NIH now requires investigators seeking large grants to address plans for data sharing in their applications. Data sets that are shared should be de-identified according to HIPAA standards. The date for release of shared data should be no later than the acceptance for publication of the main findings from the final data set. This policy provides an incentive for researchers to carry out secondary analyses in a timely manner. The original investigators are expected to benefit from first and ongoing use of the data, but not prolonged, exclusive use. From the perspective of a research sponsor, such sharing multiplies the benefits gained from the original grant.

PRESS COVERAGE OF PUBLICATIONS

Many journals will not publish research that has already been published elsewhere. This restriction may include an embargo on press coverage before the article is published online or in print. Authors commonly question what they are permitted to say before publication. Presentation of an abstract at a professional meeting is acceptable as a time-honored means of disseminating research findings in a timely manner. Presentation of abstracts should be disclosed to the journal. Authors are permitted to talk with the press after an abstract presentation, provided that they discuss only the findings in the presentation. Many meetings also post slides from presentations on their website, which is also acceptable. If authors have questions about what is permitted, they should contact the journal.

Journals generally welcome press coverage of articles they publish. Typically, journals set an embargo date for press coverage and send prepublication copies of the issue to reporters. Investigators should not be deterred by an embargo from speaking with reporters before publication. Reporters need time to write their stories, and they and their organizations promise to respect the embargo. It is prudent for the researcher to confirm with the journalist at the beginning of the interview that the embargo will be respected.

Many universities have a public affairs office that will work with researchers to prepare a press release when important articles are published. When writing a press release, investigators need to explain their study in simple, lay language.

TAKE HOME POINTS

1. Authorship involves responsibility as well as prestige.
2. Researchers should understand the criteria for authorship, and all authors listed on a manuscript should meet those criteria.
3. Disputes and ethical problems regarding authorship are common. Researchers should understand how to respond to disputes.

ANNOTATED BIBLIOGRAPHY

DeAngelis CD, Drazen JM, Frizelle FA, et al. Is this clinical trial fully registered? A statement from the International Committee of Medical Journal Editors. *N Engl J Med* 2005;352:2436–2438.
  Explanation of the requirement by journal editors that clinical trials be registered in a clinical trials registry.
Moffatt B, Elliott C. Ghost marketing: pharmaceutical companies and ghostwritten journal articles. *Perspect Biol Med* 2007;50:18–31.
  Analysis and critique of practice of ghostwritten articles in medical journals.

REFERENCES

1. Eastwood S, Derish P, Leash E, et al. Ethical issues in biomedical research: perceptions and practices of postdoctoral research fellows responding to a survey. *Sci Eng Ethics* 1996;2:89–114.
2. Flanagin A, Carey LA, Fontranarosa PB, et al. Prevalence of articles with honorary authors and ghost authors in peer-reviewed medical journals. *JAMA* 1998;280:222–224.
3. Shapiro DW, Wenger NS, Shapiro MS. The contributions of authors to multiauthored biomedical research papers. *JAMA* 1994;271:438–442.
4. Moffatt B, Elliott C. Ghost marketing: pharmaceutical companies and ghostwritten journal articles. *Perspect Biol Med* 2007;50:18–31.
5. Mathews AW. Ghost story: at medical journals, writers paid by industry play big role. *Wall St J (East Ed)* 2005: A1, A8.
6. Ross JS, Hill KP, Egilman DS, et al. Guest authorship and ghostwriting in publications related to rofecoxib: a case study of industry documents from rofecoxib litigation. *JAMA* 2008;299:1800–1812.
7. Fugh-Berman A. The corporate coauthor. *J Gen Intern Med* 2005;20:546–548.
8. Tierney WM, Gerrity MS. Scientific discourse, corporate ghostwriting, journal policy, and public trust. *J Gen Intern Med* 2005;20:550–551.
9. von Elm E, Poglia G, Walder B, et al. Different patterns of duplicate publication: an analysis of articles used in systematic reviews. *JAMA* 2004;291:974–980.
10. Rennie D. Fair conduct and fair reporting of clinical trials. *JAMA* 1999;282:1766–1768.
11. Kahn JO, Cherng DW, Mayer K, et al. Evaluation of HIV-immunogen, an immunologic modifier, administered to patients infected with HIV having 300 to 549 $\times$ 10^6/L CD4 cell counts. *JAMA* 2000;284:2193–2202.
12. DeAngelis CD. Conflict of interest and the public trust. *JAMA* 2000;284:2237–2238.
13. Davidoff F, DeAngelis CD, Drazen JM, et al. Sponsorship, authorship, and accountability. *JAMA* 2001;286: 1232–1234.
14. DeAngelis CD, Drazen JM, Frizelle FA, et al. Is this clinical trial fully registered? A statement from the International Committee of Medical Journal Editors. *N Engl J Med* 2005;352:2436–2438.
15. Bhandari M, Busse JW, Kulkarni AV, et al. Interpreting authorship order and corresponding authorship. *Epidemiology* 2004;15:125–126.
16. Browner WS. *Authorship. Publishing and Presenting Clinical Research.* 2nd ed. Philadelphia: Lippincott Williams & Wilkins; 2006:137–144.
17. Wright V. An audit of excuses. *BMJ* 1994;309:1739–1740.
18. National Research Council. *Sharing Publication-Related Data and Materials: Responsibilities of Authorship in the Life Sciences.* Washington, DC: National Academies Press; 2003.
19. Vogeli C, Yucel R, Bendavid E, et al. Data withholding and the next generation of scientists: results of a national survey. *Acad Med* 2006;81:128–136.
20. Campbell EG, Clarridge BR, Gokhale M, et al. Data withholding in academic genetics: evidence from a national survey. *JAMA* 2002;287:473–480.

Patenting and Commercialization of Discoveries

T o benefit patients, scientific discoveries need to be translated into clinical tests and therapies. Because universities have had little success in developing commercially successful tests and therapies, for-profit companies play a crucial role in translating scientific discoveries to new tests and therapies. To encourage such product development, the Bayh-Dole Act of 1980 encouraged federally funded researchers and research institutions to patent and license their discoveries and retain licensing fees. As a result, many university-based researchers have patented discoveries and founded biotechnology companies to develop products. However, such patents and licenses raise a number of ethical, public policy, and practical issues. Researchers need to be aware of these issues and help ensure that licensing and material transfer agreements are consistent with the goals of developing clinical tests and treatments and fostering additional research.

STUDY 14.1   **Patent for human embryonic stem cells.**

After researcher James Thompson of the University of Wisconsin isolated and cultured human embryonic stem cells, the university in 1998 obtained patents on the lines and the technique to derive them. The Wisconsin Alumni Research Foundation (WARF) required scientists who wished to use the cells and methods to provide an up-front fee plus royalties from sales of any products that would result from their research. In addition, the WARF materials transfer agreements limited the scope of research use, sharing with additional researchers, and intellectual property rights (1). These "reach through" provisions conflicted with scientific norms for sharing of materials. The journal Science, which published the original research, requires research materials to be made available without "unreasonable restrictions." WARF granted the Geron company exclusive rights to develop diagnostic and therapeutic products using neural stem cells, cardiomyocytes, and pancreatic islet cells. Under strong criticism from stem cell researchers and universities, WARF eased restrictions for research at universities. In January 2007, WARF waived the licensing fees for university-based researchers.

In July 2006, consumer advocacy organizations challenged these patents, arguing that Thompson's work, while of immense importance, was "obvious" in light of previous publications on the derivation of mouse embryonic stem cells. In April 2007, a preliminary ruling invalidated the patents.

This case illustrates how patents may stifle rather than encourage additional research. The embryonic stem cell patents covered basic techniques that would be used by any researcher deriving a human embryonic stem cell line. Furthermore, researchers who wished to work with the Wisconsin-derived stem cell lines would be subject to costs and paperwork, and would have to agree to assign intellectual property rights on discoveries they made using the lines to Wisconsin. Such a loss of intellectual property would be a disincentive to other researchers working in a rapidly developing field of research. The term "reach through" refers to the situation in which a patent holder requires as a condition of licensing his patented discovery that other researchers promise to share intellectual property rights to additional discoveries they make when using the patented invention (3). If the patent is for an essential upstream research tool, such as methods or materials (including assays and markers), the patent holder might have considerable leverage over other researchers who have no other options for carrying out their work.

WHAT IS THE PURPOSE OF THE PATENT SYSTEM?

The patent system encourages invention by awarding patent holders a period of exclusive use (currently 20 years) to develop and market new products. During this period, competitors may not use, make, or sell the patent holder's invention (4). Patent holders and their investors are protected from competition as they try to recover the costs of product development and clinical trials. Patent holders may license their inventions to others in exchange for royalties. An exclusive license grants one party sole use of the invention for a particular purpose.

Without patent protection and the prospect of a return on their investment, investors are unlikely to fund product development. In exchange for patent protection, inventors must publicly disclose sufficient information so that others can make and use the invention. Such disclosure diffuses new knowledge and promotes further discoveries by allowing other scientists to "invent around" the patent and find other approaches to achieve the results of the invention.

To be patentable, an invention must be

- Novel. The invention could not be wholly anticipated by prior art or information in the public domain.
- Non-obvious. The invention must go beyond the abilities of a skilled "artisan" who is knowledgeable in the field. As discussed later, the implementation of this requirement is predicated on opinions by experts in the field.
- Useful. The invention must have some practical purpose.

The Bayh-Dole Act allows institutions to patent discoveries made under federal research grants and to grant exclusive licenses for others to develop those discoveries. Universities may retain licensing and royalty fees, which they generally share with the scientists who developed the patented invention. This law has led to a dramatic increase in university patent applications, licensing agreements, and royalties (5). Blockbuster patents are rare. Less than one-half of licenses have generated royalties, and less than 1% earned an income of more than $1 million in 2000 (5).

The stem cell patents in Study 14.1 illustrate a crucial difference between patenting and licensing. Academic researchers and their universities did not object to the patenting and licensing of discoveries for the development of commercial products. However, they argued that onerous licensing requirements would thwart other researchers (1).

WHAT ARE THE ETHICAL CONCERNS ABOUT PATENTS?

There are several ethical concerns regarding the patenting of biomedical discoveries (2).

PATENTING HUMAN LIFE

In the United States, patents may be granted for living organisms that have been isolated, purified, or modified. This includes patents on genes and their products. Some critics contend that patenting human and animal life degrades it by treating it as an inanimate object (3). In their view, nature is violated when it is used exclusively as a means to human ends. Genes have been called the common heritage of mankind, with the implication that no one should own or control them.

However, patents are only awarded for genes and proteins that have been purified, isolated, or modified—not as they exist in nature. There is a long history of awarding patents for the purification and isolation of naturally occurring chemicals, and such patents are not regarded as conferring ownership over nature. Furthermore, societies permit people to own plants and animals, and do not regard it as being disrespectful of nature.

PATENTS DETER FURTHER RESEARCH

Society benefits if researchers build on patented information to make additional discoveries. However, patents can deter future basic science research in several ways.

Burdens on Other Researchers

Patents make further research less efficient. In a complex biomedical research project, it would require considerable time and expense for a university to try to identify multiple patents applicable to the project, and to negotiate licensing and material transfer agreements with many patent holders. This effort, licensing costs, and uncertainty would greatly discourage research that might build on previous discoveries (6). These transaction costs are inconsistent with the scientific ideal of free sharing of research materials and knowledge. Lost opportunities are particularly great if broad patents are issued for basic discoveries that offer powerful new methods for future research (6). Furthermore, royalties and other restrictions on the use of patented discoveries may be prohibitive for other researchers. The negative impact on future research has been characterized as the "tragedy of the anticommons" (7). Although it is in society's interest as a whole to promote upstream basic research, it is in the self-interest of each individual patent holder to maximize his royalty income even if it discourages other researchers from carrying out further basic research based on his discovery.

Inability to Invent Around the Patent

For many patents, other inventors can "invent around" the discovery, achieving the same goals in a new way that does not use the patented discovery. However, researchers cannot invent around patents on DNA sequences or on fundamental research processes. Some patent applications claim the information in a DNA sequence, as well as a specific use of a gene. Thus, any future research or product based on the genomic sequence would infringe on the patent. In contrast to other patents, it is impossible for other scientists to invent around a patent on a DNA sequence or, as in Study 14.1, a fundamental research process for deriving embryonic stem cells. Because genes interact, researchers may need to work with long genomic sequences that include several patented sequences.

In response to these concerns, the U.S. Patent Office has tightened patent requirements, rejecting patents for small regions in the active part of the gene (called expressed sequence tags or ESTs) whose function or utility has not been established (4).

PATENTS MAKE TESTS AND THERAPIES UNAFFORDABLE

Patent holders may set the price of products so high that patients cannot afford them. However, people who donate their biomaterials and data to a biobank commonly expect that new tests and therapies will be available and affordable. In the case of several new genetic tests, these expectations were not met.

STUDY 14.2	BRCA testing (4).

When BRCA1, a gene that increases susceptibility to breast and ovarian cancer, was identified, the inventor and his university patented the genes and granted an exclusive license to a biotechnology company he helped found, called Myriad Genetics. A second breast cancer gene, BRCA2, was identified by this inventor and a group in the United Kingdom. Both research groups applied for patents for BRCA2. Myriad enforced its patent rights

---

STUDY 14.2 **(Continued).**

against university laboratories that were offering tests that included more mutations at a lower cost (8,9). After receiving criticism from academic researchers, Myriad agreed to give NIH-funded investigators a discount to use the test for research, in exchange for access to resulting data.

STUDY 14.3 **Canavan disease.**

Canavan disease is a progressive, fatal neurological disease that afflicts infants. Families of children with this rare disease helped to collect materials for research. After the gene for Canavan disease was identified and patented, a diagnostic test was developed (2). The research institution holding the patent charged high royalties or licensing fees, which made the test unaffordable for many families. Advocacy groups sued, but the appellate court ruled against them, declaring that under state law "the property right in blood and tissue samples . . . evaporates once a sample is voluntarily given to a third party." Advocacy groups and the research institution and researchers reached an out-of-court settlement, the terms of which are confidential.

In Study 14.2, Myriad's policies discouraged other researchers from conducting studies to identify additional genetic variations and to correlate genotypes with clinical phenotypes (4). In addition, the development of more comprehensive or lower-cost diagnostic tests, which would benefit patients, was impeded (10). In another, similar example, the holder of the patent for the hemachromatosis gene charged such high royalty fees that many clinical laboratories stopped developing or discontinued tests for that condition (11). These cases raise concerns about patents for genomic discoveries.

The case of cystic fibrosis (CF) testing provides an illustrative counter-example (3). The patent holders for the CF transmembrane conductance regulator (*CFTR*) gene allowed free access for the development of diagnostic testing and collected royalties only from makers of commercial test kits. Because of competition among different manufacturers of test kits, CF testing is readily available at a modest cost. Thus the key policy issue is not whether a discovery is patented, but whether the licensing arrangements are strict and rigid or further research is fostered.

There are several reasons why unaffordable prices are a particular concern with biomedical discoveries.

First, as discussed above, other researchers cannot invent around a patent on a DNA sequence and its use. Thus, market forces that would drive down the price of other products do not operate in this context.

Second, researchers may depend on the efforts of disease advocacy groups and patients with diseases to collect materials with unique characteristics, without which research could not be carried out. As a matter of reciprocity, researchers may owe these indispensable partners a commitment to provide fair access to tests and therapies resulting from the research. In Study 14.3, families of children with a rare disease helped to collect samples, without which the research could not be done, only to find that the diagnostic test resulting from the research was beyond their economic means. Similarly, some persons have a special susceptibility or resistance to a disease, which makes their materials particularly valuable for scientists. Analogous concerns about fair access to the fruits of research arise when scientists work with biologics and seeds that have been used for centuries by indigenous cultures. These populations might not benefit from patents obtained for isolating the active ingredients in traditional remedies or identifying the genetic basis of traditional crops. Indigenous peoples may even need to pay royalties to continue to use their traditional materials. Such royalties have been criticized as exploitative.

Third, the cost of developing DNA-based diagnostic tests may be very low once the genomic sequence associated with a gene and its alleles are identified. With high-throughput DNA chips, little additional intellectual effort is needed to develop a diagnostic test. Thus, the high prices for these tests seem excessive in terms of the resources needed to develop the product.

STUDY 14.1   (Continued).

The European patent court overturned the Myriad patent for BRCA2 because the British group had filed its claim first. The U.K. researchers made the genomic sequence available to the public for free, allowing the development of many diagnostic test kits. Myriad's European patents on BRCA1 were also struck down or narrowed because of errors in the original sequence and the lack of an inventive step.

Still another issue arises if the research that leads to a discovery is publicly funded. In return for providing funding, the public may expect that no patient will be denied tests or treatments developed from patents arising from that funded research because of financial or insurance reasons.

RESEARCH EXEMPTION FROM PATENT RESTRICTIONS

Many universities assumed that they could use patented discoveries for further noncommercial, "pure" research without concerns about patent infringement. In the case of *Madey v. Duke University*, however, the Supreme Court rejected this exception, holding that such researchers could be liable for patent infringement (12). The court ruled that it is irrelevant that the research was noncommercial or carried out at a nonprofit institution. In light of this decision, how can the freedom of researchers to pursue basic, noncommercial research be maintained?

In Study 14.1, researchers successfully weakened stringent licensing and materials transfer agreements, and patents were successfully overturned in court. However, resolving patent disputes through the courts and by putting pressure on patent holders is inefficient. Delays in the adjudication of patent disputes create uncertainty, which deters further research. In a rapidly progressing field, it would be a serious setback if researchers could not obtain upstream research tools for a few years while a case is adjudicated.

One approach to make patented discoveries widely available to noncommercial researchers is for universities that hold patents to write into exclusive licensing agreements that academic or nonprofit research institutions have the right to use those inventions. The rationale for this approach is based on reciprocity: a university cannot in fairness expect its faculty to have access to discoveries patented by other universities unless it grants other researchers access to its patents. These agreements, however, do not address the issue of university researchers wanting to use discoveries patented by for-profit companies.

Reform of the patent system is another way to allow researchers greater access to patented discoveries. In 2005, the National Academy of Sciences (NAS) issued a consensus-based, peer-reviewed report entitled "A Patent System for the 21st Century" (4). This report recommended that inconsistencies among U.S., European, and Japanese patent systems be reduced. The report also recommended reinvigorating the non-obviousness standard. In Study 14.1, stem cell patents were challenged because other scientists believed that the discovery was obvious in light of previous work on embryonic stem cells in animals. The key legal issue is whether other scientists would have found the innovation to be obvious at that time. Resolving this issue requires expert scientific testimony. The NAS panel recommended instituting an open review procedure in which third parties can challenge patents before an administrative law judge. These procedures would include expert testimony.

The NAS report further recommended federal legislation to exempt noncommercial research using patented inventions from liability for patent infringement. The exemption would cover research on the validity and scope of the patents, the characteristics of the invention, novel methods of making or using the invention, and novel alternatives, improvements, or substitutes (4). A federal law allowing an exemption from patent infringements for university-based and nonprofit researchers would promote the public policy goal of advancing scientific knowledge, which would in the long run benefit society.

ACCESS TO NEW PRODUCTS DEVELOPED FROM PATENTS

For biomedical patents to be useful to society, new tests and therapies need to be developed and patients must have access to them. Several stakeholders can take steps to ensure that the benefits of research are shared with patients in need.

DONORS OF MATERIALS

Consent documents for donating biological materials typically specify that individual donors will not share in the intellectual property, licensing fees, or profits from any products that are developed. This is reasonable because often many samples will be studied during the process of making a discovery, and researchers often cannot identify which particular samples were used.

However, benefit sharing with a broader group of donors is feasible. National biobanks have negotiated payments from commercial companies to the government, as in Iceland. Several groups representing patients or indigenous peoples have also insisted on a share of royalties in exchange for providing materials (2). Furthermore, in the wake of Study 14.3 (involving Canavan disease), patient advocacy groups can be expected to negotiate explicit agreements for sharing royalties or accessing clinical products as a condition of helping researchers recruit donors and supporting the research. Making such agreements public would help identify best practices and set standards (13).

ADVOCACY GROUPS

Advocacy groups may promote research by raising funds, publicizing the research, and helping to recruit donors of biological materials. They are becoming savvier about making these arrangements explicit at the beginning of a research project. It is likely that disease advocacy groups will become tougher negotiators, learn from the experience of previous negotiations by other groups, and increase their bargaining power relative to that of researchers.

NONPROFIT FUNDERS OF RESEARCH

Current NIH policy allows grantees to patent discoveries and retain royalty and licensing payments with no return to the federal treasury, even for blockbuster patents. However, there are precedents for public sponsors of biomedical research to insist on some public return on highly profitable patents.

The California Institute for Regenerative Medicine (CIRM), which will award $3 billion in state funding for stem cell research, is making it a condition of receiving an award that the public will have both a share of the revenues for blockbuster patents and affordable access to tests and therapies (see http://www.cirm.ca.gov/policy/policy.asp).

CIRM has established an innovative revenue-sharing agreement that is both tiered (below a threshold level of revenue from the patent, no sharing is required; the threshold allows institutions to recover the costs of obtaining a patent and supporting an intellectual property office) and progressive (higher payments are made for blockbuster patents). Caps in payments would be tied to the size of the original grant.

This conceptual framework tries to strike a balance between competing interests, including encouraging the development of commercial products, fostering additional research in an emerging field, and providing a return to taxpayers. Negotiations over the provisions of the policy involved a variety of interest groups, including research institutions, public interest groups, disease advocacy groups, venture capitalists, and for-profit biotechnology firms (14).

Another issue is access to treatments resulting from patented discoveries for patients who are uninsured or who receive care through public funding. In the case of publicly funded stem cell research, there was a strong feeling that in exchange for the research funding that led to the discovery, the public should have some assurance that new therapies would be accessible to those who need them. There are different approaches to this issue. A disease advocacy group might insist as a condition of supporting the research and helping to recruit donors of biological materials that some percentage of revenue from new drugs developed from the research should be set aside for a patient assistance program for those who cannot afford the drug. The percentage might apply only after a certain level of revenue is attained, so that the costs of product development and testing can be recovered. A nonprofit sponsor of research might set a similar requirement as a condition of funding. In state-funded research, there could be a requirement that patients in state-funded health insurance programs, such as Medicaid, should receive the lowest price negotiated by other health payors for the drug.

TAKE HOME POINT

1. Although patents are an important step in translating scientific discoveries into new tests and treatments, they raise ethical concerns regarding access to resulting products and barriers to downstream research.

ANNOTATED BIBLIOGRAPHY

Brody B. Intellectual property and biotechnology: the U.S. internal experience—Part I. *Kennedy Inst Ethics J* 2006;16:1–37.
Brody B. Intellectual property and biotechnology: the U.S. internal experience—Part II. *Kennedy Inst Ethics J* 2006;16:105–128.
> Lucid, thoughtful articles on the development of U.S. intellectual property law regarding biotechnology discoveries.
National Research Council. *Reaping the Benefits of Genomic and Proteonomic Research: Intellectual Property Rights, Innovation, and Public Health*. Washington, DC: National Academies Press; 2005. Available at http://www.nationalacademies.org/publications/.
> Comprehensive, in-depth report on the topic.

REFERENCES

1. Murray F. The stem-cell market—patents and the pursuit of scientific progress. *N Engl J Med* 2007;356: 2341–2343.
2. Brody B. Intellectual property and biotechnology: the U.S. internal experience—Part I. *Kennedy Inst Ethics* J 2006;16:1–37.
3. Soini S, Ayme S, Matthijs G. Patenting and licensing in genetic testing. *Eur J Hum Genet* 2008;16:S10–S50.
4. National Research Council. *Reaping the Benefits of Genomic and Proteonomic Research: Intellectual Property Rights, Innovation, and Public Health*. Washington, DC: National Academies Press; 2005.
5. Thursby JG, Thursby MC. Intellectual property. University licensing and the Bayh-Dole Act. *Science* 2003; 301:1052.
6. Eisenberg RS, Nelson RR. Public vs. proprietary science: a fruitful tension? *Acad Med* 2002;77:1392–1399.
7. Heller MA, Eisenberg RS. Can patents deter innovation? The anticommons in biomedical research. *Science* 1998;280:698–701.
8. Andrews LB. Genes and patent policy: rethinking intellectual property rights. *Nat Rev Genet* 2002;3:803–808.
9. Brody B. Intellectual property and biotechnology: the U.S. internal experience—Part II. *Kennedy Inst Ethics* J 2006;16:105–128.
10. Cho MK, Illangasekare S, Weaver MA, et al. Effects of patents and licenses on the provision of clinical genetic testing services. *J Mol Diagn* 2003;5:3–8.
11. Merz JF, Kriss AG, Leonard DG, et al. Diagnostic testing fails the test. *Nature* 2002;415:577–579.
12. Sewell DG. Rescuing science from the courts: an appeal for amending the patent code to protect academic research in the wake of Madey v. Duke University. *Georgetown Law J* 2005;93:759–782.
13. Korobkin R. *Stem Cell Century*. New Haven: Yale University Press; 2007.
14. Lo B. Can public policy keep pace with stem cell science? *Cell Stem Cell* 208;2:203–204.

15

Conflicts of Interest

Funding from for-profit companies is essential to develop new therapies from scientific discoveries and to fund clinical trials. Before passage of the 1980 Bayh-Dole Act, when the federal government held patents resulting from publicly funded research, very few patents were licensed for commercial development. Hence few discoveries were translated into new therapies. The Bayh-Dole Act gives universities control over patents resulting from federally funded research. It is intended to promote technology transfer from universities to industry, so that more discoveries will lead to therapeutic products. Collaboration between academic researchers and drug, device, and biotechnology companies is essential to develop new tests and therapies.

Since the passage of Bayh-Dole, universities and investigators have developed close relationships with for-profit companies, including founding companies, holding stock and options, establishing long-term consulting arrangements, and obtaining research funding from industry (1). Industry funding for clinical trials now exceeds public funding. Although these ties with industry are essential, they also raise concerns about conflicts of interest.

WHAT IS A CONFLICT OF INTEREST?

A conflict of interest is a situation in which a person entrusted with the interests of a client, a dependent, or the public tends to be unduly influenced by a secondary interest (1,2). The primary interests of a researcher should be to obtain and present valid, generalizable data and protect research participants. These primary interests should take precedence over the researcher's self-interest or the interests of a third party, such as the manufacturers of the study drug. University-based researchers play an important public role as impartial and independent agents, distinct from the role of employees of drug manufacturers (3).

Practicing physicians, government officials, and judges also encounter conflicts of interest. For instance, a judge is not permitted to sit in a case in which he, a relative, a close friend, or a former business associate is a party. Even if the ultimate decision is fair, it is considered unacceptable that the judge might take into account inappropriate factors or make rulings about motions and objections that no evenhanded decision-maker would make. The possibility of procedural errors would be disturbing even if the final ruling were impartial. Moreover, conflicts of interest undermine public trust in the judicial system. These are important considerations even if there is no indication that a particular case was managed improperly.

HOW IS CONFLICT OF INTEREST DEFINED?

People often use the term "conflict of interest" without defining it clearly.

Compromise of the Researcher's Primary Interest

The narrowest definition of conflict of interest is that the researcher has reached an invalid conclusion because of bias caused by a secondary interest. However, it is extremely difficult to determine the cause of an invalid finding, which may also result from unintentional error, carelessness, or inadequate skill or knowledge. Moreover, bias may be unconscious rather than intentional. Furthermore, it is time-consuming to focus backward on the cause of biased conclusions, rather than look forward to prevent bias in research studies and thereby maintain the trust of research participants and the public.

Bias in Researcher's Decisions or Actions

More broadly, the researcher's judgment or decision-making process might be compromised, even though the conclusions are not biased. A researcher must exercise discretion in many ways, such as when determining eligibility, cleaning data, and carrying out statistical analyses. It would be prohibitively difficult and intrusive for someone else to review or oversee these innumerable decisions for evidence of bias.

Unacceptable Risk for Bias and Loss of Trust

A still broader definition of conflict of interest includes situations in which there is an unacceptable tendency for secondary interests to unduly influence the primary interest. This definition does not require evidence of *actual* bias or compromised judgment in a particular situation (1,2). Several arguments support this broader definition. First, it is usually impractical to determine whether bias occurred or discretion was inappropriately exercised in any given study. As a matter of public policy, it is prudent to require researchers to avoid situations that offer a significant possibility of bias, even if no misbehavior can be proven in a particular study. Avoiding such situations also reduces the occurrence of bias, which may be preferable to determining after the fact whether bias occurred. Second, allowing situations in which there is a tendency to compromise the validity of research may undermine public trust in medical research, even if there is no actual bias. Third, this broader definition is consistent with how conflicts of interest are handled in other professions (e.g., the judiciary).

Reasonable and independent people should determine whether there is potential undue influence in a research situation, not the individual researcher. Physicians and researchers tend to view themselves as being insusceptible to bias from financial relationships, although they regard others as being prone to such bias. This determination should take into account many factors, including the nature of the relationship and the likelihood and seriousness of the potential compromise of the primary interest (1,2). Value judgments must be made regarding what kinds of responses are appropriate in different situations. Individual research participants often are not in position to determine whether the researcher's clinical judgment and decision-making process are likely to be compromised. However, patient advocacy groups or public interest groups can play an important role in setting policies regarding conflicts of interest.

MISCONCEPTIONS ABOUT CONFLICTS OF INTEREST
Perceived or Apparent Conflicts of Interest

Certain situations sometimes are described as only *perceived* or *apparent* conflicts of interest, with the implication that there is no harm and not even a significant potential for harm. For example, many researchers believe that their judgment is not compromised by participating in a speakers bureau of a drug company that provides slides, text, and training for talks. However, the public might view such a researcher as a company spokesperson rather than an independent judge of the evidence. A critic might also question whether a person who suspends critical thinking in one context can be trusted to act independently in other situations. Recently, some commentators have argued that the concept of perceived or apparent conflict of interest is misguided because all conflicts of interest represent an unacceptable tendency for bias in the study, not a demonstration that bias has actually occurred (1,2).

The concept of perceived conflict of interest is also flawed because not every perception that a conflict of interest exists should be regarded as credible. A conflict of interest should be judged by reasonable people in light of their past experience and available facts about the situation. For example, it is not a conflict of interest for a researcher to invest in a mutual fund involving drug companies, since she has no control over the purchase or sale of individual stocks in the fund.

Competing Versus Conflicting Interests

The interests of the patient and physician never coincide completely. *Conflicting* interests, as we have defined them, should be prioritized in a certain way. The validity of data and conclusions should be regarded as paramount, and the self-interest of the physician should be secondary. In contrast, *competing* interests have equivalent claims to priority. For example, a researcher has important competing interests in continuing medical education, teaching, and family responsibilities. Such competing interests can usually be accommodated without undermining the integrity of research.

Implications About Unethical Behavior

Some physicians might be offended because concerns about potential or perceived conflicts of interest apparently impugn their integrity and imply they are acting unethically. Doctors need to understand that the public is not singling them out for censure, but simply treating them as human and therefore fallible, just like public officials and judges. It is the situation that is problematic, not the person.

EXAMPLES OF CONFLICTS OF INTEREST

Several highly publicized recent incidents have heightened public concerns about conflicts of interest in clinical research (4–6).

STUDY 15.1   Cardiac effects of rofecoxib.

In November 2000, a randomized controlled trial (RCT), the VIGOR study, showed that the selective COX—2 inhibitor rofecoxib caused fewer gastrointestinal complications than naproxen (2.1 vs. 4.5 per 100 patient-years), while providing similar efficacy against arthritis. The rofecoxib arm also had more heart attacks (0.4% vs. 0.1%), which was attributed to the protective effect of naproxen. Because of this study, rofecoxib was widely prescribed, with sales of more than $2.5 billion annually.

Before the article was published, three additional heart attacks in the rofecoxib arm were reported to the Food and Drug Administration (FDA), but not to the university-based authors of the paper or to the journal that published it. Two authors who were employees of the manufacturer knew of these additional cases.

A 2005 RCT (the APPROVe study) clearly showed that rofecoxib caused heart attacks and strokes (1.50 thrombotic events per 100 patient-years vs. 0.78 in the placebo group). The manufacturer voluntarily withdrew the drug from market. The article reported that the cardiac risk increased only after 18 months. However, the study counted only adverse events that occurred while the participant was on rofecoxib or within 14 days of stopping the drug, and did not count events throughout the follow-up period.

The university-based authors of the study claimed they were just following the definition of endpoints in the protocol. However, the manufacturer presented all thrombotic events to FDA in May 2006, showing that the risks increased after 4 months, not 18.

Many patients who had taken rofecoxib and suffered a heart attack sued the manufacturer. The drug manufacturers commonly argued that the plaintiff had not taken the drug long enough to experience cardiac toxicity. In a deposition, an editor of the New England Journal of Medicine, which published both studies, made several revelations. First, the journal sold over 900,000 reprints of the VIGOR article, gaining an income of $697,000. Second, peer reviewers raised serious concerns about the APPROVe paper, noting that "[the paper] is going out on limb by emphasizing the 18 month issue . . ., [the] hand of sponsor is too evident . . ., [it is] written consistently in manner designed to support the company's public positions . . .," and "[the article] aggressively promotes safety of up to 18 months of use . . . beyond the data of the study." Originally, the editors had asked the authors to drop all references to the 18-month threshold.

The rofecoxib clinical trials illustrate several conflicts of interest. First, the withholding of unfavorable data by for-profit sponsors undermined the evidence base for clinical practice and caused grave harm to patients. An estimated 160,000 heart attacks and strokes were attributed to rofecoxib.

Second, the VIGOR authors who were employees of the manufacturer knew of the additional heart attacks but failed to notify their co-authors or the journal. Scientific publications should present complete and valid data. Although negative data may be detrimental to the financial interest of the manufacturers, intentionally omitting clinically significant unfavorable data from scientific publications is a form of research misconduct.

Third, a medical journal might not zealously follow up on concerns raised during the peer review process. The VIGOR incident may have been caused not by an error, a difference of opinion, or lack of investigative resources, but by a financial conflict of interest.

HOW COMMON IS THE WITHHOLDING OF NEGATIVE RESULTS?

The withholding of significant unfavorable data by the sponsor in Study 15.1 is by no means an isolated case (7).

- The manufacturer of valdecoxib, another selective COX-2 inhibitor, also withheld information on serious unexpected adverse events, including deaths, from the FDA and the public. The company contended that data collected in studies of a medical indication for which it was not seeking FDA approval were trade secrets.
- The manufacturer of the antidepressant paroxetine withheld from the public information on an increased risk of suicide in adolescents taking the drug (8,9). The company argued that because the FDA had not approved the drug for use with this population, they could not release such data to physicians. Although published trials suggest that selective serotonin reuptake inhibitors are beneficial in children with depression, a meta-analysis revealed that when unpublished data are considered, the risks appear to outweigh the benefits for all but one drug in this class (10).
- The manufacturer of an implantable cardioverter-defibrillator allegedly failed to report critical, potentially fatal design defects for more than 3 years (11).
- The manufacturer of aprotinin, an antifibrinolytic drug used in cardiac surgery to decrease bleeding, withheld data that the drug increased renal failure, heart attack, and congestive heart failure (12).
- The manufacturer of PolyHeme, a blood substitute, failed to release results from a clinical trial showing increased mortality until news stories about the delay appeared 5 years after the conclusion of the trial (13,14).
- The manufacturer of cervistatin, a lipid-lowering drug, did not process adverse event reports on cases of rhabdomyolysis associated with the drug. An internal memo stated, "If the FDA asks for bad news, we have to give it, but if we don't have it, we can't give it to them" (7,15).
- In a pivotal trial of celecoxib, another selective COX-2 inhibitor, only 6-month data on outcomes were presented, even though the original protocol called for a longer duration of the trial and outcomes at 12 months were available when the manuscript was submitted. The 6-month outcomes showed an advantage for the study drug, but the 12-month outcomes showed no advantage compared to control drugs (16,17,18).
- The manufacturer of a brand-name thyroid hormone attempted to block the publication of an article showing that a generic thyroid replacement had similar bioavailability as the brand-name preparation (18).
- The manufacturer of a novel immune modulator for the treatment of HIV infection refused to provide a complete data set to investigators in a randomized clinical trial that showed that the investigational agent was ineffective (19).

In the first six cases, withholding information on adverse events exposed research participants or patients taking the drug to potentially fatal consequences.

Empirical studies show that withholding of negative findings is widespread. A study of materials submitted to the FDA in support of successful new drug applications found that clinical trials with statistically favorable results were three times more likely to be published. Overall, over half of clinical trials submitted to the FDA remained unpublished more than 5 years after the drug was approved (20).

Surveys of investigators also suggest that the withholding of unfavorable results may be widespread. One survey of faculty in the life sciences found that about 20% had delayed publication of their research results by more than 6 months during the previous 3 years. They did so for a number of reasons, including filing a patent application, trying to protect their scientific lead, or slowing the dissemination of undesired results. Faculty members with industry ties were significantly more likely to delay publication (21).

Other types of conflicts of interest may also occur in research. Researchers may have a desire for fame or an intellectual commitment to an approach or idea. Such conflicts are inherent to a competitive enterprise and are more difficult to identify and respond to than financial relationships. Institutions as well as individuals may have conflicts of interest. Research institutions may have a financial stake in the products being tested, or in future grants and contracts from sponsors.

Another concern regarding conflicts of interest is bias in the study design, as we discuss next.

IS DRUG COMPANY SPONSORSHIP OF CLINICAL TRIALS ASSOCIATED WITH POSITIVE RESULTS?

Clinical trials are more likely to have positive results if a drug manufacturer sponsors them or if the investigators have financial relationships with manufacturers. One meta-analysis (22) indicated that studies with such ties to drug manufacturers were 3.6 times more likely to find that the tested drug was effective compared to studies without such ties. Similarly, a Cochrane review found that studies sponsored by pharmaceutical companies were 4.05 times more likely to have outcomes favoring the sponsor than studies by nonprofit sponsors (23).

Despite individual examples of flawed studies, three systematic reviews have found that the quality of industry-sponsored trials is comparable to that of studies funded by nonprofits (22). However, these studies did not take into account such issues as the appropriateness of the control intervention and the clinical relevance of the research question (24). Thus the possibility of bias needs to be evaluated on a case-by-case basis.

The interpretation of these data is complicated. The studies show only an association, not a causal relationship. There are several possible explanations for the association. For-profit companies may fund trials only for highly promising compounds and may be more risk-adverse than nonprofit sponsors. Furthermore, investigators may develop financial relationships with trial sponsors because their research persuades them that a drug is efficacious. For instance, an investigator in a trial that shows a drug is effective may be asked to join the company's speakers bureau to give talks on the study results. Furthermore, there may be selection bias against negative studies by journals. Finally, any bias may be unconscious rather than a result of malicious motives.

In addition, critical reviews that look at meta-analyses rather than individual clinical trials as the unit of analysis also find an association between industry funding and conclusions that favor the sponsor's product. Another study, a review of meta-analyses of clinical trials for hypertension (25), found that meta-analyses with financial ties to a single drug company were not more likely than meta-analyses funded from other sources to report results that favored the sponsor's drug. However, the authors of the meta-analyses with financial ties to a single company did report favorable conclusions. Among meta-analyses that had financial ties to one drug company, 27 of 49 (55%) reported favorable results from the meta-analysis, but 45 of 49 (92%) reported favorable conclusions. The authors of the review (25) suggested that there is "a discordance between the data that underlie the results and the interpretation, or 'spin,' of these data that constitute the conclusions."

DO RESEARCH SUBJECTS CARE ABOUT FINANCIAL CONFLICTS OF INTEREST?

According to a recent study (26), most participants in cancer clinical trials are not highly concerned about financial conflicts of interests by investigators. More than 70% of the respondents still would have enrolled in the clinical trial even if the researcher had financial ties to the drug company sponsoring the trial or received royalty payments. Only 31% wanted disclosure of the researcher's financial interests. Only about one-fourth of the respondents believed that a researcher in a clinical trial should be forbidden from receiving a patent royalty or holding stock in the company sponsoring the study.

However, this study had a number of limitations. The respondents were not knowledgeable about conflicts of interest. Most said that previously they had heard little or nothing about financial relationships in clinical trials. The investigators did not provide any background information about the potential consequences of financial ties, such as withholding negative findings from clinical trials. Thus it is not clear whether respondents understood how conflicts of interest might compromise study designs and contribute to bias in the reporting of results. Finally, the study did not include persons who had declined to enter trials, who might be more concerned about conflicts of interest.

HOW ARE CONFLICTS OF INTEREST CURRENTLY HANDLED?

When conflicts of interest arise in other areas, the three most common responses are disclosure, management, and prohibition (1).

DISCLOSURE

A requirement to disclose financial relationships might deter researchers and organizations from establishing inappropriate arrangements with sponsors. If the researcher or sponsor would find it difficult to justify a relationship to an oversight committee, research participants, or the public, the situation may well be ethically unacceptable.

Disclosure to the Research Institution

The National Institutes of Health (NIH) requires investigators applying for grants and contracts to disclose significant financial interests that would reasonably appear to be affected by the research (27), including:

- payments, such as salary and consultation fees, exceeding $10,000 a year;
- stock and stock options totaling over $10,000; and
- more than 5% ownership in a company.

"Significant financial interests" are those that reasonably appear to be affected by the research for which funding is sought, and relationships with entities whose financial interests might be affected. Amounts below these thresholds are regarded as *de minimus*, too small to influence researchers' judgment or actions. Disclosure need not include publicly traded mutual funds over which the investigator has no control. All "key personnel" on the grant are required to submit financial disclosures. Investigators must also disclose the financial interests of their spouses and dependent children. These disclosures must be made to the institution submitting the grant application, which is required to "manage, reduce or eliminate" any conflicts of interest (27).

These NIH requirements have been expanded in several ways. Most medical schools require such disclosure for all research, regardless of the funding source. Many institutions also require that conflicts of interest be disclosed directly to the institutional review board (IRB) when a protocol is submitted for review, as well as to department chairs or deans.

Disclosure to Research Participants

Disclosure of conflicts of interest might encourage more informed decisions by potential participants, leading them to consider the risks of the clinical trial more carefully. However, skeptics point out that potential participants are in a poor position to judge the impact of financial relationships on the risks of research or their own well-being (26). Furthermore, disclosure does not address the underlying problems of undue risk to participants or bias in the design of the study. The greatest value of such disclosure may be to deter researchers from relationships that they would find difficult to explain to the public.

Disclosure to Journals

Many leading medical journals require that researchers disclose any financial conflicts of interest when submitting a manuscript (28). Furthermore, journals may also disclose them to readers when the article is published. Such disclosure may encourage more careful scrutiny of the article by reviewers and readers.

MANAGEMENT

Although disclosure is a necessary response to conflicts of interest, it may be insufficient in some situations. Some financial relationships have such a high likelihood of resulting in bias or harm that they are not acceptable even if conflicts of interest are disclosed (1).

Under NIH regulations, research institutions must "manage, reduce or eliminate" any conflicts of interest (27). The American Association of Medical Colleges (AAMC) has published more specific and stringent recommendations on how academic health centers should manage conflicts of interest in clinical trials, where bias can seriously harm participants and future patients (29). These AAMC guidelines established a general rule that investigators conducting clinical trials should have no significant conflicts of interest. Significant conflicts of interest include equity interest in a start-up company manufacturing a product being studied. Exceptions to this rule are permitted for compelling reasons; however, the default position is that investigators may not have significant conflicts, and the burden of argument is on the investigator who seeks to retain such interests with respect to a particular clinical trial. For instance, in some clinical trials an investigator who holds a patent related to the investigational intervention may be in a unique position to carry out a clinical trial safely. In such cases, the institution should consider, on a case-by-case basis, additional oversight, such as:

- allowing an investigator with a conflict to serve as a consultant but not the principal investigator;
- not allowing an investigator with a conflict to obtain informed consent, perform the data analysis, or write the abstract, results, or discussion sections of the manuscript;
- establishing an independent data and safety monitoring board with no financial ties to the sponsor or close relationship with the researchers.

In other clinical trials, the scientist may be asked to either dissociate herself from the competing relationship or to turn the investigator's role over to someone else, while serving as a consultant to the trial.

PROHIBITION

A few situations present such strong conflicts of interest that they should be prohibited, not merely disclosed or managed (1).

Restrictions on Access to Data or Publication

Researchers should not accept conditions in research contracts and grants that undermine their ability to obtain and publish valid, generalizable knowledge. Investigators at universities should not accept grants and contracts that compromise their academic freedom to present all valid findings, both favorable and unfavorable. Some medical journals require authors submitting manuscripts to certify that they have access to all study data, control over data analysis, and the right to publish findings. The sponsor may request to see and comment on manuscripts, but must not censor publications or insist on changes.

These guarantees are sometimes omitted when academic health centers sign contracts for industry-sponsored research. In a 2005 study (30), almost 15% of academic health centers did not forbid contracts that gave industry sponsors the authority to revise manuscripts or decide whether results should be published. The study reported that 50% of the centers allowed the sponsor to draft the manuscript, while 40% forbade it; 17% of institutions reported disputes over control or access to data.

Falsifying Data

Intentionally omitting or altering data to support a hypothesis is falsification, which falls under the definition of scientific misconduct (see Chapter 12). When allegations of scientific misconduct in federally funded research are raised, the research institution must conduct an inquiry and, if necessary, an investigation. Many universities extend scientific misconduct policies and procedures to all research. However, research organizations that do not receive federal funding are not required to have similar scientific misconduct policies and procedures.

Disclosure to Clinical Trials Databases

Many medical journals, the NIH, and the FDA require that clinical trials be registered in a clinical trials registry (such as http://www.clinicaltrials.gov) before their inception. This prevents investigators from changing parts of the study design, such as the primary endpoint, after they have looked at the data. Furthermore, the public and other researchers will be able to identify trials that were started but subsequently not published, and thus have some indication of unpublished trials whose results might be unfavorable.

In addition, the FDA is now requiring that the results of clinical trials that are submitted to it must be posted on an online clinical trials registry. This requirement addresses the problem of failure to publish negative findings. However, this requirement does not affect clinical trials that are carried out but not used to support an investigational new drug application or a new indication for an approved drug.

ADDITIONAL RESPONSES TO RESEARCH CONFLICTS OF INTEREST

Current oversight of conflicts of interest in clinical trials is problematic because it fails to address the most serious problems. The emphasis on front-end disclosure of financial relationships does not prevent the serious back-end consequences of withholding negative data. What can be done to prevent future incidents similar to those described above?

Actions by IRBs

IRBs could require sponsors and investigators who submit clinical trials to promise to submit the findings, including negative findings, for timely publication in a peer-reviewed journal. If the sponsor or investigator is unwilling to make such a promise, the IRB should require this to be disclosed to participants during the consent process. Moreover, IRBs could require that clinical trials receive independent scientific peer review to reduce the possibility of bias. If the design of a clinical trial is so flawed that no valid conclusions can be drawn, it is unethical to subject participants in the trial to any risk or inconvenience. The IRB would fail in its mission to protect human subjects if it approved clinical trials whose design was seriously flawed. However, many IRB members lack the expertise and time to perform a scientific peer review. Rather than carrying out their own review, IRBs should ensure that clinical trials undergo an independent scientific review equivalent to those carried out by the NIH, FDA, professional scientific societies, leading nonprofit foundations, and collaborative research networks. Alternatively, the department or institution conducting the trial can assume responsibility for performing an independent peer review. The goal is to ensure that some organization can vouch for and be held accountable for the design of each clinical trial. Because external reviews do not usually need to be repeated, this requirement should not delay major clinical trials.

Actions by Medical Journals

Journals should require investigators and sponsors who submit manuscripts regarding clinical trials to attest that they have not withheld clinically significant negative findings. In addition, journals should require that authors of accepted articles update their manuscripts to include pertinent outcomes data that become available before publication. At a minimum, authors should provide to the journal any negative findings that are presented to the FDA before publication of the manuscript.

Journals should report to the appropriate authority, such as the medical school dean or department chair, any author who violates their conflict of interest policy. One leading journal requires the offending author to submit a letter to the editor in which he or she provides full disclosure and apologizes to the readers. For severe violations, the author may be banned from publishing articles in that journal (31).

TAKE HOME POINTS

1. Conflicts of interest are common and may be associated with serious bias in research projects.
2. Disclosure of a conflict of interest is required but may not be sufficient to prevent bias or loss of trust by the public. Management or prohibition of some relationships may be required.

ANNOTATED BIBLIOGRAPHY

AAMC-AAU Advisory Committee on Financial Conflicts of Interest in Clinical Research. *Protecting Patients, Preserving Integrity, Advancing Health: Accelerating the Implementation of COI Policies in Human Subjects Research.* Washington, DC: American Association of Medical Colleges; 2008.
> Report from a committee that included executives from pharmaceutical manufacturers. Available at https://services.aamc.org/Publications/index.cfm?fuseaction=Product.displayForm&prd_id=220&cfid=1&cftoken=8612A038-5DED-4BDE-8850E70F6DA1DE2E.

DeAngelis CD, Fontanarosa PB. Impugning the integrity of medical science: the adverse effects of industry influence. *JAMA* 2008;299:1833–1835.
> Editorial calling for reforms in research funding, authorship, and publication to address the problem of conflicts of interest.

Lo B, Field MJ. *Conflicts of Interest in Medical Research, Education, and Clinical Practice.* Washington, DC: National Academies Press; 2009.
> Consensus report from the Institute of Medicine on conflicts of interest. Text available at http://www.nap.edu/.

REFERENCES

1. Lo B, Field MJ. *Conflicts of Interest in Medical Research, Education, and Clinical Practice.* Washington, DC: National Academies Press; 2009.
2. Emanuel EJ, Thompson DF. The concept of conflicts of interest. In: Emanuel EJ, Grady C, Crouch RA, et al, eds. *The Oxford Textbook of Clinical Research Ethics.* New York: Oxford University Press; 2008:758–766.
3. Moses H, Martin JB. Academic relationships with industry: a new model for biomedical research. *JAMA* 2001; 285:933–935.
4. Krumholz HM, Ross JS, Presler AH, et al. What have we learnt from Vioxx? *BMJ* 2007;334:120–123.
5. Ross JS, Hill KP, Egilman DS, et al. Guest authorship and ghostwriting in publications related to rofecoxib: a case study of industry documents from rofecoxib litigation. *JAMA* 2008;299:1800–1812.
6. Hill KP, Ross JS, Egilman DS, et al. The ADVANTAGE seeding trial: a review of internal documents. *Ann Intern Med* 2008;149:251–258.
7. Kesselheim AS, Avorn J. The role of litigation in defining drug risks. *JAMA* 2007;297:308–311.
8. Turner EH, Matthews AM, Linardatos E, et al. Selective publication of antidepressant trials and its influence on apparent efficacy. *N Engl J Med* 2008;358:252–260.
9. Healy D. Did regulators fail over selective serotonin reuptake inhibitors? *BMJ* 2006;333:92–95.
10. Whittington CJ, Kendall T, Fonagy P, et al. Selective serotonin reuptake inhibitors in childhood depression: systematic review of published versus unpublished data. *Lancet* 2004;363:1341–1345.
11. Hauser RG, Maron BJ. Lessons from the failure and recall of an implantable cardioverter-defibrillator. *Circulation* 2005;112:2040–2042.

12. Avorn J. Dangerous deception—hiding the evidence of adverse drug effects. *N Engl J Med* 2006;355:2169–2171.
13. Burton TM. Amid alarm bells, a blood substitute keeps pumping. *Wall Street Journal* February 22, 2006.
14. Northfield Laboratories. Northfield Laboratories releases summary observations from its elective surgery trial. Available at: http://phx.corporate-ir.net/phoenix.zhtml?c=91374&p=irol-newsArticle&ID=833808&highlight=. Accessed April 25, 2008.
15. Psaty BM, Furberg CD, Ray WA, et al. Potential for conflict of interest in the evaluation of suspected adverse drug reactions: use of cerivastatin and risk of rhabdomyolysis. *JAMA* 2004;292:2622–2631.
16. Juni P, Rutjes AWS, Dieppe PA. Are selective COX-2 inhibitors superior to traditional nonselective nonsteroidal anti-inflammatory drugs? *BMJ* 2002;324:1287–1288.
17. Wright JM, Perry TL, Bassett KL, et al. Reporting of 6-month vs 12-month data in a clinical trial of celecoxib. *JAMA* 2001;286:2398–2400.
18. Rennie D, Flanagin A. Thyroid storm. *JAMA* 1997;277:1238–1243.
19. Kahn JO, Cherng DW, Mayer K, et al. Evaluation of HIV-immunogen, an immunologic modifier, administered to patients infected with HIV having 300 to 549 × 10^6/L CD4 cell counts. *JAMA* 2000;284:2193–2202.
20. Lee K, Bacchetti P, Sim I. Publication of clinical trials supporting successful new drug applications: a literature analysis. *PLoS Med* 2008;5:e191.
21. Blumenthal D, Campbell EG, Anderson MS, et al. Withholding research results in academic life science. Evidence from a national survey of faculty. *JAMA* 1997;277:1224–1228.
22. Bekelman JE, Li Y, Gross CP. Scope and impact of financial conflicts of interest in biomedical research: a systematic review. *JAMA* 2003;289:454–465.
23. Lexchin J, Bero LA, Djulbegovic B, et al. Pharmaceutical industry sponsorship and research outcome and quality: systematic review. *BMJ* 2003;326:1167–1170.
24. Hampson LA, Bekelman JE, Gross CP. Empirical data on conflicts of interest. In: Emanuel E, ed. *Oxford Textbook of Research Ethics*. New York: Oxford University Press; 2008:767–779.
25. Yank V, Rennie D, Bero LA. Financial ties and concordance between results and conclusions in meta-analyses: retrospective cohort study. *BMJ* 2007;335:1202–1205.
26. Hampson LA, Agrawal M, Joffe S, et al. Patients' views on financial conflicts of interest in cancer research trials. *N Engl J Med* 2006;355:2330–2337.
27. Responsibility of Applicants for Promoting Objectivity in Research for Which PHS Funding is Sought. 2000. Available at: http://grants.nih.gov/grants/compliance/42_CFR_50_Subpart_F.htm. Accessed December 8, 2008.
28. van Kolfschooten F. Conflicts of interest: can you believe what you read? *Nature* 2002;416:360–363.
29. AAMC-AAU Advisory Committee on Financial Conflicts of Interest in Clinical Research. *Protecting Patients, Preserving Integrity, Advancing Health: Accelerating the Implementation of COI Policies in Human Subjects Research*. Washington, DC: American Association of Medical Colleges; 2008.
30. Mello MM, Clarridge BR, Studdert DM. Academic medical centers' standards for clinical-trial agreements with industry. *N Engl J Med* 2005;352:2202–2210.
31. DeAngelis CD, Fontanarosa PB. Impugning the integrity of medical science: the adverse effects of industry influence. *JAMA* 2008;299:1833–1835.

Vulnerable Participants

CHAPTER 16

Persons With Impaired Decision-Making Capacity

It is ethically troubling to carry out research with persons who are unable to give informed consent. Because such persons may not understand the research procedures and risks, they might be subjected to risks that competent persons would avoid. Thus they might be treated primarily as a means to advance the goals of research rather than as persons who are respected for their own sake. Historically, serious research abuses have been committed against persons who were institutionalized because of severe psychiatric illness and dementia (1). Recently, research involving drug discontinuation and symptom provocation in persons with serious psychiatric illness has raised ethical controversies (2–5).

One approach to these ethical concerns is to protect such persons by restricting their participation in research. However, research is needed to ameliorate or cure the very conditions that impair their capacity, such as major depression, severe schizophrenia, advanced dementia, and delirium. Some important research can only be carried out with persons with advanced illness who lack decision-making capacity.

This chapter discusses research with adults who lack decision-making capacity. Research with children is discussed in Chapter 17.

STUDY 16.1 Placebo controlled study of a new antidepressant.

Researchers propose a randomized controlled trial (RCT) of a new drug for depression, which is intended to have fewer side effects than currently used drugs. Eligible participants will meet standard diagnostic criteria for major depression. The trial will have two control arms: a placebo arm and an arm receiving a serotonin reuptake inhibitor that is widely used in clinical practice.

There are strong scientific reasons to use a placebo control in clinical trials of antidepressants (6). In several RCTs, established antidepressants were found to be no more effective than the placebo, even though they had been shown to be effective in many other trials. From one trial to another there is considerable variation in the percentage of participants with depression who respond to either an active drug or placebo. Thus, if a clinical trial showed only that a new drug for depression was equivalent to a standard drug, it would be unclear whether either drug was more effective in that trial than a placebo.

Study 16.1 illustrates several ethical concerns regarding research with persons who lack decision-making capacity. Persons with major depression may have impaired decision-making capacity and therefore not appreciate several key features of the study. Drugs known to be effective for this condition will be withheld in the placebo arm but are readily available in standard clinical care. There are serious risks to withholding therapy for major depression, including the development of suicidality.

When a person has impaired or questionable decision-making capacity, several ethical issues need to be addressed:

- How should decision-making capacity be assessed?
- How may persons who lack decision-making capacity be ethically enrolled in research studies?
- What additional protections should be put in place for research with persons who lack decision-making capacity?
- How should researchers respond when such a participant does not cooperate with study procedures?

We use the term "competent" to refer to patients who have the capacity to make informed decisions about medical interventions. Strictly speaking, all adults are considered competent to make such decisions unless a court has declared them "incompetent." In everyday clinical practice, however, physicians usually make de facto determinations as to whether patients lack decision-making capacity without involving the courts (7,8). We avoid the term "impaired decision-making capacity" because although impairments in decision-making capacity lie on a continuum, there must be a threshold beyond which a person's decision will not be accepted as informed.

HOW PREVALENT IS IMPAIRED DECISION-MAKING CAPACITY?

Impaired decision-making capacity is common in many neurological and psychiatric conditions, but not universal. Persons with Alzheimer's disease and schizophrenia score lower on assessments of decision-making capacity than normal controls, particularly regarding comprehension of disclosed information (9). Studies have reported that 34% of persons with mild to moderate Alzheimer's disease, and between 10% and 52% of persons with schizophrenia lack decision-making capacity (10,11). Cognitive impairment is the strongest predictor of a lack of decision-making capacity in persons with Alzheimer's disease and schizophrenia. The severity of psychopathology in schizophrenia is not as strong a predictor.

Patients with schizophrenia or depression may fail to appreciate how information about their condition applies to their situation. In one study of inpatients with schizophrenia, 35% did not acknowledge their symptoms and diagnosis, and 13% of the patients denied the potential benefit of treatment (12). Psychiatric illness may also impair decision-making capacity more subtly (13). Patients who are depressed may overemphasize the risks of treatment, underestimate the benefits, believe that treatment is less likely to be successful for them than for others, or feel unworthy of the intervention.

Thus certain diagnoses should trigger a more detailed individual assessment of decision-making capacity. However, having a particular diagnosis does not mean that an individual lacks decision-making capacity. Many persons with psychiatric or neurological illnesses are competent to make decisions about their medical care or participate in research.

HOW TO EVALUATE DECISION-MAKING CAPACITY

Under federal regulations, persons who consent to participate in research must have adequate decisional capacity. However, the regulations do not specify how capacity should be assessed.

In some situations it is obvious that a person lacks decision-making capacity, such as a person who is comatose. More commonly, there is only a suspicion that a person lacks decision-making capacity, as in the following examples:

- The person has a condition in which impaired decision-making capacity is common, such as dementia, cognitive impairment, delirium, stupor, schizophrenia, or substance abuse.
- A family member or friend reports that the person is confused.
- The person is confused when interacting with research staff.

Because such a person may lack decision-making capacity, closer scrutiny of his decision-making capacity is appropriate. However, not everyone with these conditions has impaired decision-making capacity. Physicians need to assess each individual's ability to give informed consent to enroll in a specific research project (7,8,14).

COMPONENTS OF DECISION-MAKING CAPACITY

Decision-making capacity requires a cluster of abilities (15). It is specific to the decision under consideration, i.e., a person may be capable of making informed decisions about some issues but not others. The person should be able to perform the following functions.

Understand Pertinent Information

To make an informed decision about whether to participate in a research study, a participant needs to understand his medical situation and prognosis, the nature of the proposed research, the risks and benefits, the alternatives, and the likely consequences of each alternative.

Appreciate the Relevance to his Situation

In addition to comprehending this information, the participant needs to appreciate how the disclosed information applies to him. For example, a participant who believes that he will definitely receive the active intervention in an RCT does not appreciate how randomization applies to him.

Use Reasoning to Make a Decision

A participant should be able to process information logically and assess the advantages, disadvantages, and consequences of participating or not participating in the research project. If the study is an RCT, he also should be able to assess the advantages, disadvantages, and consequences of each arm. This requires the ability to make comparisons and to judge the consequences of decisions. Although this process of decision-making should be reasonable, the actual decision may differ from what most people would do in the situation. Unconventional decisions do not necessarily imply lack of decision-making capacity.

Make and Communicate a Choice

The participant must appreciate that he—and not the researcher, personal physician, nurses, or family members—has decision-making power regarding his participation in research.

Some writers have suggested a sliding scale for judging decision-making capacity: a participant in a research project that has great risk and little prospect of personal benefit should meet higher standards for decision-making capacity than a participant in a very low-risk research project, such as a questionnaire study (8,14). This suggestion is intuitively appealing because it protects participants by preventing persons with borderline decision-making capacity from consenting to high-risk studies. However, implementing a sliding scale is challenging because people might disagree over what level of decision-making capacity should be required for a particular set of research risks. To prevent such problems, researchers should define explicitly what criteria they are using to assess a participant's decision-making capacity in a specific study. The IRB application should describe who will conduct the assessment, how prospective subjects' decisional capacity will be evaluated, and what criteria will be used to identify incapable subjects.

WHAT QUESTIONS SHOULD RESEARCHERS ASK TO ASSESS DECISION-MAKING CAPACITY?

There are several instruments for determining decision-making capacity in the research setting (14,16–18). Because decision-making capacity is specific to the situation and decision, researchers need to adapt existing instruments for their particular study. The questions in Table 16.1 are useful for assessing decision-making capacity.

| TABLE 16.1 | Questions for Assessing Decision-Making Capacity |

Question	Sample Phrasing
Does the person understand the nature of the research study?	"What is the purpose of the research project I just described to you?"
Does the person appreciate the consequences of her choices?	"Do you believe that you have been asked to be in this study primarily for your benefit?"
	"What do you believe would happen if you were to decide not to be in this study any longer?"
Does the person use reasoning to make a choice?	"What is it that makes [the subject's choice] seem better than [the nonchosen options]?"

These questions presuppose that the participant has received adequate information about her condition and the interventions involved in the study. If there is any doubt about whether this has occurred, the researcher needs to repeat the information.

Researchers who use any of these instruments need to decide (and justify to the IRB) how they will interpret responses to the questions they ask. There are no standard passing scores for any of these questions, and no standard methods to combine performance across different domains into an overall determination of adequate/inadequate decision-making capacity.

The MacArthur Competence Assessment Tool for Clinical Research (MCAT-CR) is the most widely used instrument, but it requires 15–20 minutes to administer and extensive staff training. A brief screening instrument that asks three simple questions regarding the purpose, benefits, and risks of the study is useful to identify individuals who require a more detailed evaluation (19).

THE ROLE OF MENTAL STATUS TESTING

Clinicians often use mental status tests to assess whether a patient has the capacity to make medical decisions. Such tests evaluate the subject's orientation, attention span, immediate recall, short-term and long-term memory, ability to perform simple calculations, and language skills (20). However, in the research context, mental status tests are less useful than direct assessments of whether the patient understands the nature of the study, the risks and benefits, the alternatives, and the consequences (21).

Mental status testing is a useful screening tool for identifying individuals who need a more extensive evaluation of their decision-making capacity. For persons with Alzheimer's disease, a Mini Mental Status Exam (MMSE) score of less than 19 accurately identifies persons who lack decision-making capacity, and a score above 23 accurately identifies persons who have adequate decision-making capacity. In the intermediate range of scores, a more detailed, protocol-specific assessment of capacity is needed (22).

INTERVENTIONS TO IMPROVE DECISION-MAKING CAPACITY

Several educational interventions have been shown to improve comprehension in research participants with psychiatric illness and cognitive impairment (9,23), as listed below:

- Assessing the participant's comprehension and providing feedback to correct misunderstandings.
- Repeating and simplifying the consent process.
- Using a stepwise consent process.
- Using multimedia presentations, such as PowerPoint slides that are read aloud by a staff member.

In some studies, such participants had levels of comprehension similar to those of normal controls. Researchers should use such techniques with persons who have impaired decision-making capacity.

ENROLLING PERSONS WHO LACK DECISION-MAKING CAPACITY IN RESEARCH

Persons who lack decision-making capacity may be enrolled in research studies on the basis of surrogate permission or advance directives, provided that appropriate safeguards are in place. Two questions must be addressed when persons lack decision-making capacity:

- Who should make decisions for such persons?
- What standards should be used in making decisions?

Our discussion in this chapter excludes children and emergency research, since there are separate guidelines for research in these areas, which are covered in Chapters 17 and 19.

WHO SHOULD SERVE AS THE SURROGATE DECISION-MAKER?

The Common Rule allows the "legally authorized representative" of an incapacitated person to give permission for research. We use the term "permission" rather than "consent" in this context to emphasize that the surrogate is deciding that someone else may participate in the research project. Under federal guidance, persons who have authority to make clinical decisions for the incapacitated person may give permission for research. State laws determine who may serve as the legally authorized representative for research participants (24). Although most state laws have some provision for proxy decision-making in this context, these laws are often not specific or clear. Researchers need to understand the laws in their state. The resulting legal uncertainty has led IRBs to reject some ethically sound studies with persons who lack decision-making capacity.

Ethically, the surrogate should be someone who is familiar with the person who lacks decision-making capacity, and has the person's best interests at heart. There is a hierarchy of persons who are generally considered appropriate to serve as surrogates. The typical order of preference is as follows:

- A guardian or conservator appointed by the courts.
- A proxy appointed by the person when still competent (for example, a health care proxy).
- The person's spouse or domestic partner.
- Adult children.
- Other close relatives.

Persons who lack decision-making capacity usually do not have a legally appointed guardian or proxy. Generally family members are allowed to make decisions for them. Most people want their family to make such decisions for them if they lose the ability to do so (25). Close family members also are likely to know what the person would want, and generally they can be trusted to act in the person's best interests (26).

A few states have formalized the hierarchy of family decision-makers through legislation. Researchers need to know the legal requirements in their state.

WHAT STANDARDS SHOULD BE USED IN SURROGATE DECISION-MAKING?

The federal regulations do not specify what standards a surrogate should use in making decisions about the incapacitated person's participation in research. Ethically, the hierarchy of standards for surrogate decision-making is ordered as follows (24,26):

Research Advance Directives

When still competent, people may indicate whether they would want to participate in research if they lose the ability to make informed decisions. Although advance directives are more commonly used for decisions about clinical treatment, some persons also use them to provide directives regarding research participation (27). For instance, persons with depression, schizophrenia, and bipolar disease might indicate while in remission that they are wiling to participate in research if they relapse and are no longer capable of giving consent. Persons with mild dementia might indicate that they would want to enroll in a clinical trial of new drugs for dementia if they lost decision-making capacity. There is a strong ethical justification for entering such persons into such research. Following advance directives respects the participant's preferences and values, provided there is no evidence that he has changed his mind. Advance directives are particularly useful for sensitive or controversial research, such as psychiatric research involving medication-free periods, symptom-provocation studies, and placebo-controlled trials. The permission of a surrogate who can act in the best interests of the participant serves as an additional protection.

Advance directives need to be completed while the person still has the capacity to make informed decisions. Written advance directives are generally more trustworthy than oral statements because the participant is more likely to have carefully considered his decision. For advance directives to be practical, research centers need to recruit cohorts of individuals who have conditions to be studied and who are likely to relapse or progress.

Substituted Judgment

In the absence of clear advance directives, surrogates should try to decide what the person would want under the circumstances, using all information that they know about him. Although substituted judgments are intended to respect the person's values, they may be speculative or inaccurate. Surrogates are commonly mistaken about the person's preferences, particularly when his wishes have not been discussed explicitly.

Best Interests

When the person's preferences are unclear or unknown, decisions should be based on his best interests. People generally take into account their quality of life when making decisions for themselves. It is understandable that surrogates would also consider the quality of life of persons who lack decision-making capacity. Judgments about quality of life are appropriate if they reflect the patient's own values. Bias or discrimination may occur, however, if others project their values onto the patient or weigh the perceived social worth of the patient.

Conflicts Among Standards

A person's previously expressed preferences may conflict with his current best interests regarding participation in a research study. Several studies suggest that most persons with Alzheimer's disease or at risk for Alzheimer's disease are willing to grant proxies the authority to enroll them in a clinical trial, even if that decision differs from what the participant said previously (28,29).

Empirical studies show that surrogates commonly do not follow the incapacitated person's previously stated or current preferences regarding research (30). Proxies report that they would override an advance directive and enroll a person in a clinical trial if they thought it would maximize his or her well-being (30). Surrogates also may decide not to enroll people who previously expressed a desire to participate in research (31). Reasons for such a refusal include the surrogates' opinion that the potential subject had unrealistic expectations, the research would increase their own caregiving burdens, the surrogate would not want to participate in such a study, or the study would disturb or upset the potential subject.

SEEK CONSENT FROM PARTICIPANTS WHO REGAIN DECISION-MAKING CAPACITY

Some participants who have been entered into a research study by a surrogate may regain decision-making capacity. For example, they may experience a remission in their psychiatric condition or recover from an acute medical condition, such as respiratory failure or major head trauma. If they recover decision-making capacity, participants should be asked whether they agree to be in the study; if they decline to participate, they should be withdrawn from the study and no additional data should be collected from them.

PROTECTING PARTICIPANTS WHO LACK DECISION-MAKING CAPACITY

Vulnerable participants need additional protections. Minimal risk research presents no serious ethical dilemmas, provided that an IRB has approved the study and an appropriate surrogate has given permission. For studies that present more than minimal risk, Table 16.2 suggests steps to protect participants who lack decision-making capacity. More steps should be taken if the risk is greater or there is less direct benefit to participants (24).

STUDY 16.2   **Pathophysiology study in Alzheimer's disease.**

Researchers wish to study the effects of Alzheimer's disease drugs on brain function. The researchers propose to carry out cognitive function testing and functional magnetic resonance imaging (fMRI) when the participants are on a medication and when they are off the drug. These findings would also be correlated with blood levels of drugs drawn through an intravenous line. During the study, participants would be admitted to the inpatient clinical research center. This kind of research may help identify surrogate endpoints to screen potential drugs or to predict their effectiveness in individual patients.

One woman, whose husband gave consent for her to participate in the study, turns away from a researcher who wishes to draw blood for tests and refuses to straighten her arm. One investigator suggests that they get the husband to talk her into cooperating. Another researcher suggests that they simply hold her arm down for a moment to start the intravenous line.

Another participant, a man who had completed an advance directive stating his willingness to be in any study concerning Alzheimer's disease, becomes agitated during the MRI scan, shouting, "I'm being crushed!"

HEIGHTEN IRB REVIEW

The IRB should include persons familiar with the condition that is impairing the participant's decision-making capacity. Examples include persons with the condition who have been successfully treated, their relatives, or advocates for them. Such persons will help the IRB understand how the study may put participants at risk, and whether the proposed safeguards will be effective.

IRBs should also give greater scrutiny to the balance of risks and potential benefits when participants lack decision-making capacity, as we next discuss.

RESTRICT SOME TYPES OF RESEARCH

IRBs should first consider whether the research could be carried out with participants who have decision-making capacity and can give informed consent themselves.

TABLE 16.2	**Protections for Participants Who Lack Decision-Making Capacity**
Heighten IRB review.	
Restrict some types of research.	
Provide specific safeguards to mitigate risks.	
Respect dissent by participants.	

Next, the IRB should assess the level of risk and benefit. When research presents more than minimal risk, ethics experts suggest that persons who lack decision-making capacity should participate only if certain benefits are likely (24,32). The federal guidelines for pediatric research provide a framework for doing so (see Chapter 17). If there is no prospect of direct benefit, the level of risk permitted should be titrated to the type of potential benefit. If the research presents only a minor increase over minimal risk, the research may be permitted if it is designed to increase understanding of the condition causing impaired decision-making capacity or the adverse clinical effects of that condition. This requirement precludes using primarily persons with impaired decision-making capacity to study conditions that also occur in persons who have decision-making capacity.

STUDY 16.2   **(Continued).**

MRI scans pose greater than minimal risk for patients with dementia because the scans often cause agitation. The risk may be considered a minor increase over minimal risk because such agitation is transient. The researchers have taken appropriate steps to minimize the risk. Such research on the pathophysiology of Alzheimer's disease is directed toward the condition that impairs participants' decision-making capacity. Such research may lead in the long run to better methods to evaluate potential therapies, or better ways to identify persons who will respond to treatments.

If the research involves more than a minor increase over minimal risk, it should offer more benefit, such as the prospect of gaining vital knowledge about the participant's condition. The terms "small increase over minimal risk" and "vital knowledge" are difficult to define precisely and involve difficult value judgments. Interpretations of these terms should take into account the perspectives of persons with the condition. This is another reason why the IRB should include persons who can articulate these perspectives.

PROVIDE SPECIFIC SAFEGUARDS TO MITIGATE RISKS

Depending on the particular protocol and the level of risk involved, it may be appropriate to apply the following additional safeguards to reduce risks or their impact (24,33):

- *Assess the surrogate's understanding* of key features of the study and ensure that they do not have a therapeutic misconception. Investigators can administer a questionnaire to assess the surrogate's comprehension of what has been disclosed.
- Have a *consent monitor*, someone independent of the research team, monitor the evaluation of the participant's decision-making capacity or discussions with a surrogate decision-maker.
- Have a *subject advocate*, a family member, friend, or mental health professional independent of the research team with the authority to withdraw the participant from the study if continued participation is not in the participant's best interests (34).
- *Closely monitor* for adverse effects, because participants who lack decision-making capacity may not spontaneously report symptoms they develop.

RESPECT DISSENT BY PARTICIPANTS

Persons who lack decision-making capacity may still have preferences regarding what is done to them, and may express these preferences by words or by actions. Some persons may indicate that they do not want to participate in a research study by making gestures, such as shaking their heads or holding up their hand. Alternatively, the subject may physically refuse to cooperate with the study procedures, such as by not holding still, not swallowing a pill, or pulling out an intravenous line.

In patients with impaired decision-making capacity, MRI scans, PET scans, or other imaging studies may illuminate pathophysiology in ways that may lead to better therapies, better methods to evaluate potential therapies, or better ways to identify persons who are likely to respond to treatments. However, such imaging studies may entail greater than minimal risk for patients with dementia or schizophrenia, who are more likely to become agitated during such procedures. On the one hand, the increase over minimal risk is small. Discomfort is transient and will not lead to worsening or relapse of the underlying disease. On the other hand, there are strong reasons to respect such dissent by participants. It is an infringement on their freedom to force people to do something that they do not want to do, causes discomfort, and is not for their own benefit.

Persons at a higher level of functioning, although unable to make informed decisions, may be able to give positive assent to participate in research. That is, they may indicate they are willing to participate by saying that they want to participate or through their actions, such as by holding out their arms for phlebotomy. Some have suggested that positive assent should be required as an additional safeguard in research that presents substantially more than minimal risk and no prospect of person benefit, such as a pathophysiology study that requires an invasive procedure.

Researchers and surrogates must keep in mind that research primarily benefits science and future patients. Research differs from clinical care, where the objections of patients who lack decision-making capacity may be overridden because they are expected to benefit from the intervention.

Researchers should respond to this situation in several ways.

Anticipate Problems With Dissent

In Study 16.2, the timing of blood draws and imaging studies needs to be coordinated with the administration of medications. Researchers need to anticipate that participants with dementia may not cooperate with procedures as scheduled, and may become more confused when they are in unfamiliar surroundings or when they are rushed. The protocol should explain how these situations will be handled.

Use Measures That Are Routinely Employed In Patient Care To Reduce Distress

Researchers should use procedures that are routinely used in clinical practice to reduce patient distress and enhance cooperation. Research staff should continually remind the participant where she is. The family should be encouraged to bring in familiar objects from home, such as photographs or music, to prevent disorientation.

Try To Persuade The Participant To Cooperate

In clinical practice, dissent by patients who lack decision-making capacity can often be reversed through persuasion, cajoling, assistance of family members and friends, or deferring care. For example, a dementia patient may refuse phlebotomy one day but agree to it when asked again the next day. In clinical care, where treatment is in the best interests of the patient, family members and hospital staff may be justified in taking additional steps to provide highly beneficial interventions, such as holding a patient's arm to start antibiotics for an infection. However, the use of force cannot be justified in research because interventions are not intended to directly benefit the participant. The research protocol should specify what kinds of attempts at persuasion are permissible—for example, how many times cooperation with a research procedure may be requested.

Anticipate Complications Of The Underlying Disease

In addition to problems with study procedures, research staff should anticipate behavioral problems due to the underlying disease. Nurses in a clinical research center, who may not be used to taking care of persons with dementia, may not be familiar with how to manage patients who wander or refuse to eat. The protocol should include a plan for responding. If a person tries to leave the research unit, one possible approach is for a relative, friend, or staff member to simply accompany him to ensure his safety.

STUDY 16.2   (Continued).

Because precise timing of research procedures is necessary, the researcher might enroll only patients who have a relative, friend, or caretaker who can remain with them during procedures and persuade them to cooperate. It would be appropriate to compensate these companions a modest amount for their time, such as payment at the minimum wage rate. These companions should also have the authority to withdraw the participant from a study procedure at any time.

Researchers should also reduce the risk of neuroimaging studies. Persons who have become anxious or agitated at previous imaging studies, or have refused such studies in the past, should be excluded from the study. As in standard clinical practice, persons undergoing imaging studies should be offered music to reduce anxiety or mild sedatives if needed. If a subject objects or becomes agitated, the radiologist directing the imaging study, who should be independent of the research team, should terminate the procedure. The threshold for stopping the procedure during a research study should be lower than in clinical care, where the study is intended to benefit the patient.

TAKE HOME POINTS

1. In projects where many individuals in the target population lack decision-making capacity, researchers should specify in the protocol how they will assess the participants' decision-making capacity.
2. Participants who lack decision-making capacity may be enrolled in research on the basis of a surrogate's permission or research advance directives.
3. Participants who lack decision-making capacity may need additional protections.

ANNOTATED BIBLIOGRAPHY

Dunn LB, Nowrangi MA, Palmer BW, et al. Assessing decisional capacity for clinical research or treatment: a review of instruments. *Am J Psychiatry* 2006;8:1323–1334.
    Practical review of methods to assess decision-making capacity.
Saks ER, Dunn LB, Wimer J, et al. Proxy consent to research: the legal landscape. *Yale J Health Policy Law Ethics* 2008;8:37–92.
    Comprehensive summary and thoughtful analysis of legal and policy issues regarding proxy consent to research. Contains comprehensive tables summarizing state laws on proxy consent.

REFERENCES

1. Katz J. *Experimentation with Human Beings*. New York: Russell Sage Foundation; 1972.
2. Schooler NR. Implications for future research of "medication-free research in early episode schizophrenia." *Schizophr Bull* 2006;32:297–298.
3. McGlashan TH. Rationale and parameters for medication-free research in psychosis. *Schizophr Bull* 2006;32:300–302.
4. Shore D. Ethical issues in schizophrenia research: a commentary on some current concerns. *Schizophr Bull* 2006;32:26–29.
5. Miller FG, Rosenstein DL. Psychiatric symptom-provoking studies: an ethical appraisal. *Biol Psychiatry* 1997;42:403–409.
6. Kupfer DJ, Frank E. Placebo in clinical trials for depression: complexity and necessity. *JAMA* 2002;287:1853–1854.
7. President's Commission for the Study of Ethical Problems in Medicine and Biomedical and Behavioral Research. *Making Health Care Decisions*. Washington, DC: U.S. Government Printing Office; 1982.
8. Buchanan AE, Brock DW. *Deciding for Others*. Cambridge: Cambridge University Press; 1989.
9. Jeste DV, Saks E. Decisional capacity in mental illness and substance use disorders: empirical database and policy implications. *Behav Sci Law* 2006;24:607–628.

10. Kim SY, Karlawish JH, Caine ED. Current state of research on decision-making competence of cognitively impaired elderly persons. *Am J Geriatr Psychiatry* 2002;10:151–165.
11. Jeste DV, Depp CA, Palmer BW. Magnitude of impairment in decisional capacity in people with schizophrenia compared to normal subjects: an overview. *Schizophr Bull* 2006;32:121–128.
12. Appelbaum PS, Grisso T. The MacArthur Treatment Competence Study. I: Mental illness and competence to consent to treatment. *Law Hum Behav* 1995;19:105–126.
13. Bursztajn HJ, Gutheil TG, Brodsky A. Affective disorders, competence, and decision making. In: Gutheil TG, Bursztajn HJ, Brodsky A, et al, eds. *Decision Making in Psychiatry and the Law.* Baltimore: Williams & Wilkins; 1991:153–170.
14. Grisso T, Appelbaum P. *Assessing Competence to Consent to Treatment: A Guide for Physicians and Other Health Professionals.* New York: Oxford University Press; 1998.
15. Kim SY. When does decisional impairment become decisional incompetence? Ethical and methodological issues in capacity research in schizophrenia. *Schizophr Bull* 2006;32:92–97.
16. Applebaum PS, Grisso T. Assessing patients' capacities to consent to treatment. *N Engl J Med* 1988;319:1635–1638.
17. Applebaum PS, Grisso T, Frank E, et al. Competence of depressed patients for consent to research. *Am J Psychiatry* 1999;156:1380–1384.
18. Dunn LB, Nowrangi MA, Palmer BW, et al. Assessing decisional capacity for clinical research or treatment: a review of instruments. *Am J Psychiatry* 2006; 8:1323–1334.
19. Palmer BW, Dunn LB, Appelbaum PS, et al. Correlates of treatment-related decision-making capacity among middle-aged and older patients with schizophrenia. *Arch Gen Psychiatry* 2004;61:230–236.
20. Kane RL, Ouslander JG, Ibrass IB. *Essentials of Clinical Geriatrics.* 2nd ed. New York: McGraw-Hill; 1989.
21. Grisso T, Appelbaum P. *Assessing Competence to Consent to Treatment: A Guide for Physicians and Other Health Professionals.* New York: Oxford University Press; 1998:90–91.
22. Karlawish JH, Casarett DJ, James BD, et al. The ability of persons with Alzheimer disease (AD) to make a decision about taking an AD treatment. *Neurology* 2005;64:1514–1519.
23. Eyler LT, Jeste DV. Enhancing the informed consent process: a conceptual overview. *Behav Sci Law* 2006;24: 553–568.
24. Saks ER, Dunn LB, Wimer J, et al S. Proxy consent to research: the legal landscape. *Yale J Health Policy Law Ethics* 2008;8:37–92.
25. Kim SY, Kim HM, McCallum C, et al. What do people at risk for Alzheimer disease think about surrogate consent for research? *Neurology* 2005;65:1395–1401.
26. Lo B. *Resolving Ethical Dilemmas: A Guide for Clinicians.* 4th ed. Philadelphia: Lippincott Williams & Wilkins; 2009.
27. Karlawish JH. Research involving cognitively impaired adults. *N Engl J Med* 2003;348:1389–1392.
28. Wendler D, Martinez RA, Fairclough D, et al. Views of potential subjects toward proposed regulations for clinical research with adults unable to consent. *Am J Psychiatry* 2002;159:585–591.
29. Stocking CB, Hougham GW, Danner DD, et al. Speaking of research advance directives: planning for future research participation. *Neurology* 2006;66:1361–1366.
30. Karlawish J, Kim SY, Knopman D, et al. The views of Alzheimer disease patients and their study partners on proxy consent for clinical trial enrollment. *Am J Geriatr Psychiatry* 2008;16:240–247.
31. Karlawish JH, Casarett D, Klocinski J, et al. How do AD patients and their caregivers decide whether to enroll in a clinical trial? *Neurology* 2001;56:789–792.
32. Kim SY, Appelbaum PS, Jeste DV, et al. Proxy and surrogate consent in geriatric neuropsychiatric research: update and recommendations. *Am J Psychiatry* 2004;161:797–806.
33. Wendler D, Prasad K. Core safeguards for clinical research with adults who are unable to consent. *Ann Intern Med* 2001;135:514–523.
34. Stroup TS, Appelbaum PS. Evaluation of "subject advocate" procedures in the Clinical Antipsychotic Trials of Intervention Effectiveness (CATIE) schizophrenia study. *Schizophr Bull* 2006;32:147–152.

17

Research With Children

R esearch with children is essential but also ethically problematic (1). Without research, there can be no rigorous evidence base for pediatric care. Research findings from adults may not apply to children for a number of reasons. Some diseases are more common or occur exclusively in children, or have different manifestations, trajectories, and responses to therapy in children. As children mature, the bioavailability, metabolism, excretion, and pharmacodynamics of their medications may change. Drugs for young children must be given in elixir or as chewable tablets, whose bioavailability must be ascertained. Several federal policies provide incentives to include children in clinical trials (2). Manufacturers who voluntarily conduct studies of drugs in children can obtain an additional 6 months of patent exclusivity. Also, the FDA may require drug manufacturers to test drugs in children that are already approved for use in adults.

Research with children inevitably raises ethical dilemmas because young children cannot provide informed consent. It is troubling to expose people to risks to which they have not consented so that others may benefit. Furthermore, children, who lack experience and cannot control their environment, often cannot avoid or mitigate risks. Hence children historically have been excluded from research to protect them from harm. As a result of these exclusions, however, the effectiveness and safety of many pediatric therapies remain uncertain.

Subpart D of the federal regulations for research with human subjects addresses research with children. The following legal case illustrates the ethical tension between protecting research participants and carrying out research to benefit children.

ACCEPTABLE RISKS IN RESEARCH INVOLVING CHILDREN

A recent highly publicized case dramatized ethical issues in pediatric research (3–6).

STUDY 17.1	Kennedy Krieger study of lead abatement.

This study compared three different methods of low-cost partial lead abatement in two control groups. The low-cost lead abatement measures were feasible for landlords to adopt without raising rents beyond the means of low-income families. The control groups lived in housing built after 1978, when lead-based paint was banned indoors, or in housing from which the lead had been completely abated. Lead levels were measured in blood samples from children and in dust samples from the homes. At the time of the study, 95% of private low-income housing in inner-city Baltimore had lead-based paint. The study was carried out by the Kennedy Krieger Institute.

Two parents in this study sued the researchers and the research institution after their children developed elevated lead levels while enrolled in the study. The plaintiffs contended that (i) the subjects were placed at unacceptable risk, (ii) mothers were not adequately informed

STUDY 17.1	**(Continued).**

of the risks associated with the study, and (iii) mothers were not notified promptly of ele-vated levels of lead in their home.

In 2001, the Maryland Court of Appeals, the highest court in the state, reversed a sum-mary judgment in favor of the defendants. The ruling harshly criticized this study and the research oversight process.

The court stated that participants place "profound trust . . . in investigators, institutions, and the research enterprise . . . to protect them from harm." Parents expect that their chil-dren will be protected from unreasonable harms and rely on researchers to fully inform them of hazards in their home and risks to their child's health related to the topic of research. The parents should have been informed that "as a result of the experiment, it was possible that there might be some accumulation of lead in the blood of the children."

The court held that a parent or guardian cannot consent to enroll a child in "nontherapeu-tic" research in which there is any risk to the child. "Parents, whether improperly enticed by trinkets, food stamps, money or other items, have no more right to intentionally and unnec-essarily place children in potentially hazardous nontherapeutic research surroundings, than do researchers. In such cases, parental consent, no matter how informed, is insufficient." The court later clarified that it would allow in research "the minimal kind of risk that is inherent in any endeavor."

According to the ruling, parents must make decisions that are in the best interest of the child: "[I]t is. . .not in the best interest of any healthy child to be intentionally put in a nonther-apeutic situation where his or her health may be impaired, in order to test methods that may ultimately benefit all children."

WHAT IS "THERAPEUTIC" RESEARCH?

As in the Kennedy Krieger ruling, some philosophers have argued that children should not be per-mitted to participate in "nontherapeutic" research, but only in "therapeutic" research. However, the terms "therapeutic research" and "nontherapeutic research" are logically inconsistent because all research is "intended to develop general knowledge," whereas therapy is "for the benefit of an individual and therefore does not involve any generalizable component" (7). Also, the term "ther-apeutic research" might be used to justify risky interventions simply because some aspects of the protocol offer a prospect of therapeutic benefit (7).

WHAT ARE THE BEST INTERESTS OF THE CHILD?

In the United States, parents are presumed to act in the best interest of their children and are granted considerable discretion to decide what is best for them (8). Parental childrearing decisions generally are protected from government interference. However, the government may set limits on parental autonomy to protect children from grave harm; for instance, parents may not neglect or abuse their children. The justification for government intervention is that the parent is no longer acting in the best interests of the child.

The concept of best interests is intuitively appealing. However, legal scholars point out that the best interests of a child are ambiguous and often "indeterminate and speculative" (9,10). Well-intentioned, reasonable persons may disagree over what is in the best interests of a particular child in a specific situation. Furthermore, parents are permitted to make decisions that conflict with a child's best interests to promote the interests of the family as a whole or another family member. For example, children may work in the family business rather than attending enrichment classes at school. Also, parents may require a child to help other people, even at some risk to the child (11). For instance, parents may require that their children help neighbors by shoveling snow from their sidewalks or mowing their lawns, which do not directly benefit the child and entail some small risk. An empirical study found that most parents were willing to have their child participate in a study that offered no prospect of direct benefit, and that they were as willing for the child to participate in such research as in a charitable activity (12). Thus, in other contexts, society interprets "best interests" broadly to allow parents to have their children participate in activities that are not in their self-interest as narrowly defined.

WHAT IS THE JUSTIFICATION FOR RESEARCH THAT DOES NOT BENEFIT THE CHILD PARTICIPANT?

Some people argue that children have a moral duty to help others. However, adults have no such duty, even though they can understand the importance of altruism and have more opportunities to help than do children. Others argue that participating in research benefits children by teaching them altruism. However, altruism, while praiseworthy, is considered optional rather than mandatory.

The most convincing justification is that all children benefit from previous research in which other children participated but did not benefit directly. It is unfair to enjoy the benefits of others' contributions without also contributing to research. Thus, research to benefit other children may be ethically permissible provided that the risks are not too great and the participants are adequately protected.

SPECIAL PROTECTIONS FOR CHILDREN IN SUBPART D

Subpart D of the federal regulations for human subjects research provides special protections for child participants in research and restricts the level of risk permitted relative to the benefits (1,13). Table 17.1 presents the different types of research that may be approved, which are often referred to by the number of the section of Subpart D that applies to them.

In these categories, more protections are required as the risk increases and the benefit to participants decreases. Research under sections 404, 405, and 406 may be approved by local IRBs. Research in Section 407 may only be approved by a national review and approval process. These regulations contain several terms that are not defined explicitly and are difficult to interpret.

TABLE 17.1	**Types of Research With Children That May Be Approved**			
Section of Subpart D	**Section 404**	**Section 405**	**Section 406**	**Section 407**
Type of benefit	*Not specified*	*Prospect of direct benefit to participants*	*Knowledge of vital importance about a participant's disorder or condition*	*Understand, prevent, or alleviate a serious problem affecting children*
Level of risk	*Minimal risk*	*Greater than minimal risk*	*Minor increase over greater than minimal risk*	*More than minor increase over minimal risk*
Who may approve protocol	*Local IRB*	*Local IRB*	*Local IRB*	*Secretary of HHS after consultation with expert panel*
Parental consent	*From one parent*	*From one parent*	*From both parents*	*From both parents*
Child assent needed?	*Yes*	*No*	*Yes*	*Yes*

WHAT IS MINIMAL RISK RESEARCH?

Intuitively, it makes sense to allow IRBs to approve research that involves very small risk to participants, such as observations of children's play, review of medical records, standard physical examinations, and questionnaires about nonsensitive topics.

According to these regulations, in a minimal risk study "the probability and magnitude of harm or discomfort anticipated in the research are not greater . . . than those ordinarily encountered in daily life or during the performance of routine physical or psychological examinations or tests." This definition contains several ambiguities that need to be clarified (1,13–16).

First, "daily life" should refer to healthy individuals in safe environments. When children have serious illness, such as leukemia, their daily experience as patients includes invasive tests such as bone marrow biopsy or lumbar puncture. Similarly, children with socioeconomic disadvantages may face daily risks because of violence. If minimal risk were defined in terms of the daily lives of individuals who are ill or disadvantaged, such children might be allowed to assume greater risks than healthy persons. However, this interpretation is ethically problematical because persons who already face greater risks need more protection, not less.

Second, the everyday experience of healthy persons needs to be viewed as an upper limit for minimal risk that should not be exceeded. Some children may be more susceptible to adverse effects, for example, because of underlying illness; an intervention that involves minimal risk for other children may pose greater than minimal risk for such children.

Third, the risks under consideration need to be regarded as socially acceptable in the research context. The physical risks of contact sports are generally considered acceptable in light of the direct benefits of athletic participation, but the same level of risk may not be regarded as acceptable in research that does not offer direct benefits. The standard of what a "reasonable parent" would allow has been proposed as the criterion for what risks are permissible.

IRBs vary greatly in how they interpret "minimal risk." For example, one study reported that 23% of IRB chairs considered allergy skin testing to be of minimal risk, 43% judged it to be a minor increase over minimal risk, and 27% considered it more than a minor increase over minimal risk (17). This variation is troublesome because some IRBs may be allowing children to be subjected to inappropriate risks in research, while other IRBs may be rejecting valuable research whose risks are ethically acceptable. To reduce unwarranted variation in the use of the term, the Health and Human Services (HHS) Secretary's Advisory Committee on Human Research Protections (SACHRP) recommended that giving a medical history or undergoing venipuncture, chest x-ray, or MRI without sedation should be considered minimal risk.

SECTION 405: PROSPECT OF DIRECT BENEFIT

Section 405 allows IRBs to approve research that involves *greater than minimal risk* but presents a prospect of *direct benefit* to participants. Research that offers a prospect of direct benefit may offer a favorable balance of benefits and risk even if the risks are greater than minimal. An example would be a clinical trial of a potential new therapy for a participant's illness. Section 405 requires that the benefit/risk balance must be at least as favorable as alternative approaches. There must also be appropriate permission from one parent or guardian. Assent from the child is not necessary.

SECTION 406: MINOR INCREASE OVER MINIMAL RISK

Section 406 allows IRBs to approve research that involves a *minor increase over minimal risk* and no prospect of direct benefit, but is likely to yield *knowledge about the subject's disorder or condition*. The knowledge gained must be generalizable and of vital importance to understanding or ameliorating the subject's disorder or condition. In addition, the research must present experiences that are "reasonably commensurate with the participants' actual or expected medical, . . . psychological, social, or educational situations." There must also be appropriate permission from parents or guardians and assent from the child participants.

The rationale for Section 406 is that research that does not offer a direct benefit to the child may be ethically acceptable provided that the risks are very small and the knowledge gained is very important for the participant's own illness or condition (18). For example, a better understanding of the pathophysiology of a condition may ultimately lead to better tests or treatments. Two undefined terms in Section 406—"minor increase over minimal risk" and "the subject's disorder or condition"—need to be clarified.

With regard to *minor increase over minimal risk*, SACHRP has proposed several criteria (13):

- Any experimentally induced pain, discomfort, or stress must not be experienced as severe.
- Any potential harms must be transient and reversible.
- Investigators must be appropriately qualified to perform the procedures.
- The setting for procedures must be appropriate.

SACHRP classified indwelling IV catheterization, nasogastric tube, bone marrow biopsy, lumbar puncture, and CT or MRI scan with sedation as a minor increase over minimal risk. Organ biopsy was considered a greater than minor increase over minimal risk.

Empirical research using hypothetical vignettes has indicated that the majority or parents and children would agree to the child's participation in some research that would not benefit the child directly and posed greater than minimal risk. In one study, parents and children were equally willing to have the child help others by participating in such research as a charitable activity (12). However, extrapolation to what parents and children would do in actual situations that excite strong emotional responses may be problematic (19).

The term "disorder" can be interpreted according to established clinical criteria for a physical or mental illness. The term "condition" is more difficult to interpret. It is intended to include healthy children who are at risk for developing illness or poor health (13). Several national panels have proposed that "disorder" should refer to specific physical, psychological, developmental, or social characteristics that negatively affect children's well-being or increase their risk of a future health problem (1,13,18). There should be an established body of scientific evidence or clinical knowledge that documents the increased risk. Interpreting "disorder or condition" narrowly to include only actual illness, disease, or injury would discourage research with "children who are currently healthy but at risk of serious illnesses that could potentially be prevented or mitigated through early interventions" (1). At the other extreme, a very broad interpretation of disorder or condition that includes "almost any social, developmental, or other characteristic" would allow most children to be exposed to greater risk (1). It is particularly controversial if children's social, economic, racial, ethnic, and environmental characteristics or circumstances are used to justify exposing them to greater than minimal risk. Investigators who define a research population on the basis of such nonmedical "conditions" need to show that the condition has a negative impact on children's health that is relevant to the research question (1).

The requirement that the research experience be "reasonably commensurate" with the subject's actual or expected situation is also ambiguous. Research procedures should be similar enough to the experience of parents and participants that they have a basis for making an informed decision about whether to participate in the study (1,13).

Section 406 is often invoked in research on the pathophysiology of diseases affecting children, particularly with regard to children who serve as normal controls in the study.

STUDY 17.2   Pathophysiology of diabetes.

To study how glucose regulation is affected by daily activities, researchers propose to place an intravenous catheter into children with Type I diabetes to measure levels of blood sugar and hormones that regulate blood sugar levels. As controls, the investigators will study healthy children of similar age, weight, and level of usual physical activity. The study will help scientists better understand how those levels are affected by daily activities such as exercise.

In Study 17.2, the researchers need to persuade the IRB that the requirements of Section 406 are being met. An indwelling intravenous catheter presents risks that are greater than minimal but are still relatively low. The discomfort is transient and not severe. Serious risks, such as infection and thrombosis, are rare and can be minimized by taking precautions and paying strict attention to technique. SACHRP classifies an indwelling catheter as a minor increase over minimal risk. Although the study offers no direct benefit to the study participants, it is very important for understanding the pathophysiology of diabetes. An indwelling catheter is commensurate with the experience of children with diabetes, who are subjected to multiple fingersticks and blood draws and may have had an intravenous catheter if they have been hospitalized. Thus, the study meets the criteria in Section 406 for participants who are children with diabetes.

The criteria in Section 406, however, are problematic for control participants who do not have diabetes. The requirement regarding the child's "disorder or condition" could be met by using as controls healthy children who have a sibling with Type I diabetes and therefore are at increased risk for diabetes themselves. The requirement that the research procedures be "commensurate" might also be fulfilled because such siblings are familiar with needlesticks. However, there may be scientific disadvantages to using as controls siblings who are at increased risk for diabetes because their glucose metabolism may differ from that of children with no predisposition to diabetes.

SECTION 407

Section 407 allows research that presents a greater than minor increase over minimal risk with no prospect of direct benefit to be approved, but only after a national review process (20). The secretary of HHS must approve the study after consultation with a panel of experts and a period of public comment. The research must also have the potential to provide knowledge to understand, prevent, or ameliorate a serious problem affecting children. There must also be appropriate permission from parents or guardians and assent from the child participants. Because of the need for federal review and public comment, protocols submitted for Section 407 approval may face considerable delays.

The federal regulations for research with children are complex. A recent study suggested that IRB members at institutions that provide comprehensive pediatric care have a limited knowledge of Subpart D, even though they rated themselves as well prepared to review such research (21). Researchers would be wise to explain explicitly how their protocol meets each of the requirements in the applicable section of Subpart D.

PARENTAL PERMISSION AND THE CHILD'S ASSENT

Free and informed consent is a fundamental requirement of research. However, young children lack the capacity to make informed decisions and thus cannot give informed consent to participate in research. Two ethical issues must then be addressed: Who should make decisions for young children, and how should the preferences of young children be taken into account?

AT WHAT AGE ARE CHILDREN CAPABLE OF MAKING INFORMED DECISIONS?

Empirical studies show that by age 14 or 15, adolescents generally are similar to adults in terms of comprehending information about research, although their judgment may not be as mature (1). Younger children (between the ages of 6 and 10) can understand the more practical aspects of research, but have difficulty appreciating the more abstract features of research. Children below age 10 may understand what they are expected to do, but not the risks of the study or their right to decline to participate.

WHY IS PARENTAL PERMISSION REQUIRED?

Because young children cannot make informed decisions, their parents or guardians make decisions on their behalf. Parents are permitted to enroll their children in research. However, the types of permissible research are limited, according to the level of risk and benefit, as we have discussed.

Only one parent needs to give permission if the research is minimal risk or offers the prospect of direct benefit to the child. For other types of research, where the balance of benefits and risks is less favorable, the permission of both parents is required unless there is only one parent or the other parent is incompetent, not known, or not reasonably available.

WHEN MAY PARENTAL PERMISSION BE WAIVED OR MODIFIED?

Parental permission is not required in situations where an exception to consent is permitted (see Chapter 6):

- The study falls outside the definition of human subjects research (for example, research with existing data or records) if the data are publicly available or recorded in such a way that the subjects cannot be identified.
- The study qualifies for a waiver or modification of informed consent. This is the case for much survey and interview research.
- Parental permission is not a reasonable requirement to protect the subjects (for example, if the children have been abused or neglected by their parents). There must be an alternative procedure for protecting the children in the study, such as having a relative or a counselor give permission and provide support.

Researchers sometimes use so-called "passive consent." Children are allowed to participate in research unless their parents opt out of the study (for example, by returning a refusal form). This term is a misnomer because there is no actual consent or permission given. Passive consent is sometimes used in school-based research because it can be difficult to obtain written permission from parents. Students may not give the permission forms to their parents, or the parents may not sign them even though they are willing for their children to participate. Passive consent is ethically acceptable only if the study qualifies for a waiver of parental permission, as a means to respect parental preferences. It should not be used to avoid parental opposition to controversial research.

WHY IS ASSENT BY THE CHILD REQUIRED?

In addition to parental permission, generally the child must also assent to participate in the research when this is developmentally appropriate. Requiring children's assent shows respect for them as persons, even though they are not capable of making autonomous decisions. Seeking their assent allows children to participate in decisions to the extent that they are capable of doing so and understanding what is at stake (22). It is intrusive to subject children to unwanted interventions that will not benefit them. It is also inhumane to override a child's vigorous and sustained dissent, such as active refusal to cooperate. Finally, seeking assent promotes the child's moral growth and development (23).

In some circumstances the child's assent is not required. Participants may not be capable of providing assent for various reasons, including age, maturity, or mental state. Alternatively, a waiver of consent may be permitted (for example, to review existing medical records). As we next discuss, the procedures for obtaining assent should be consistent with these requirements.

HOW SHOULD THE CHILD'S ASSENT BE SOUGHT?

The federal regulations do not specify how assent should be sought. Empirical studies show that IRBs vary greatly in their policies and judgments regarding assent (24–26). Usually assent is obtained after the parents have decided that their child may be involved. Most IRBs have an age threshold for assent, which is most commonly 7 years, but is sometimes up to 12 years. A minority of IRBs require an assent form that is separate from the parents' consent form and written in age-appropriate language. Only a few IRBs require different assent forms for different age groups. Many IRBs simply have an extra line for the child to sign on the parental permission form. There is similar variation in what information must be provided to children. Most IRBs require children to be told the purpose of the research, what will be done, and that they may choose not to participate. Only a minority of IRBs require children to be told of rare but serious risks.

Assent procedures need to be individualized to the developmental stage of the child and to the communication and decision-making patterns of the family (22,23). It makes little sense to provide children with information they cannot comprehend or expect them to make decisions in ways that are inconsistent with how the family usually decides an issue. Investigators should keep in mind that children usually have little experience in exercising their rights and are likely to be unfamiliar with research.

Researchers should specify in the protocol how they will seek assent and what behaviors they will accept as assent. At a minimum, children should be told what they are being asked to do and that they do not have to do it. The information disclosed regarding the purpose and risks may be less extensive than that provided during informed-consent discussions.

Investigators need to explain to the IRB how they will operationally define assent in the study. Will they require affirmative agreement to participate in the study, or just lack of objection? Affirmative agreement makes sense if the study procedures are complicated or lengthy, and if the child is capable of comprehending the procedures.

There is no point in seeking the child's assent if the researcher and IRB agree that parental permission suffices to enroll the child in a study. It is disrespectful to ask children to assent if their dissent will be overridden. However, even if children will not have a choice about participating in research, they should be told what will happen to them—for example, that they will get a shot or a needlestick.

Finally, documentation of assent also needs to be considered. Asking for a signature may be developmentally inappropriate for children younger than 9 or 10 years (1). Such a request may be confusing or even perceived as coercive because they do not appreciate that they may decline.

WHAT PERMISSION IS REQUIRED FOR RESEARCH IN SCHOOLS?

STUDY 17.3   School-based questionnaire study.

A researcher proposes to study how diet, weight, and exercise change during middle school. The researcher wishes to administer a questionnaire that deals with these issues and also assesses smoking, popularity, and perceptions of peer pressure. The 10-minute questionnaires will be filled out during science class. The scientists want to correlate the students' grades and disciplinary records with responses on the questionnaire. The principal and teachers support the study. It is sponsored by the National Institutes of Health.

To tell parents about the study, the researchers will put a notice in the school newsletter and give the students a flyer to take home to their parents. Parents who do not want their child to participate may mail back a refusal form, or call or e-mail the researchers.

Carrying out research in schools allows survey researchers to gather data from large numbers of children. However, such research may also raise special concerns regarding parental permission and control. Several federal laws may apply.

The 2002 No Child Left Behind Act requires some parental control over survey research on sensitive topics that is carried out in schools. The sensitive topics include political affiliations; mental and psychological problems; sex behaviors and attitudes; illegal, self-incriminating, or demeaning behaviors; critical appraisals of close family members; religious affiliations and beliefs; and income (27).

If the school receives any funding from the Department of Education, parents have the right to ask to inspect surveys that address these sensitive topics and must have an opportunity to exclude their child from the survey. Almost all public school districts receive some funding from the Department of Education. If the survey research is sponsored by the Department of Education, parents must give permission for minors to participate in surveys addressing these sensitive topics.

The Family Educational Rights and Privacy Act requires written parental permission for a school to release to researchers identifiable information from a student's record, including test scores, grades, or disciplinary status (27). The ethical rationale is that parents, who have responsibility for their children, should have control over whether their child provides such sensitive information. If the confidentiality of responses on these sensitive topics is breached, the children might suffer loss of privacy, embarrassment, or even legal liability.

STUDY 17.3 **(Continued).**

This study addresses a sensitive topic because smoking at this age is illegal. Researchers need to allow parents to request to review the questionnaire and to refuse their child's participation. To obtain access to students' grades and records, they need explicit parental permission.

The researchers decided that it would not be feasible to obtain active parental permission from a representative sample of students. They considered carrying out the study in private schools that receive no federal funding and thus are outside the scope of the No Child Left Behind Act and the Family Educational Rights and Privacy Act. However, the researchers decided that they wanted to study children from diverse socioeconomic backgrounds. Hence they decided to eliminate the analysis of student records.

PAYMENTS FOR PARTICIPATION IN RESEARCH

Although any payments to research participants may raise ethical concerns (see Chapter 9), concerns about undue influence are particularly serious in pediatric research. Payments to children may be problematic because they may not appreciate the value of money. Payments to parents may also raise concerns because it is the children who bear most of the risks of research participation. The following study illustrates concerns regarding payments in pediatric research (26).

STUDY 17.4 **Drugs in hypertension.**

In a multisite study, children with hypertension who responded to high dose of a medication were randomized to either placebo or a low, medium, or high dose of the same drug. The study required 19 clinic visits and daily procedures at home during the early phases of the trial. At the sites participating in the study, the maximum compensation allowed varied about eightfold, from $500 to $4000. On a per-hour basis, the rate varied from $7.50 to almost $60 per hour of participation in the study.

This large variation in payment from one site to another highlights the questions of what level of payment is appropriate, and what levels are too little or too much. Such substantial variation needs to be explained and justified.

ETHICAL CONCERNS ABOUT PAYMENT

Children, who lack the ability to make informed choices, might be induced by financial considerations to accept inappropriate risks. A recent empirical study found that children under age 9 did not appreciate the value and role of money. They asked for an excessive amount that bore no relation to what participation involved, and had no concept of what money could buy (28). In contrast, children over age 9 showed an appreciation of the role and value of money. The authors concluded that paying children under age 9 for their time and inconvenience was inappropriate.

Payments to parents beyond reimbursement of out-of-pocket expenses may raise concerns that the children are being regarded as sources of income. A consensus Institute of Medicine (IOM) panel recommended that parents not be paid "for the use of their child in research" (1). Moreover, parents should not be paid more to encourage participation in riskier research. Although it is morally acceptable to pay adults more for high-risk work, the IOM committee rejected large incentives in pediatric research because children cannot make informed decisions regarding risk.

As discussed in Chapter 9, it is helpful to distinguish different models of payment, or different rationales for payment. Reimbursement for out-of-pocket expenses, such as parking, bus fares, or childcare, raises no ethical concerns because the participants and parents receive no net financial gain. Small tokens of appreciation, such as t-shirts, stuffed animals, and movie coupons, are also unproblematic.

STUDY 17.4 **(Continued).**

In Study 17.4, the higher payment levels are greater than token gifts or reimbursement for actual expenses. Are these payments designed under a wage-payment model or a market model? Payments to compensate participants for time and inconvenience usually are set at minimum-wage levels to address concerns about undue influence. Thus the higher payments in Study 17.4 are consistent with a market model to attract participants, and raise concerns that such high levels are needed because the level of risk or inconvenience is unacceptable to families.

IRB POLICIES REGARDING PAYMENT

IRB policies and practices regarding payments to parents and children vary considerably (25,29). Many IRBs do not have written policies on these topics. Most allow reimbursement to parents for time and expenses related to their children's involvement in research. A few permit payment of "incentives" or "inducements" to parents who enroll their children in research.

With respect to payments to child subjects, policies range from prohibiting to encouraging such payments. A few IRBs discourage monetary payments to children and suggest instead giving toys, gift certificates, or books. In one study (29), the maximum cash amount approved by IRBs in pediatric studies varied from $10 to $1000 ($11.74 to $1174 in 2007 dollars), with a median level of $100.

Another study (30) found that in 36% of studies, the entire payment was meant to be an incentive to enroll in the study, whereas in 26% of studies, all payment was meant as reimbursement for expenses. When payment was made, 93% of investigators said that the amount of payment was not influenced by the risks in the study.

RECOMMENDATIONS REGARDING PAYMENT

No bright line separates acceptable payments from unacceptable payments. Researchers need to anticipate potential criticisms about payment and be prepared to explain how they chose the level and method of payment, and how they decided that the amount was neither too high nor too low.

STUDY 17.4 **(Continued).**

The researchers need to address several ethical issues regarding payment. Is it fair for some families to receive much greater payments for the same time and procedures? Why were families unwilling to participate at lower rates of payment? How did the researchers ensure that the higher payment levels were not an undue inducement?

The variation in payment among sites raises questions regarding fairness. In addition, researchers need to explain why the highest payment rates are not an undue influence.

TAKE HOME POINTS

1. Research with children is essential but raises important ethical concerns.
2. Special federal regulations, known as Subpart D, govern research with children. They classify research according to the level of risk and benefit to participants.
3. Parental permission and the assent of the child are generally required.
4. Payments for participation should not be so high as to be an undue inducement.

ANNOTATED BIBLIOGRAPHY

Field MJ, Behrman RE. *Ethical Conduct of Clinical Research Involving Children*. Washington, DC: National Academies Press; 2004.
> Comprehensive consensus report from the Institute of Medicine. Available at http://www.nap.edu/catalog.php?record_id=10958.

Fisher CB, Kornetsky SZ, Prentice ED. Determining risk in pediatric research with no prospect of direct benefit: time for a national consensus on the interpretation of federal regulations. *Am J Bioethics* 2007;7:5–10.
> Proposal from SACHRP regarding research with children that does not offer the prospect of direct benefit to participants.

Kon AA. Assent in pediatric research. *Pediatrics* 2006;117:1806–1810.
> Analysis of the concept of assent by children, taking into account that for many decisions children defer to parents and other adults.

REFERENCES

1. Field MJ, Behrman RE. *Ethical Conduct of Clinical Research Involving Children*. Washington, DC: National Academies Press; 2004.
2. Steinbrook R. Testing medications in children. *N Engl J Med* 2002;347:1462–1470.
3. Hoffmann DE, Rothenberg KH. Whose duty is it anyway? The Kennedy Krieger opinion and its implications for public health research. *J Health Care Law Policy* 2002;6:109–147.
4. Buchanan DR, Miller FG. Justice and fairness in the Kennedy Krieger Institute lead paint study: the ethics of public health research on less expensive, less effective interventions. *Am J Public Health* 2006;96:781–787.
5. Kopelman LM. Pediatric research regulations under legal scrutiny: Grimes narrows their interpretation. *J Law Med Ethics* 2002;30:38–49.
6. Nelson RM. Appropriate risk exposure in environmental health research. The Kennedy-Krieger lead abatement study. *Neurotoxicol Teratol* 2002;24:445–449.
7. National Commission for the Protection of Human Subjects of Biomedical and Behavioral Research. *Report and Recommendations: Research Involving Children*. Washington, DC: U.S. Government Printing Office; 1977.
8. Mnookin RH, Weisberg DK. *Child, Family, and State*. 4th ed. Gaithersburg: Aspen Law & Business; 2000.
9. Mnookin RH. The enigma of children's interests. In: Mnookin RH, ed. *In the Interest of Children*. New York: W.H. Freeman and Company; 1985:16–24.
10. Mnookin RH. Two puzzles. *Arizona State Law J* 1984;4:667–684.
11. Wendler D, Belsky L, Thompson KM, et al. Quantifying the federal minimal risk standard: implications for pediatric research without a prospect of direct benefit. *JAMA* 2005;294:826–832.
12. Wendler D, Jenkins T. Children's and their parents' views on facing research risks for the benefit of others. *Arch Pediatr Adolesc Med* 2008;162:9–14.
13. Fisher CB, Kornetsky SZ, Prentice ED. Determining risk in pediatric research with no prospect of direct benefit: time for a national consensus on the interpretation of federal regulations. *Am J Bioethics* 2007;7:5–10.
14. National Bioethics Advisory Commission. *Ethical and Policy Issues in Research Involving Human Participants*. Rockville, MD: National Bioethics Advisory Commission; 2001.
15. Wendler D, Varma S. Minimal risk in pediatric research. *J Pediatr* 2006;149:855–861.
16. Nelson RM. Minimal risk, yet again. *J Pediatr* 2007;150:570–572.
17. Shah S, Whittle A, Wilfond B, et al. How do institutional review boards apply the federal risk and benefit standards for pediatric research? *JAMA* 2004;291:476–482.
18. Lo B, O'Connell ME, eds. *Ethical Considerations for Research on Housing-Related Health Hazards Involving Children*. Washington, DC: National Academies Press; 2005.
19. Reynolds WW, Nelson RM. Empirical data and the acceptability of research risk: a commentary on the charitable participation standard. *Arch Pediatr Adolesc Med* 2008;162:88–90.
20. Kopelman LM. Ethical concerns about federal approval of risky pediatric research studies. *Pediatrics* 2004;113:1783–1789.
21. Stroustrup A, Kornetsky S, Joffe S. Knowledge of regulations governing pediatric research. *IRB* 2008;30:1–7.
22. Kon AA. Assent in pediatric research. *Pediatrics* 2006;117:1806–1810.
23. Miller VA, Nelson RM. A developmental approach to child assent for nontherapeutic research. *J Pediatr* 2006;149:S25–S30.
24. Whittle A, Shah S, Wilfond B, et al. Institutional review board practices regarding assent in pediatric research. *Pediatrics* 2004;113:1747–1752.
25. Wolf LE, Zandecki J, Lo B. Institutional review board guidance on pediatric research: missed opportunities. *J Pediatr* 2005;147:84–89.

26. Kimberly MB, Hoehn KS, Feudtner C, et al. Variation in standards of research compensation and child assent practices: a comparison of 69 institutional review board-approved informed permission and assent forms for 3 multicenter pediatric clinical trials. *Pediatrics* 2006;117:1706–1711.

27. Hicks L. Research in public schools. In: Bankert EA, Amdur RJ, eds. *Institutional Review Board Management and Function*. 2nd ed. Sudbury, MA: Jones and Bartlett Publishers; 2006:341–345.

28. Bagley SJ, Reynolds WW, Nelson RM. Is a "wage-payment" model for research participation appropriate for children? *Pediatrics* 2007;119:46–51.

29. Weise KL, Smith ML, Maschke KJ, et al. National practices regarding payment to research subjects for participating in pediatric research. *Pediatrics* 2002;110:577–582.

30. Iltis AS, DeVader S, Matsuo H. Payments to children and adolescents enrolled in research: a pilot study. *Pediatrics* 2006;118:1546–1552.

CHAPTER 18

Research With Adolescents

Adolescents are at high risk for many serious health problems, including alcohol and drug use, depression, sexually transmitted diseases, and unintended pregnancy (1). Research on these issues is important to establish more effective prevention programs and therapies. However, research with adolescents is challenging for several reasons. First, despite their developing maturity, the law generally requires people to be at least 18 years old before they may decide for themselves to participate in research. Below that age, parental permission is generally necessary. However, adolescents may not be willing to participate in research on sensitive topics if their parents will know about their participation. Second, adolescents vary in their maturity, independence, and ability to make informed decisions. Although they may wish to make their own decisions, adolescents usually benefit from parental guidance. Third, the federal regulations for the protection of human subjects do not take into account how adolescents and younger children differ in their ability to make decisions. Hence IRBs and researchers often are unsure how to apply Subpart D to adolescents. Finally, many of the public health risks that adolescents face are politically charged, and research on these problems is often socially controversial.

ADOLESCENT DEVELOPMENT

The ability to make informed, voluntary decisions increases with age and varies from child to child (2). Research suggests that children aged 14 or over generally are similar to adults in their understanding of research and their ability to make decisions about participation in research. Below this age, children usually have difficulty weighing alternatives, seeing the value of others' perspectives, and thinking abstractly. However, many younger children are able to understand some aspects of research participation, particularly the practical issues of what might happen to them and what they are expected to do. As children mature, they seek greater decision-making power relative to parents. Thus discussions with adolescents regarding research participation should be individualized and designed to reinforce the crucial concepts that participation is voluntary and refusal will not be penalized.

Adolescents and parents tend to disagree on how decisions about research participation should be made. Adolescents are much less likely than parents to believe that parental permission should be required for them to participate in surveys on risk behaviors (3). Furthermore, adolescents with asthma are more willing to participate in research that presents some risk than their parents are willing to allow (4). Both adolescents and parents are willing to be influenced by a physician's opinion when considering participation in research. Thus, the researcher can play an important role in discussions about research participation by helping both adolescents and parents understand the risks and benefits of the study, and encouraging adolescents' participation in decisions to the extent they are capable of doing so.

WHEN MAY ADOLESCENTS AGREE TO RESEARCH PARTICIPATION?

The federal guidelines for research on children generally require both parental permission and the assent of the child, as Chapter 17 discusses in detail. When dealing with adolescents who are capable of making informed decisions, researchers should seek their informed consent rather than just assent. That is, they should be given more information about the research than younger children—the same amount as adults receive. Furthermore, the affirmative agreement of the adolescent should be required, not just the absence of dissent.

Parental permission is not required under three circumstances, as described below.

WHEN IS CONSENT NOT REQUIRED?

Consent is not required if a study is not considered research under the Common Rule or does not involve human subjects, or if the IRB has approved a waiver of consent (see Chapter 6). These provisions hold for all research, not just for research with adolescents. The Society for Adolescent Medicine recommends that parental permission not be required for minimal risk research, such as survey research on risk behaviors (1). The justification is that research on sensitive topics is not practicable if parental permission is required, because many adolescents might not participate or give candid information. Furthermore, bias would occur because high-risk adolescents would be more likely to be denied parental permission or to withhold information. Thus the prevalence of high-risk behaviors would be underestimated.

Some parents fear that surveys about sensitive topics such as sexual behaviors and alcohol and substance use may promote or induce unhealthy behaviors, perhaps by suggesting them or appearing to sanction them. However, there is little evidence that asking about unhealthy behaviors induces adolescents to engage in them (5). Hence it is appropriate to consider anonymous surveys regarding sensitive subjects as minimal risk.

WAIVER OF PARENTAL PERMISSION

Subpart D recognizes that in some circumstances parental permission "would not be a reasonable requirement to protect subjects." For example, victims of abuse or neglect would be at risk if their parents had to give permission for them to participate in research on the prevalence and consequences of abuse.

STATE LAWS ALLOWING ADOLESCENT CONSENT

Subpart D defers to state laws regarding the "legal age to consent to treatments or procedures involved in the research" under state law. Persons over 18 years old are considered adults. Laws vary from state to state regarding the circumstances under which younger children are permitted to make health decisions for themselves (1). Depending on the specific situation, different laws may apply, including laws on age of majority, emancipation, mature minors, consent for medical care, and consent for care for specific sensitive conditions (6). For example, most states permit adolescents less than 18 years of age to consent to treatment for mental health conditions, substance and alcohol abuse, sexually transmitted infections, pregnancy care, and contraception. Furthermore, many states allow children who are functioning as adults and meeting their basic needs without parental support to consent to treatment. Many IRBs therefore allow adolescents to consent for themselves to participate in research under these conditions. However, few states have explicit laws regarding a minor's agreement to participate in research without parental permission (6).

Researchers need to justify to the IRB and, if necessary, to the public why they propose to enroll adolescents without parental permission. Researchers also should explain why parental permission is not practicable, why it might be harmful to participants, or how it might lead to serious bias in the study.

CONFIDENTIALITY

Adolescents commonly wish to keep certain information confidential from their parents. Assurances of confidentiality increase the willingness of adolescents to disclose sensitive information to physicians and to seek health care (7). It is likely that assurances of confidentiality will encourage adolescents to participate in research and provide information candidly. Thus, researchers need to pay particular attention to maintaining confidentiality and explaining to participants how the information they provide will be kept confidential. Adolescents are particularly concerned about whether their parents will know about their participation. However, researchers also need to explain that confidentiality is not absolute and will be overridden in certain situations, for example to report child abuse, sexual assault, domestic violence, and sexually transmitted diseases (8). Generally adolescents support these exceptions to confidentiality.

ADDITIONAL PROTECTIONS
FOR ADOLESCENT PARTICIPANTS

In studies where adolescents may consent for themselves, without parental consent, the investigators should consider what additional protections might be appropriate. Adolescents may not be completely autonomous and mature. Even though the permission of parents is not required, their involvement may be beneficial to the adolescents. Hence researchers should generally try to encourage adolescents to involve their parents whenever that is feasible and unlikely to harm the adolescent (5). Often an adolescent's fears about parental opposition or rejection are unfounded. If parental involvement would not be in an adolescent's best interests, the investigators should try to have another adult, such as a relative, teacher, religious leader, or social worker, serve as an advocate and counselor.

Researchers should also provide participants the opportunity to seek confidential advice and counseling if the research raises any concerns or questions. Furthermore, researchers can refer participants to social or medical services in the community.

Investigators should meet with community representatives and organizations that provide services to adolescents to help determine whether the study and the enrollment and consent procedures are appropriate, and whether additional measures to protect adolescent participants might be appropriate.

INTERNET RESEARCH WITH ADOLESCENTS

The majority of adolescents participate in social networking sites on the Internet. Researchers use the Internet to conduct research in several ways. They may recruit subjects for research studies through Internet sites, they may carry out observational research on the information posted on those sites, and they may use a social networking intervention as part of a clinical or prevention trial. Such use of social networking sites raises several ethical issues (9). The information on the sites is public, and the participants have implicitly chosen not to restrict access to their information. Thus there is no invasion of privacy when a research records information from the website. However, there are confidentiality concerns; as with any research, when researchers present or publish data they must ensure that the participants cannot be identified, particularly if they are studying risky, embarrassing, or illegal activities. Another ethical concern is informed consent. If researchers are recruiting participants for a study on a social networking site, they need to follow the same rules for consent and parental permission as when they are recruiting participants in face-to-face or telephone encounters. Researchers need to keep in mind that on the Internet people may assume a different persona. If researchers are obtaining research data from social network or Internet postings, they may ask whether they should seek the concurrence of the people on the site. It is misleading to think that formal consent needs to be obtained from people using the site, since no one has the authority to speak on behalf of all users. Some might argue that users of social networks already know that there are risks—for example, bullies, sexual predators, or potential employers may be accessing their data—and they have implicitly accepted those risks (9). Nonetheless, it is desirable for researchers to be respectful of the participants they are studying. Researchers may not want to announce that they are doing a study, lest people change their behaviors and undermine the validity of the study. It is not clear whether such concerns are warranted. There are other steps researchers could take to show respect, such as announcing afterward that the study was done and posting the results on the site.

TAKE HOME POINTS

1. Confidentiality and independence from parents are important issues for adolescents.
2. Researchers should maximize informed decision-making by adolescents, to the extent that they are capable of doing so. In certain situations, parental permission for adolescents to participate in research is not required and may even pose risks.

REFERENCES

1. Santelli JS, Smith Rogers A, Rosenfeld WD, et al. Guidelines for adolescent health research. A position paper of the Society for Adolescent Medicine. *J Adolesc Health* 2003;33:396–409.
2. Field MJ, Behrman RE. *Ethical Conduct of Clinical Research Involving Children*. Washington, DC: National Academies Press; 2004.
3. Pasternak RH, Geller G, Parrish C, et al. Adolescent and parent perceptions on youth participation in risk behavior research. *Arch Pediatr Adolesc Med* 2006;160:1159–1166.
4. Brody JL, Scherer DG, Annett RD, et al. Family and physician influence on asthma research participation decisions for adolescents: the effects of adolescent gender and research risk. *Pediatrics* 2006;118:e356–e362.
5. Society for Adolescent Medicine. Guidelines for adolescent health research. *J Adolesc Health* 2003;33:410–415.
6. Campbell AT. State regulation of research with children and adolescents. In: Field MJ, Behrman RE, eds. *Ethical Conduct of Clinical Research Involving Children*. Washington, DC: National Academies Press; 2004:320–387.
7. English A, Ford CA. More evidence supports the need to protect confidentiality in adolescent health care. *J Adolesc Health* 2007;40:199–200.
8. Society for Adolescent Medicine. Confidential health care for adolescent: position paper of the Society for Adolescent Medicine. *J Adolesc Health* 2003;21:408–415.
9. Moreno MA, Fost NC, Christakis DA. Research ethics in the MySpace era. *Pediatrics* 2008;121:157–161.

CHAPTER 19

Emergency and Intensive Care Research

Clinical trials are required to determine how best to care for patients who require emergency and critical care. For conditions such as cardiac arrest, respiratory failure, traumatic brain injury, hemorrhagic shock, and status epilepticus, current treatment is often not successful, and unless critical care and emergency research is carried out, patients with such life-threatening conditions will receive only unproven or unsatisfactory treatments (1). Therefore, such patients might potentially benefit from research. However, such trials raise ethical dilemmas because the participants usually cannot give informed consent (2). Moreover, because there is a narrow therapeutic window, surrogates commonly cannot be contacted to provide permission to enroll the patient in research. Furthermore, it is not feasible to identify in advance persons who will develop these conditions and obtain their prospective consent to join a future research study. However, carrying out research on people without their knowledge and consent requires special justification because it violates the ethical principle of respect for persons. Such persons are particularly vulnerable: not only are they unable to consent to participate in research, they cannot actively refuse enrollment. Being enrolled in research without consent may be particularly objectionable to groups who have suffered abuses in research and discrimination in clinical care, such as African-Americans.

EMERGENCY RESEARCH

To allow such important emergency research to be carried out, the Food and Drug Administration (FDA) allows an exception to informed consent, provided that additional safeguards are in place (available at http://www.access.gpo.gov/nara/cfr/waisidx_04/21cfr50_04.html). This waiver applies only to research with a new drug or medical device for which an FDA Investigational New Drug (IND) application or Investigational Device Exemption (IDE) is required.

WHEN DOES THE EMERGENCY EXCEPTION TO CONSENT APPLY?

Several criteria must be met for the exception for emergency research to apply (3). First, the participants must be in a life-threatening situation for which available treatments are unproven or unsatisfactory. Second, obtaining informed consent is not feasible because the participants are not able to give informed consent, the intervention under investigation must be administered before permission can be obtained from surrogates, and the participants cannot be identified prospectively. Third, participation in the research offers the prospect of direct benefit to participants, and the risks associated with the investigation are reasonable. Fourth, it would not be feasible to carry out the research without the waiver of consent. Fifth, there is a therapeutic window within which the intervention must be initiated to be effective.

MEASURES TO RESPECT PATIENT AUTONOMY

Even when obtaining informed consent is not feasible, researchers must take steps to respect patients (2). During the therapeutic window, they must attempt to contact a surrogate to obtain permission for the participant to enter the clinical trial. This surrogate must be a person who is legally authorized to make medical decisions on behalf of the participant.

Furthermore, at the earliest opportunity, researchers must inform the participant (if his condition improves) or his surrogates that he has been entered into the study. They must also provide information about the study and notify the participant or surrogates that they may discontinue participation.

COMMUNITY CONSULTATION

One requirement for an exception from informed consent is that the researchers must consult with representatives of the communities in which the clinical investigation will be conducted and from which the subjects will be drawn (3).

Empirical Studies

Empirical reports indicate that community consultation is interpreted in different ways in different studies and requires extensive time and effort. Critics have charged that this requirement stifles emergency and intensive care unit (ICU) research (4,5).

One study compared different methods for carrying out community consultation, including community meetings, telephone surveys, and interviews with patients in the waiting room, in a low-risk study involving infusion of L-arginine in persons with traumatic brain injury (6). More than 20% of the respondents said they would not be willing to participate in that study. Fewer than 60% approved of the waiver of consent. Willingness to participate varied by demographic characteristics, by the method of seeking community consultation, and by the framing of questions. The respondents stated whether they agreed or disagreed with five aspects of the study; however, they stated their views before they had the opportunity to ask questions and hear the investigators' responses. Hence, their preferences probably were not informed. However, the crucial ethical issue is not their objections to the study when they first heard of it, but rather their objections after hearing the investigators respond to concerns about the study. Other studies have reported that researchers can overcome the vast majority of objections to a study by listening to concerns and providing more information about the study and the rationale for starting interventions without consent (4).

Telephone surveys have the advantage of being cost-effective and enabling researchers to reach people who are representative of the community from which participants will be drawn. However, telephone surveys are problematic because they do not allow discussion between members of the public and researchers (2). According to the Food and Drug Administration (FDA), community consultations "should provide opportunities for representatives of the communities involved in the research to discuss the proposed clinical investigation . . . with the IRB [institutional review board] and investigators." Thus community consultation should be a dialogue, not just an elicitation of opinions about the study.

Best Practices for Community Consultation

Best practices for community consultation have been suggested (3,7). Community meetings, appearances on radio talk shows, and telephone hot lines, which are commonly employed, are reasonable de facto standards for community consultation in emergency research. The type and extent of community consultation should be "titrated" to the risk of the study (3,4,8). Studies raise heightened ethical concerns if the study intervention is riskier than standard care, the intervention is invasive, vulnerable persons are disproportionately enrolled, or some persons or groups can be predicted to object to being included in study (for instance, because of religious objections to transfusion). For these kinds of studies, multiple meetings should be convened and presentations given to community groups, public forums, and city governments. Feedback should be sought via the Internet or telephone. Investigators should also meet with groups that would likely object to being in the study. It is advisable to use multiple methods of communication and to involve a public relations department and event planner to handle the logistics of organizing meetings (9). Investigators should be prepared to respond to inaccurate news reports or rumors about the study. The IRB might appoint additional community members as consultants to review the study, and open its meetings on such studies to the public. In addition, the IRB might make its reasoning available to the public, for example, by posting summaries of the deliberation on the Internet.

Researchers need to keep in mind that the goal of community consultation is to assess the acceptability of the study so that improvements can be made to the protocol. The investigators should make it clear that the community does not have veto power, cannot provide community consent, and does not substitute for individual consent when that is feasible.

ADDITIONAL PROTECTIONS FOR EMERGENCY RESEARCH

Under federal regulations, a study must incorporate several additional protections (2). Before a study begins, the investigators must publicly disclose to communities where the study will be conducted, the plans for the investigation, and its risks and expected benefits. After the study is completed, there must be public disclosure of the results. In addition, the trial must have an independent data monitoring committee.

ICU RESEARCH

In clinical practice, ICU physicians vary substantially in how they manage the details of clinical care. Unless well-designed clinical trials are carried out, it will not be known which management strategies are more effective and safer. However, it is impossible to conduct such studies if informed consent is required from participants or their surrogates. These management decisions need to be made immediately on admission to the ICU, when patients cannot give informed consent and surrogates are often not available.

THE ARDS NET CLINICAL TRIALS

Patients with acute respiratory distress syndrome (ARDS) have a mortality rate of between 30% and 50% despite treatment in the ICU. The ARDS Network (ARDS Net) carried out a series of multicenter randomized controlled trials (RCTs) on the effectiveness and safety of intensive care interventions for ARDS (10–12).

| STUDY 19.1 | Clinical trials on ARDS. |

The first ARDS Net trial examined the use of a lower tidal volume compared to the larger tidal volume that has traditionally been used in mechanical ventilation. It found that the low-volume group had significantly lower mortality than the high-volume group (31% vs. 40%). A second ARDS Net RCT compared different approaches to the use of intravenous fluids and catheters. The trial compared conservative vs. liberal fluid management strategies, and pulmonary artery catheter vs. central venous catheter.

Two critical care physicians at the National Institutes of Health (NIH) Clinical Center sharply criticized these studies and triggered investigations of ARDS Net by the NIH and the Office for Human Research Protections (OHRP). These critics charged that the control group in the study of tidal volumes did not receive "the current best practice standards of the time." Furthermore, the critics alleged that both trials used as a comparison extremes of practice rather than how cases are most commonly managed, which may be safer. They concluded that the trials were both unethical and scientifically flawed.

STUDY 19.1   (Continued).

In response, in July 2002 the National Heart, Lung, and Blood Institute (NHLBI) put the fluid-and-catheters trial on hold. Five external consultants who were asked to review the studies concluded that the study was "well designed, safe and likely to result in important results for ARDS patients."

In October 2002, OHRP raised concerns about the control group in the tidal volume study and asked for additional data comparing participants in the study with patients with ARDS who were not enrolled or who were treated before the study was carried out. The OHRP made its report in July 2003. OHRP consultants agreed that risks in the trial were minimized and appropriate. OHRP requested no changes in the protocol. However, OHRP raised concerns that many IRBs failed to obtain enough information to make these determinations and approved consent forms that did not provide sufficient information about the study, its purpose, and its design. OHRP asked IRBs at institutions participating in the study to re-review and approve the protocols and a revised consent process.

In June 2006, the results of the trial of fluids and catheters were published. The conservative strategy of fluid management shortened the duration of mechanical ventilation and intensive care without increasing failure of organs other than the lung. There was no difference in mortality between the two strategies. Pulmonary artery catheter (PAC)-guided management did not improve survival or organ function, but was associated with more complications than central venous catheter (CVC)-guided therapy. These results support a conservative strategy of fluid management in patients and suggest that the PAC should not be routinely used in patients with acute lung injury.

These ARDS Net studies dramatized ethical issues regarding clinical trials in ICU settings, consent for such trials, and the oversight of such trials. Defenders of the trials objected that these important studies, which had been approved by IRBs and the NIH peer review process, were delayed by extensive investigations. Moreover, they objected that requirements for additional informed consent procedures were misguided because in routine clinical care, physicians manage ventilator settings, fluids, and catheter placement without discussing management options with patients. The IRBs were unclear about how they were supposed to pay more attention to scientific and design concerns. IRBs need to consider scientific and design concerns to carry out their mandate to assess the risks of studies. However, they lack the expertise to conduct in-depth scientific reviews.

IS INFORMED CONSENT NECESSARY IN ICU CLINICAL TRIALS?

Some RCTs of intensive and emergency care may not quality for the emergency exception to informed consent discussed in the previous section. To qualify for this exception, the trial must be carried out under an IND or IDE from the FDA. However, the ARDS Net trials did not evaluate new technologies; rather, they compared treatments that could be provided outside the trial as part of standard care, without obtaining specific informed consent or discussing alternative management strategies.

How can such clinical trials be conducted without informed consent before enrollment? In the early 1980s, trials of brain resuscitation after CPR were carried out under a theory of "deferred consent." Subjects were asked after they regained decision-making capacity to give retrospective permission to participate in the trial. This idea that consent after the fact could justify participation in the trial was sharply criticized. Furthermore, because many patients did not recover, in practice there often was no consent (13).

Some ethics experts proposed other reasons why participants may be enrolled into trials like the ARDS Net trials without consent. They noted that such trials add little additional risk to ordinary clinical care for ARDS. The interventions tested are widely used in routine care. The collection of data poses no incremental risk or burden because it is merely a more systematic use of the kinds of data and samples that are commonly collected in the course of clinical care. The key difference from ordinary care is that the choice of management options is selected by randomization rather than by the treating physician; however, there is no rigorous evidence to help the physician determine which option offers the most benefit or least risk. Indeed, the risks of participating in an RCT might be less than the risks of care outside the trial, because in a trial greater attention is paid to procedures and closer monitoring of clinical data. Of course, when a surrogate becomes available or the patient regains decision-making capacity, they should be informed of their enrollment in the trial and asked to consent to continue in the trial.

The following considerations justify an exception to informed consent (14–17):

First, all the treatments offered in a trial are available outside the trial without the specific consent of the patient or surrogate.

Second, there should be clinical equipoise between the arms of the trial. Experts in the field should be uncertain and disagree about which arm is superior. No reasonable patient or surrogate or primary care physician should have a preference for one treatment over the other. In the ARDS Net trials, the patient and family would have had the same subjective experience regardless of which ventilator setting, fluid strategy, or choice of catheter was adopted.

Third, there should be no known treatment with a more favorable risk/benefit profile available outside of the trial. Thus, the RCT compares what experts in the field believe are the best options for management.

Fourth, the treating ICU physician may remove the patient from the trial and alter the management strategy if it is in the best interests of the patient to do. For example, the treating physician could alter a patient's fluid management if the patient developed hypotension or pulmonary congestion.

Fifth, patients and their surrogates should be informed, if and when it is feasible, that they were entered into the clinical trial, what the rationale of the trial is, that interventions in the trial are commonly ordered by ICU physicians without consulting patients or surrogates, that doctors do not know which arm of the trial is safer or more effective, and that in their case the choice of treatment was determined by randomization.

Sixth, patients and surrogates should have the option of withdrawing from the trial if they choose. In fact, if they understand the nature of the trial, there should be little reason to do so, because the treating physician already has the option to alter management if it is in the participant's best interests. Nonetheless, the principle of respecting autonomy means that people should have the authority to refuse for idiosyncratic reasons.

There is one regulatory issue that needs to be addressed. There is a compelling argument that these six criteria provide a strong justification for allowing RCTs like ARDS Net to enroll patients without consent. However, it is not clear that the Common Rule permits this. Several writers use the term "minimal risk" to refer to such studies, in the sense that the incremental risk of participating in the study compared to ordinary clinical care is extremely small. However, in the Common Rule, "minimal risk" is a requirement for a waiver of informed consent to be granted, and the regulatory definition of minimal risk (see Chapter 5) requires a comparison with the daily experience of healthy persons, not patients with serious medical illness. It would be more intellectually sound for the Department of Health and Human Services to issue additional regulations for ICU research that would allow RCTs like the ARDS Net trials without imposing burdensome layers of additional regulation. The determination that the arms of the trial are in clinical equipoise should be made during the scientific peer review process; local IRBs lack the expertise and experience to make such judgments. A model of centralized IRB review may be appropriate in such trials (see Chapter 4).

TAKE HOME POINTS

1. Clinical trials in emergency and intensive care present dilemmas because patients in these situations commonly lack decision-making capacity, and treatment often must begin before surrogates can be contacted.

2. Such clinical trials may be carried out with a waiver of informed consent under certain conditions, provided that investigators try to obtain consent to continue in the study from surrogates and from patients upon recovery.

ANNOTATED BIBLIOGRAPHY

Halperin H, Paradis N, Mosesso V Jr, et al. Recommendations for implementation of community consultation and public disclosure under the Food and Drug Administration's "Exception from informed consent requirements for emergency research": a special report from the American Heart Association Emergency Cardiovascular Care Committee and Council on Cardiopulmonary, Perioperative and Critical Care: endorsed by the American College of Emergency Physicians and the Society for Academic Emergency Medicine. *Circulation* 2007;116:1855–1863.
    Comprehensive report from a consensus panel.
Steinbrook R. How best to ventilate? Trial design and patient safety in studies of the acute respiratory distress syndrome. *N Engl J Med* 2003;348:1393–1401.
Steinbrook R. Trial design and patient safety—the debate continues. *N Engl J Med* 2003;349:629–630.
    Analysis of controversies surrounding ethical issues in the ARDS Net clinical trials.

REFERENCES

1. Baren JM, Biros MH. The research on community consultation: an annotated bibliography. *Acad Emerg Med* 2007;14:346–352.
2. Lo B. Strengthening community consultation in critical care and emergency research. *Crit Care Med* 2006; 34:2236–2238.
3. Halperin H, Paradis N, Mosesso V Jr, et al. Recommendations for implementation of community consultation and public disclosure under the Food and Drug Administration's "Exception from informed consent requirements for emergency research": a special report from the American Heart Association Emergency Cardiovascular Care Committee and Council on Cardiopulmonary, Perioperative and Critical Care: endorsed by the American College of Emergency Physicians and the Society for Academic Emergency Medicine. *Circulation* 2007;116:1855–1863.
4. Mosesso VN Jr, Cone DC. Using the exception from informed consent regulations in research. *Acad Emerg Med* 2005;12:1031–1039.
5. Sanders AB, Hiller K, Duldner J. Researchers' understanding of the federal guidelines for waiver of and exception from informed consent. *Acad Emerg Med* 2005;12:1045–1049.
6. Contant C, McCullough LB, Mangus L, et al. Community consultation in emergency research. *Crit Care Med* 2006;34:2049–2052.
7. Richardson LD, Quest TE, Birnbaum S. Communicating with communities about emergency research. *Acad Emerg Med* 2005;12:1064–1070.
8. Ernst AA, Fish S. Exception from informed consent: viewpoint of institutional review boards—balancing risks to subjects, community consultation, and future directions. *Acad Emerg Med* 2005;12:1050–1055.
9. Salzman JG, Frascone RJ, Godding BK, et al. Implementing emergency research requiring exception from informed consent, community consultation, and public disclosure. *Ann Emerg Med* 2007;50:448–455, 455 e1–4.
10. Steinbrook R. How best to ventilate? Trial design and patient safety in studies of the acute respiratory distress syndrome. *N Engl J Med* 2003;348:1393–1401.
11. Steinbrook R. Trial design and patient safety—the debate continues. *N Engl J Med* 2003;349:629–630.
12. Drazen JM. Controlling research trials. *N Engl J Med* 2003;348:1377–1380.
13. Bircher NG. Resuscitation research and consent: ethical and practical issues. *Crit Care Med* 2003;31:S379–S384.
14. Truog RD, Robinson W, Randolph A, et al. Is informed consent always necessary for randomized, controlled trials? *N Engl J Med* 1999;340:804–807.
15. Morris MC, Nelson RM. Randomized, controlled trials as minimal risk: an ethical analysis. *Crit Care Med* 2007;35:940–944.
16. Luce JM, Cook DJ, Martin TR, et al. The ethical conduct of clinical research involving critically ill patients in the United States and Canada: principles and recommendations. *Am J Respir Crit Care Med* 2004;170:1375–1384.
17. Silverman HJ, Luce JM, Lanken PN, et al. Recommendations for informed consent forms for critical care clinical trials. *Crit Care Med* 2005;33:867–882.

CHAPTER 20

Research With Ethnic and Minority Populations

HISTORICAL BACKGROUND

Egregious misconduct in clinical research has often involved ethnic and minority populations, as exemplified by the Nazi "experiments" and the Tuskegee study (see Chapter 1). Such scandals may make members of ethnic and minority groups reluctant to participate in research. As a legacy of Tuskegee, many African-Americans mistrust medical research, fear that by signing consent forms they are waiving their rights, and believe that researchers would deceive them and expose them to unnecessary risks (1–4). Furthermore, African-Americans tend to place research in the context of broader concerns about racism and remain skeptical that research could benefit them (4,5). Ethnic and minority communities may also fear that research will support political and social policies that will harm them. For example, many genetics researchers in the late 19th and early 20th centuries supported eugenicist public policies, including immigration restrictions and forced sterilization (6).

This chapter focuses on research in the United States. Chapter 22 discusses international research in resource-poor countries, which often have predominantly non-Caucasian populations.

REASONS FOR RESEARCH ON ETHNIC AND MINORITY POPULATIONS

Today the burden of many diseases falls disproportionately on certain ethnic groups. In the United States, new cases of HIV, end-stage renal disease, lead poisoning, and several other conditions are significantly more common among African-Americans than among other ethnic groups (7). In the United States, racial and ethnic minorities tend to have poorer health care outcomes, lower quality of care, and worse access to care than others (7). These disparities in health outcomes persist even when minorities have similar access to health care. Thus, research is essential to clarify the reasons for these disparities.

Researchers sometimes target ethnic and minority groups to study or ameliorate a serious condition that disproportionately afflicts them. Studies targeting ethnic and minority groups are justified when they are designed to improve the circumstances that lead to serious risks, illness, or health disparities in their lives (8). However, even when the disproportionate inclusion of persons from ethnic and minority groups is justified, it might lead to concerns about inequitable selection of subjects (5). For example, in the context of HIV research, minority persons might be concerned that they will be used as research subjects to test vaccines or drugs that they will not have access to afterward (9).

Ethnic and racial minorities generally are underrepresented in research (1,10). As a result, evidence regarding the safety and efficacy of therapies in these populations is weaker than in Caucasians, and consequently clinical recommendations for such populations are also based on less robust evidence. For example, in the United States, HIV infection in Caucasians most commonly results from men having sex with other men, whereas HIV infection in persons of color primarily results from injection drug use or heterosexual intercourse with injection drug users. Research that enrolls primarily Caucasian participants may not be applicable to the minority communities who are most affected by HIV.

What are the reasons for such underrepresentation? One study found that the consent rate among persons who were invited to participate in research was the same in minorities and non-minorities. The authors concluded that lower participation rates may be a result of lack of access to clinical trials rather than minority attitudes toward research (11). However, it is possible that minority persons are reluctant to even receive information about a research project or to meet with researchers—steps that are a prerequisite for being invited to participate.

STUDY 20.1   Cancer screening in minority populations.

A research team at a university-based cancer center wants to carry out a study to increase the rate of mammography among low-income Chinese-speaking women. Rates of screening are lower in this population than in Caucasian women. Previous research identified misunderstandings about breast cancer, poor transportation, and lack of familiarity with hospitals as barriers to screening. The intervention group will receive mailed brochures about cancer screening in Chinese women, reminder postcards from participating physicians, and access to a mobile mammography van at community sites so that the women will not need to go to a hospital and find their way to the radiology department.

Community-based organizations raise several objections to Study 20.1. While recognizing the importance of research to reduce health disparities, the groups criticize the study as culturally inappropriate. Furthermore, while addressing barriers to access, such as transportation and difficulty in navigating around a hospital, the project does not address cultural and psychological barriers.

Although the university-based researchers in Study 20.1 had good intentions in trying to reduce health disparities, they failed to work with the community in ways that would have greatly strengthened the study. Community organizations were offended that they were not consulted while the study was being planned; this is particularly serious in a culture where "losing face" is important. There are several reasons why researchers working with minority populations should work with community organizations. As in Study 20.1, the lack of support from key community groups and leaders can make a project impractical. Community representatives can suggest ways to strengthen the study, particularly by making it more culturally appropriate. Researchers cannot be expected to appreciate all the concerns that community groups might raise about a study, particularly if their own cultural background differs from that of the targeted research participants. However, it is reasonable to expect researchers to consult with people who are respected in the community and familiar with it. In Chinese communities, family associations often play a key role. In African-American communities, ministers and beauty shop operators have partnered successfully with researchers (12,13). In general, research with minority populations is best carried out as a partnership between researchers and community stakeholders that begins during the planning stages of a project.

STUDY 20.1   (Continued).

Representatives from the community pointed out that Chinese women in this community often are embarrassed to talk about their breasts or have their breasts examined, particularly by male health care workers (14). Furthermore, many are unwilling to talk about cancer explicitly. Community representatives also suggested that community-based organizations should be sought as cosponsors of the study. After these discussions, several modifications were made to the study, including framing the study as health promotion rather than cancer screening, reassuring the women that their modesty would be respected, and ensuring that all health care workers in the project, including those photographed in the study brochure, would be Chinese women.

SPECIAL ETHICAL CONSIDERATIONS IN RESEARCH WITH MINORITY POPULATIONS

The analytical framework outlined in the Belmont Report (beneficence, respect for persons, and justice; see Chapter 2) provides a useful way to think about the special ethical issues regarding research with minority populations.

RISKS AND BENEFITS OF RESEARCH

The risks of research participation may be greater for minority populations than for the general population. A person's participation in a research study may not remain confidential within a small and tightly knit community. Furthermore, some diseases and conditions (e.g., HIV infection) may be more stigmatized in minority communities.

Even if individual confidentiality is maintained, psychosocial harms may still occur. Some communities are geographically localized, have authorized political leaders, and take action as a group (15,16). For example, indigenous tribes may resemble sovereign nations in terms of political autonomy. Such groups may be harmed by the research process—for example, if researchers take samples in a way that violates the spiritual significance the group ascribes to their biological materials. Furthermore, such groups may also be harmed if the research results challenge or disparage their spiritual traditions, historical narratives, or traditional beliefs (15,17,18). For example, Native Americans may object to patenting natural materials, which may be perceived as tribal property or as something that should not be exploited for personal profit (19). Similarly, genetic studies of migration might undermine tribal members' beliefs about their creation and tribal origin (17). Some tribes have taboos against the handling of body specimens by persons of the opposite gender, or against disclosing the name and location of a particular community to outsiders, as in a research publication. Such concerns, once identified, can be readily addressed by researchers. Tribes may also suffer harm to their dignity if researchers use materials collected in one research study for another study. In one case, a tribe that gave specimens to study the genetic basis of diabetes strongly objected when the specimens were later used to study mental illness, inbreeding, and migration (17). These studies were perceived as denigrating the reputation of the tribe.

Some writers have rejected such intangible group risks as speculative or unimportant (20). However, from the perspective of the ethnic or minority group, these are serious harms because they violate core beliefs. Generally, risks should be evaluated from the viewpoint of participants, not investigators. Even a small risk of a very serious harm deserves careful attention.

Individuals who define themselves, at least in part, as members of a group may also be harmed if results from the research lead to stereotyping and discrimination. Individuals in the group may also suffer lower self-esteem and self-image (21). Such harms would be particularly troubling in groups that are already disadvantaged because of racial discrimination or low socioeconomic status.

RESPECT FOR PERSONS

Obtaining informed consent may be challenging in some minority and ethnic populations. Before deciding whether to participate in a study, individuals need to be informed about risks that might be pertinent to their decision.

The biomedical model of health and illness may not be accepted in some cultures (9). For example, some believe that disease is caused by spirits or by an individual's failure to observe prescribed rituals. Furthermore, if the authority of healers is typically not questioned, it may be difficult to explain that researchers in a clinical trial do not know whether the study drug is effective. Moreover, the idea of explaining what the research involves and asking for consent may seem bizarre in cultures where the patients do not give consent for therapy. Community groups and representatives can often suggest how to explain these concepts to participants in a particular study (5,22).

The concept of individual informed consent may be alien to some cultures because the people regard themselves primarily as members of a family, community, or culture, rather than as autonomous individuals (9). Chapter 23 discusses this topic in detail.

JUSTICE

Recruitment efforts that target specific ethnic/minority groups need to be justified, particularly if the group has additional conditions that make them vulnerable as research subjects, such as low literacy, poor education, poverty, or low social status. Mere convenience or access to subjects is not an adequate rationale. An increased burden of disease is a necessary but not sufficient condition. It also should be plausible that the research will benefit the group itself.

In addition, justice in the sense of reciprocity requires researchers and sponsors to give participating individuals and communities their due (23). Researchers need to address concerns about exploitation by providing collateral benefits to the community. The project managers can hire members of the community as staff and provide them with opportunities for training and advancement. Moreover, researchers can carry out community service, such as education and screening programs. Finally, ethnic or minority communities that are economically disadvantaged may not be able to afford the drugs that are proven effective in clinical trials. Researchers should take reasonable steps to help the groups who participate in clinical trials obtain access to the intervention after the trial (9).

GENOMICS RESEARCH WITH ETHNIC AND MINORITY POPULATIONS

In genomics research, there often is a strong scientific rationale for studying ethnic and minority populations. Genes for conditions of interest are more likely to be identified in populations that have a high prevalence of genetic disorders or low genetic diversity. Also, researchers of human population genetics need to study samples from diverse populations. As previously discussed, however, in some circumstances research may result in harm to the group being studied. The following examples further illustrate the challenges of conducting genomics research in ethnic and minority populations.

RESEARCH WITH ASHKENAZI JEWISH POPULATIONS

Over the past several decades, researchers have studied Tay-Sachs disease, BRCA1/2 genes in breast cancer, and the APC gene in colon cancer in the Ashkenazi Jewish population. Researchers have worked closely with community and religious leaders, conducting extensive community outreach and education programs, and obtaining the support of rabbis and community advisory committees for their studies (24).

These researchers have had to address concerns about stigmatization and discrimination. Persons identified as carriers of Tay-Sachs disease may have difficulty finding marriage partners (25). In cancer susceptibility research, individuals found to be at risk may experience discrimination from health insurers and employers (26). Researchers have addressed these concerns in innovative ways in conjunction with community leaders. For example, a nonprofit group called Dor Yeshorim was created to perform confidential and anonymous genetic testing for Tay-Sachs disease in Orthodox Jewish couples considering marriage, and to inform them if they are genetically incompatible (25).

STUDY 20.2   **Genetic susceptibility to breast cancer.**

After the 185 del AG mutation for BRCA1 was identified in several Ashkenazi families, breast cancer researchers directed their attention to the Ashkenazi Jewish population (24). Several teams analyzed samples left over from previous Tay-Sachs research. Other research teams sought to collect new samples, together with clinical information about breast cancer. Researchers sought the assistance of synagogues and community centers. In some communities, objections to the research were raised. Some community leaders worried that the group would be stigmatized as "bad gene" carriers or as being linked to cancer even if individual confidentiality was maintained. Others were concerned that people with Jewish surnames might encounter insurance discrimination.

Researchers spent considerable time with community groups explaining the study and its potential long-term benefits, and addressing their concerns. Many researchers were themselves Jewish, which helped to establish trust. Although Jewish communities in some cities had considerable concerns, others had relatively few (21). Researchers were therefore able to conduct studies in communities whose members believed that the potential benefits of the research outweighed the risks of group harm. As a result of this research, today Ashkenazi Jewish women are more likely to be screened for BRCA than other women and have a relatively inexpensive screening panel for BRCA mutations common in their population.

RESEARCH WITH AMISH AND MENNONITE COMMUNITIES

Amish and Mennonite communities in the United States have several characteristics that are advantageous for studying genetic diseases (27,28). They experience high rates of genetic disease because of a founder effect (many members of the community can trace their ancestry to a single individual) and inbreeding. In addition, the communities are relatively small, geographically localized, consist of large families, and keep detailed genealogical records.

While studying and treating this population, researchers must take into account that these groups shun modern technology, including automobiles and electricity. Children with severe Crigler-Najjar syndrome, a congenital disorder of bilirubin metabolism that leads to kernicterus, require extensive daily treatment with special blue lights. More advanced cases may require liver transplantation. Most families have accepted such research and therapy, although they continue to reject most other technologies (29). Often the bluish phototherapy lamps are the only electrical appliances in the home (30).

Genetics researchers have made a commitment to provide clinical care to these communities in addition to carrying out their research. One researcher lives in an Amish and Mennonite community, founded the Clinic for Special Children, and raises funds to provide care for children afflicted with serious genetic diseases (29). The clinic also holds meetings to educate the community about the diseases under study, their research findings, and potential new therapies.

THE HUMAN GENOME DIVERSITY PROJECT

Investigators proposed the Human Genome Diversity Project (HGDP) to study variations within the human genome by collecting, storing, and analyzing samples from diverse populations (31). Researchers aimed to identify alleles that cause or predispose to disease and affect response to drugs. The HGDP would also provide important information about human migration and evolution.

Critics attacked the project as biocolonialism and biopiracy because genes from indigenous peoples would be patented and developed into commercial products, yielding profits for corporations in the developed world (31). To address concerns about exploitation, HGDP investigators were urged to benefit "individual participants and their communities" by providing services such as health screening, medical care, and education (32). The project managers also promised to "work to ensure that the sampled population [would] benefit from the financial return" from any commercial products that might be developed (32).

Group consent (in addition to individual consent) was controversial. The North American investigators called for collective consent (33). Native American tribes have formal political leaders with the power to give or withhold consent for the group. However, critics objected that group consent mistakenly implied that there were significant genetic differences among populations with different cultures (20,34,35). The HGDP was never carried out because of lack of funding, disagreements over data collection, and opposition from native and aboriginal communities.

USE OF RACIAL AND ETHNIC CATEGORIES IN RESEARCH

In the United States, racial and ethnic minorities tend to have worse health care outcomes, lower quality of care, and worse access to care than non-minority populations (7). These disparities, as well as the history of racial discrimination against African-Americans, give rise to many controversies over the use of ethnic and racial categories in research. An Institute of Medicine report called for ongoing collection of racial and ethnic data in outcomes research and clinical care to monitor these disparities and evaluate measures intended to reduce them (7).

In addition to outcomes research, some clinical trials are targeted to specific ethnic populations. Historically, racial and ethnic minorities have been underrepresented in clinical trials. Hence the NIH requires grant applicants to document the expected participation of minority populations in the study, and to explain either what efforts will be made to make the study population representative of the entire U.S. population or why such representativeness is not scientifically warranted.

The most contentious ethical issues regarding racial categories concern pharmacogenomics research based on self-identified race.

| STUDY 20.3 | BiDil for congestive heart failure (CHF) in blacks. |

Clinical trials showed that the combination of hydralazine + isosorbide was ineffective for treating CHF. However, post-hoc subgroup analyses suggested that the combination was effective for CHF in blacks but not in whites. Therefore, an RCT of the combination added to standard CHF therapy in blacks with severe CHF was carried out.

The RCT was terminated on interim analysis because mortality in the BiDil arm was 6.2%, compared with 10.2% in the control arm, exceeding prespecified stopping rules. Furthermore, there was a statistically significant difference in the primary composite endpoint. The FDA approved BiDil for use only in blacks. The doses of the component drugs used in the trial were not readily available in generic format, and the combination medication cost about seven times what generics would likely cost. Many insurers are not covering the cost of BiDil.

Several objections to studying this drug only in blacks were made (36–38). First, race misclassifies CHF patients with regard to the effectiveness of BiDil. Race was used as a proxy for specific genetic variations that cause different responses to the drug but have not yet been discovered (39). Specific polymorphisms related to the effectiveness of BiDil are most likely absent in some blacks and present in some members of other self-identified racial groups. Thus, approving the drug only for blacks excludes some individuals from its benefits. Second, some critics argue that ethnic and racial categories are outmoded in the genomics era (40). To classify research participants, it is better to test individuals for specific alleles associated with disease susceptibility or response to therapy than to use self-identified ethnic and racial categories, which are fraught with lack of precision and accuracy. Such individualized testing will become increasingly possible as genomic variations become better understood and microchips for DNA sequencing become more powerful. Finally, some critics attacked the trial for reinforcing the misconception that racial categories have a sound biological basis, rather than being based on social constructs and conventions.

In response, supporters of such studies argued that race has clinical usefulness and should continue to be used until researchers elucidate the specific biological mechanisms for race-based differences in therapeutic responses or until pharmacogenomic tests are clinically available (41). For certain conditions, genetic variability accounts for medically important differences in disease frequency and outcome among racial and ethnic groups. In addition, some clinically important alleles occur almost exclusively in certain ethnic populations. Other readily ascertainable patient characteristics, such as age, are used to guide clinical decisions even though their biological mechanism is unclear and they can lead to misclassification of individual patients regarding the effectiveness of a therapy. In the case of BiDil, a previous clinical trial had shown that the drug was ineffective in the population as a whole. There was no scientific justification for carrying out a clinical trial involving Caucasians. If race were ignored completely, Study 20.3 would not have been carried out, and blacks with heart failure would not have gained the option of a drug that significantly reduces mortality (42).

RECOMMENDATIONS FOR RESEARCH WITH MINORITY AND ETHNIC POPULATIONS

COMMUNITY INVOLVEMENT IN THE RESEARCH

By seeking community involvement, researchers can show respect for the community, identify and minimize risks to participants and the community, and strengthen the informed consent process (5). In addition, community involvement can benefit researchers by enhancing enrollment in studies.

A community may be involved in research in a variety of ways (5,16). On the most basic level, researchers should provide the communities targeted for participation information about the topic of research and the purpose of the specific project. After the study is completed, researchers should communicate their findings to the community.

On the next level, researchers can discuss the study design and protocol with community representatives and obtain their feedback on the research questions, the risks and benefits of the project, ways to minimize those risks, and ways to enhance informed consent. Such discussions often strengthen a study by focusing on research questions that will make a difference in clinical decision-making and by increasing the ratio of benefits to risks. Community members often can suggest how to enhance recruitment and follow-up (5). Researchers should elicit feedback from the community regarding the proposed research project and should respond to concerns and suggestions that are raised. Researchers do not need to accept every suggestion, but they should explain why they chose not to accept them (5). This dialogue shows respect for members of the community, educates them about research, and increases their trust in the researchers and the project.

Even greater involvement occurs in community-based participatory research, in which community representatives and leaders are partners in the research. For example, community partners help to draw up the long-term research agenda.

Obtaining formal approval from the community may be feasible in ethnic or minority communities that have authorized political leaders, are geographically localized, and have clear rules for group membership (16). Native American tribes in the United States, for example, are considered sovereign nations. Formal approval from the tribal government may be required to carry out research. Community involvement is more controversial and more complex, however, if the community has no political authority, is geographically dispersed or culturally heterogeneous, or has ambiguous criteria for group membership (16). With no clear political authority, a community should not have formal veto power over individual members' decisions to participate in research (34,43,44). However, influential community leaders may have de facto veto power. Their strong opposition may make a research study impractical.

It may be difficult to determine who has a legitimate right to speak on the community's behalf, because there may be a range of views within a community. In addition, cooption may occur if researchers pick community representatives who are likely to agree with them. These problems are not specific to this situation—they also occur with any process of selecting community members, as in the selection of lay and community members for IRBs. However, potential pitfalls in implementing a policy do not justify rejecting it completely.

HEIGHTENED REVIEW BY FUNDING AGENCIES AND IRBs

Recruitment efforts targeted to specific ethnic/minority groups should trigger special scrutiny during scientific review by funding agencies and IRBs. Such targeting may be intentional or it may result from a recruitment strategy that is facially neutral regarding the recruitment of ethnic and minority groups. Questions that reviewers should ask include the following:

- What is the scientific justification for targeting these groups as research participants?
- What is the relationship of the researcher to the communities being studied?
- Are these groups at increased risk in this study?
- Does the study raise special informed consent concerns in these groups?
- Will enrollment and retention in the community be feasible?

There should be reviewers who are knowledgeable about conducting the particular type of research in the targeted populations (45). However, IRBs and peer review committees as ordinarily constituted may not have sufficient expertise among their members regarding the perspectives of the targeted ethnic or minority groups. Thus these review bodies may need to add ad hoc reviewers who are from the communities being studied or can articulate a native's perspective (5).

RESPONSIBILITIES OF RESEARCHERS

Researchers who work with minority and ethnic communities have special obligations to address community concerns and mistrust (5).

Involve the affected minority community in the planning of the research project (5). Researchers should elicit and respond to community concerns about the project. Scientists do not need to make all changes that community stakeholders request, but they should listen to their concerns and explain why they do not agree with their requests (5). This process shows respect for community members and groups, and helps to build trust.

Provide benefits to the community. Researchers can educate the community about the project and research topic. In addition, researchers ought to make reasonable efforts to use their expertise for the well-being of participants and communities. For instance, they might provide technical assistance to community groups in writing grants to fund needed social or medical services (5).

Use due care in presenting and publishing findings, particularly in light of the history of misinterpretations and abuses of research in ethnic and minority communities. Researchers need to point out the limitations of their findings. They should distinguish their empirical findings from broader speculations on controversial social issues and policy recommendations.

Help disseminate study findings in the lay media. Scientists are sometimes reluctant to give media interviews about their work, believing that peer-reviewed publications speak for themselves. However, by helping to write press releases and by practicing explaining their work in lay terms, scientists can increase the likelihood of receiving accurate coverage in the press. Scientists also have some responsibility to speak out when others misinterpret their data in ways that harm the community or the participants they studied. Although researchers cannot be responsible for how other people draw social and political implications from their work, they should use their expertise and authority to try to correct misunderstandings and distortions of their work. This may involve giving interviews to the press and testifying before government committees. Although researchers are always responsible for communicating their findings to the public, it is particularly important to do so in the context of the long-standing health disparities that vulnerable groups commonly face.

TAKE HOME POINTS

1. Ethnic and minority communities may mistrust researchers because of a history of unfavorable experiences with research projects.
2. There may be cogent reasons to target research to such communities, and research may also benefit these communities.
3. Researchers must be sensitive to the fact that research with such communities raises particular ethical issues regarding assessment of research risks and informed consent.

ANNOTATED BIBLIOGRAPHY

Hausman D. Protecting groups from genetic research. *Bioethics* 2008;22:157–165.
  Draws a distinction between harms that structured groups experience when important beliefs are disruptive and discrimination that is experienced by individual members of the group.
Lo B, O'Connell ME, eds. *Ethical Considerations for Research on Housing-Related Health Hazards Involving Children.* Washington, DC: National Academies Press; 2005.
  Recommends that researchers who target ethnic and minority populations for enrollment should elicit feedback from communities regarding the project and respond to concerns and suggestions.

Weijer C, Emanuel EJ. Protecting communities in biomedical research. *Science* 2000;289:1142–1144.
> Analyzes different types of communities that participate in research. Only those that are geographically localized and have authorized political leaders should have the power to approve or reject a research protocol.

REFERENCES

1. Braunstein JB, Sherber NS, Schulman SP, Ding EL, Powe NR. Race, medical researcher distrust, perceived harm, and willingness to participate in cardiovascular prevention trials. *Medicine (Baltimore)* 2008;87:1–9.
2. Corbie-Smith G, Thomas SB, St George DM. Distrust, race, and research. *Arch Intern Med* 2002;162:2458–2463.
3. Corbie-Smith G, Thomas SB, Williams MV, Moody-Ayers S. Attitudes and beliefs of African Americans toward participation in medical research. *J Gen Intern Med* 1999;14:537–546.
4. Freimuth VS, Quinn SC, Thomas SB, Cole G, Zook E, Duncan T. African Americans' views on research and the Tuskegee syphilis study. *Soc Sci Med* 2001;52:797–808.
5. Lo B, O'Connell ME, eds. *Ethical Considerations for Research on Housing-Related Health Hazards Involving Children*. Washington, DC: National Academies Press; 2005.
6. Kevles DJ. *In the Name of Eugenics: Genetics and the Uses of Human Heredity*. New York: Knopf; 1985.
7. Committee on Understanding and Eliminating Racial and Ethnic Disparities in Health Care. *Unequal Treatment: Confronting Racial and Ethnic Disparities in Health Care*. Washington, DC: National Academies Press; 2003.
8. Wendler D, Emanuel E. A framework for assessing the ethics of housing research with children. In: Paper commissioned by the Committee on Ethical Issues in Housing-Related Health Hazards Research in Children. National Academy of Sciences; 2004.
9. National Bioethics Advisory Commission. *Ethical and Policy Issues in International Research*. Rockville, MD: National Bioethics Advisory Commission; 2001.
10. Ford JG, Howerton MW, Lai GY, et al. Barriers to recruiting underrepresented populations to cancer clinical trials: a systematic review. *Cancer* 2008;112:228–242.
11. Wendler D, Kington R, Madans J, et al. Are racial and ethnic minorities less willing to participate in health research? *PLoS Med* 2005;3:e19.
12. Corbie-Smith G, Ammerman AS, Katz ML, et al. Trust, benefit, satisfaction, and burden: a randomized controlled trial to reduce cancer risk through African-American churches. *J Gen Intern Med* 2003;18:531–541.
13. Linnan LA, Ferguson YO. Beauty salons: a promising health promotion setting for reaching and promoting health among African American women. *Health Educ Behav* 2007;34:517–530.
14. Kwok C, Sullivan G, Cant R. The role of culture in breast health practices among Chinese-Australian women. *Patient Educ Couns* 2006;64:268–276.
15. Hausman D. Protecting groups from genetic research. *Bioethics* 2008;22:157–165.
16. Weijer C, Emanuel EJ. Protecting communities in biomedical research. *Science* 2000;289:1142–1144.
17. McGregor JL. Population genomics and research ethics with socially identifiable groups. *J Law Med Ethics* 2008;36:356–370.
18. Foster MW, Freeman WL. Naming names in human genetic variation research. *Genome Res* 1998;8:755–757.
19. Dalton R. When two tribes go to war. *Nature* 2004;430:500–502.
20. Reilly PR. Rethinking risks to human subjects in genetic research. *Am J Hum Genet* 1998;63:682–685.
21. Nelson NJ. Ashkenazi community is not unwilling to participate in genetic research. *J Natl Cancer Inst* 1998;90:884–885.
22. Woodsong C, Karim QA. A model designed to enhance informed consent: experiences from the HIV prevention trials network. *Am J Public Health* 2005;95:412–419.
23. Wertheimer A. Exploitation in clinical research. In: Emanuel EJ, Grady C, Crouch RA, Lie RK, Miller FG, Wendler D, eds. *The Oxford Textbook of Clinical Research Ethics*. New York: Oxford University Press; 2008:201–210.
24. Brandt-Rauf SI, Raveis VH, Drummond NF, Conte JA, Rothman SM. Ashkenazi Jews and breast cancer: the consequences of linking ethnic identity to genetic disease. *Am J Public Health* 2006;96:1979–1988.
25. Bach G, Tomczak J, Risch N, Ekstein J. Tay-Sachs screening in the Jewish Ashkenazi population: DNA testing is the preferred procedure. *Am J Med Genet* 2001;99:70–75.
26. Lehmann LS, Weeks JC, Klar N, Garber JE. A population-based study of Ashkenazi Jewish women's attitudes toward genetic discrimination and BRCA1/2 testing. *Genet Med* 2002;4:346–352.
27. Morton DH, Morton CS, Strauss KA, et al. Pediatric medicine and the genetic disorders of the Amish and Mennonite people of Pennsylvania. *Am J Med Genet* 2003;121C:5–17.
28. Puffenberger EG. Genetic heritage of the Old Order Mennonites of southeastern Pennsylvania. *Am J Med Genet* 2003;121C:18–31.
29. Belkin L. A doctor for the future. *New York Times Magazine* 2005 Nov 6.
30. Grady D. At gene therapy's frontier, the Amish build a clinic. *New York Times* 1999 June 29:Sect. F1.
31. Greely HT. Human genome diversity: what about the other human genome project? *Nat Rev Genet* 2001; 2:222–227.

32. Human Genome Diversity Committee of HUGO. Summary document. 1995. Available at: http://www.stanford.edu/group/morrinst/hgdp/summary93.html. Accessed September 2008.
33. North American Regional Committee of the Human Genome Diversity Project. Proposed model ethical protocol for collecting DNA samples. *Houst Law Rev* 1997;33:1431–1473.
34. Juengst ET. Groups as gatekeepers to genomic research: conceptually confusing, morally hazardous, and practically useless. *Kennedy Inst Ethics J* 1998;8:183–200.
35. National Research Council. *Evaluating Human Genetic Diversity.* Washington, DC: National Academies Press; 1997.
36. Sankar P, Kahn J. BiDil: race medicine or race marketing? Health Aff (Millwood) 2005 Jul-Dec; Suppl Web Exclusives:W5-455–463.
37. Carlson RJ. The case of BiDil: a policy commentary on race and genetics. Health Aff (Millwood) 2005 Jul-Dec; Suppl Web Exclusives:W5-464–468.
38. Bibbins-Domingo K, Fernandez A. BiDil for heart failure in black patients: implications of the U.S. Food and Drug Administration approval. *Ann Intern Med* 2007;146:52–56.
39. Bloche MG. Race-based therapeutics. *N Engl J Med* 2004;351:2035–2037.
40. Cooper R, Kaufman J, Ward R. Race and genomics. *N Engl J Med* 2003;348:1166–1170.
41. Burchard E, Ziv E, Coyle N, et al. The importance of race and ethnic background in biomedical research and clinical practice. *N Engl J Med* 2003;348:1170–1175.
42. Temple R, Stockbridge NL. BiDil for heart failure in black patients: the U.S. Food and Drug Administration perspective. *Ann Intern Med* 2007;146:57–62.
43. Juengst ET. Commentary: what "community review" can and cannot do. *J Law Med Ethics* 2000;28:3, 52–54.
44. Reilly PR. Public concern about genetics. *Annu Rev Genomics Hum Genet* 2000;1:485–506.
45. Lo B, Bayer R. Establishing ethical trials for treatment and prevention of AIDS in developing countries. *BMJ* 2003;327:337–339.

21

Research With Prisoners

Research involving prisoners has been sharply criticized because of concerns that consent may not be voluntary and informed, and the risks may be unacceptable (1). After World War II, biomedical research in U.S. prisons was widespread, particularly in Phase I clinical trials (2). Many abuses occurred (3,4). For example, prisoners were administered hallucinogenic drugs, dioxin, and radioactive isotopes (4). Because prisoners may feel that they are not free to decline to participate in research, the potential for abuse is unavoidable. To address concerns that prisoners might be used as "guinea pigs," federal regulations were enacted in 1978 to severely limit research in prisons. However, research involving prisoners is needed to understand and treat medical problems that occur only or predominantly in prisoners. Many prisoners now want access to clinical trials because of their potential personal benefits. This shift from seeking protection to regarding participation in research as a means to access potential new therapies was driven by clinical trials of antiretroviral agents in the AIDS epidemic. When antiretrovirals were available only in clinical trials, HIV-infected prisoners had no access to these potentially life-saving therapies. Rather than wanting to be protected from clinical research, some prisoners and their advocates called for greater access to research.

The challenge is how to carry out research with prisoners in an ethically acceptable manner. A recent Institute of Medicine (IOM) report analyzed the ethical issues in research with prisoners in great detail (5). The following study illustrates how some important research can only be conducted in a prison setting.

STUDY 21.1 **Case management for tuberculosis.**

After they are discharged from prison, inmates with tuberculosis often face discontinuity in their medical care. This research project will carry out a randomized clinical trial of a case-management program in which, prior to discharge, a public health nurse will meet with prisoners with tuberculosis who are soon to be released. The nurse and prisoner will work to develop a plan for postincarceration medical care and medications, and to identify barriers to taking antituberculosis medications regularly. All participants in the study will receive a physical examination, chest x-ray, sputum smear and culture, blood tests (including HIV testing), and education about tuberculosis. Participants in the intervention group will have several sessions with a counselor prior to release, as well as follow-up visits and tests afterward. Participants in the control group will receive usual postincarceration care through the public health department.

Study 21.1 illustrates the ethical dilemmas inherent to biomedical research in prisons, particularly clinical trials. Prisoners are at high risk for tuberculosis and for discontinuous care upon release. Treatment failure also has serious public health consequences. Study 21.1 is likely to benefit participants, and the medical risks in the study are similar to the risks of standard treatment for tuberculosis. Even the control group will benefit because they receive education about tuberculosis.

However, the study also poses psychosocial risks. HIV testing is a standard aspect of tuberculosis care and part of the research study. In prisons, an inmate's HIV status is highly sensitive information, and those who are known to be seropositive may be stigmatized by guards and prisoners. In some prisons, they may be segregated or limited in their work assignments. In addition, potential participants in the study need to be told what information obtained during the study might be passed on to public health officials or probation officers after discharge.

WHAT MAKES RESEARCH WITH PRISONERS ETHICALLY DIFFERENT?

Prisoners are vulnerable as research participants because their liberty is restricted in several ways (1).

First, the voluntariness of consent may be compromised in prisons. Prisoners have severely curtailed freedom and choices. Furthermore, they are subject to additional discipline and sanctions by prison guards and officials. Hence inmates may feel that declining to participate in research is not a feasible option. Furthermore, overcrowding and poor access to health care may make participation in research seem attractive, without regard to the risks.

Second, privacy and confidentiality are compromised in prisons. Which prisoners are enrolled in a research project is likely to be common knowledge, and guards and other prisoners may be able to infer a participant's medical condition from the fact of their participation. If some information is disclosed, it may lead to embarrassment, stigmatization, retaliation, or additional punishment.

Third, most IRB members have no direct experience with prisons and thus may not appreciate how daily prison life may compromise research ethics or place prisoners at risk. For instance, in Study 21.1, the risks will be higher in a prison where there is poor access to good medical care or poor training of guards regarding communicable diseases.

Fourth, it is difficult to monitor adverse events in research conducted in prisons because they are closed institutions. Participants may find it difficult to call attention to problems that arise as a research project is carried out. Monitoring to ensure that the study is actually carried out in accordance with the protocol is also difficult.

Finally, prisoners often have other characteristics that make them vulnerable, such as poor education, mental health problems, and substance abuse problems, which may impair decision-making.

CURRENT REGULATIONS INVOLVING PRISONERS

Research involving prisoners must comply with additional requirements that restrict the type of research that may be carried out and may require additional review.

WHO ARE PRISONERS?

Prisoners are defined in the regulations as individuals who are "confined or detained in a penal institution." This includes federal and state prisons as well as city and county jails. In addition, prisoners include persons who are detained in other facilities as an alternative to criminal prosecution or incarceration in a penal institution.

There are many persons who are under the control of the criminal justice system but are not incarcerated, including persons on parole or probation. The number of persons on parole or probation is more than double the number in prisons. A recent IOM committee recommended extending protections to all persons whose freedom is limited by the criminal justice system, because their ability to give free and voluntary consent may be impaired (5).

SUBPART C OF FEDERAL REGULATIONS ON RESEARCH WITH PRISONERS

Subpart C of the federal regulations for protection of human subjects deals with research involving prisoners. Although 17 agencies, including the Department of Health and Human Services (HHS), have adopted the Common Rule, only three have adopted Subpart C.

Categories of Acceptable Research

Only the following types of research are permitted in prisons:

- Research on the causes, effects, and processes of incarceration, provided that it presents only minimal risk and no more than inconvenience.
- Research on prisons as institutional structures or on prisoners as incarcerated persons. Again, the research may present only minimal risk and no more than inconvenience.
- Epidemiologic studies that involve no more than minimal risk and inconvenience may qualify for a waiver of Subpart C.

As Chapter 5 discusses in more detail, the definition of minimal risk requires a comparison with the risk in the daily lives or routine medical examinations of healthy persons. Although Subpart C does not say so explicitly, the comparison should be with healthy persons living outside of prison settings, because prisoners have a high baseline level of daily risk. This increased baseline risk should not be used to justify placing prisoners at greater risks in research than non-inmates.

- Research on conditions particularly affecting prisoners as a class. This category of studies must be approved by the secretary of HHS after consultation with experts in penology, medicine, and ethics. Examples include research on hepatitis C, HIV, drug addiction, and sexual assaults.
- Research that has the intent and a reasonable probability of improving the health and well-being of the participants. If some participants are assigned to control groups that may not benefit, the study must be approved by the secretary of HHS after consultation with experts.

STUDY 21.1   (Continued).

This study addresses conditions that affect prisoners as a group and have a reasonable likelihood of improving the participants' well-being. Even the well-being of participants in the control group will likely improve as a result of the study because they will receive education about tuberculosis. The study therefore would be permitted under Subpart C.

Requirements for IRBs

IRBs that approve research with prisoners must have a member who is a prisoner or a prisoner representative. These members help the IRB understand what the risks of the research may be in the prison and whether the prisoners' participation is voluntary.

Heightened Protections

Subpart C requires additional protections for prisoners who participate in research. IRBs must determine that:

1. The benefits of participation are not so great relative to what is otherwise available in prison that informed consent is impaired.
2. The risks of the study would be acceptable to nonprisoners.
3. The selection procedures are fair and free of arbitrary intervention by prison authorities or other prisoners.
4. Participation in research will not be considered in parole or probation decisions.
5. Adequate follow-up care will be provided if needed after the study ends.
6. The consent forms can be easily understood by prisoners.

These protections minimize the possibility of undue influence and inappropriate risk. Because of these additional requirements, IRB review of research involving prisoners may require a longer review process than other research.

FEDERAL BUREAU OF PRISONS (BOP) REGULATIONS

The BOP has issued separate regulations for research in federal prisons that are stricter than those in Subpart C.

Types of Acceptable Research

In federal prisons, nontherapeutic medical research, pharmaceutical trials, and cosmetic research are not permitted. Therapeutic medical research is allowed, including clinical trials "that may be warranted for an inmate's specific diagnosis or treatment," provided that the research conforms to Subpart C and is approved by the prison's medical director. In addition, research on disease prevalence and outcomes of accepted therapeutic or behavioral interventions and nonmedical research are permitted.

Confidentiality

Additional confidentiality protections are required in federal prisons. Personal identifiable information may not be released without the participant's written consent and may not be admitted as evidence in any judicial or administrative hearing. Identifiable information may not be entered into any electronic retrieval system. Researchers who are not employees of the BOP may not have access to identifiable information. Prospective participants must also be told that information about intent to commit a crime, harm themselves or someone else, or escape from prison will not be kept confidential.

Undue Influence

All incentives for research participants are forbidden, except for soft drinks and snacks to be consumed at the research visit. In addition, steps may be taken to avoid putting prisoners at a disadvantage for participating in research, such as by interfering with work schedules.

Review of Research

The BOP requires a more complex review process than is required by Subpart C. In addition to approval from a local research review board at the prison, approval is also required from a central IRB at the BOP, the director of the federal BOP, and the local warden.

ADDITIONAL REGULATIONS

States, counties, and cities may have additional regulations for research in jails under their jurisdiction.

ADDRESSING ETHICAL CONCERNS

The following study illustrates more complicated ethical and regulatory issues (6,7).

STUDY 21.2   Dietary supplementation to reduce violent behavior.
Dietary supplementation with omega-3 fatty acids, which are commonly found in fish, reduced aggressive behaviors and hostility in an RCT carried out in the community. Researchers propose an RCT in prison to determine whether an over-the-counter supplement containing omega-3 fatty acids would reduce antisocial behaviors and violence in prisoners. The protocol is virtually identical to the protocol used in the previous study in the community. Participants would take a daily capsule of supplement or placebo, keep a food diary for 1 week, and have their disciplinary records reviewed by the researchers.

To organize their thinking about a research project involving prisoners, investigators and IRBs should ask the following questions:

WHY ARE PRISONERS INVOLVED IN THE RESEARCH PROJECT?

There should be a compelling reason for conducting the research in a prison setting. Convenience or efficiency is not a sufficient reason to carry out research within prisons. Study 21.2 deals with a problem that is particularly common among prisoners. The RCT offers the prospect of improving the health and well-being of participants in the active arm.

WHAT ARE THE RISKS AND BENEFITS OF THE STUDY?

The study agent is available over the counter and its efficacy has been demonstrated in an RCT. The protocol for Study 21.2 is substantially the same as in previous clinical trials, where no serious unexpected adverse events were identified. Thus the medical risks of the supplement are small. However, the psychosocial risks may be considerable, particularly if confidentiality is breached. For instance, in Study 21.2, if participants are selected because of a history of antisocial behavior or violence, guards may be stricter with them or even harass them.

HOW WILL PRIVACY AND CONFIDENTIALITY BE MAINTAINED?

Prisoners identified as participants in Study 21.2 might suffer psychosocial harms because they are perceived as being prone to violent behavior. IRB members who are former prisoners or prisoner advocates would need to judge whether this is likely to occur at the study sites. For example, will correctional officers be able to hear or see the interview, or know who is eligible for the project? A federal certificate of confidentiality would be useful to protect research data from subpoena.

HOW WILL VOLUNTARY AND INFORMED CONSENT BE ENSURED?

Because participants in any RCT often misunderstand randomization and placebos, it may be helpful to assess whether the participants understand that they might not receive the study supplement and that it might not be effective. Moreover, investigators can ascertain whether participants understand the salient psychosocial risks of the study. Giving signed consent forms to participants or putting them in the prisoners' records may enable staff to infer the participants' medical conditions. Hence these aspects of standard informed consent procedures may need to be modified.

WILL PARTICIPANTS OBTAIN APPROPRIATE MEDICAL CARE?

Although the medical risks of the supplement are very small, the investigators still need to consider and describe how they will respond if participants experience adverse medical events that they ascribe to the study supplement.

ARE ADDITIONAL PROTECTIONS FOR PARTICIPANTS APPROPRIATE?

An IOM committee suggested that prisoner research subject advocates (PRSAs) can provide important additional protections in some studies (5). The PRSA would be independent of the researchers and the prison; for example, he or she could be an ombudsman or a person employed by the IRB. The task of the PRSA would be to monitor the consent process, adverse events, protocol compliance, and additional protections. To carry out these objectives, the advocate would need access to all research activities and data.

STUDY 21.2 (Continued).

This study could be designed to meet the provisions of Subpart C. It would need to be approved by the secretary of HHS after appropriate consultation. However, the more stringent BOP regulations may preclude carrying out the study in federal prisons. Participants in federal prisons must be selected because of a previous history of violent behavior; that is, the study cannot be open to all inmates. Researchers need to expect that this requirement will be widely known within the prison. Hence all inmates taking the study supplement or

STUDY 21.2   (Continued).

placebo could be identified as having a history of violence, and this could lead inmates or guards to act in ways that put participants at risk.

Of note, this RCT was carried out in prisons in Great Britain. The study found that the dietary supplements reduced violent behavior, including assaults, by over one-third.

As noted previously, people who are not incarcerated but are on parole or probation may also be vulnerable because they might feel they cannot decline a request to participate in research. Thus, it would be desirable to give heightened attention to the risks of participation, the consent process, and confidentiality. It would be useful for IRBs reviewing such research to have a member who is an advocate for potential participants and has direct experience with parole and probation.

RESEARCH PARTICIPANTS WHO BECOME INCARCERATED

Participants in research studies conducted outside prisons may become incarcerated during a study. For example, participants in a clinical trial of an experimental vaccine for HIV infection may include injection drug users and commercial sex workers. The researcher should anticipate that participants may be incarcerated and consider whether study activities should continue if this occurs.

If a participant decided to enroll in study when he or she was not incarcerated, there are no prison-specific ethical issues. However, after a participant is incarcerated, any interaction with the research project—for example, to draw blood for tests or to assess clinical outcomes—raises concerns about undue influence, confidentiality, and psychosocial risks. If the researcher will interact or intervene with participants in prison, the study needs to be reviewed and approved in accordance with the regulations for research involving prisoners.

TAKE HOME POINTS

1. Research with prisoners presents particular ethical dilemmas because of the risk of undue influence, as well as heightened threats to confidentiality.
2. Research with prisoners is subject to additional regulations and requires careful ethical justification.

ANNOTATED BIBLIOGRAPHY

Gostin LO. Biomedical research involving prisoners: ethical values and legal regulation. *JAMA* 2007;297:737–740. Summary of a consensus IOM report on the topic. The full report may be downloaded at http://www.nap.edu/catalog.php?record_id=11692.

REFERENCES

1. Gostin LO, Vanchieri C, Pope A. *Ethical Considerations for Research Involving Prisoners*. Washington, DC: National Academies Press; 2006.
2. Bonham VH, Moreno JD. Research with captive populations: prisoners, students, and soldiers. In: Emanuel EJ, Grady C, Crouch RA, Lie RK, Miller FG, Wendler D, editors. *The Oxford Textbook of Clinical Research Ethics*. New York: Oxford University Press; 2008:461–474.
3. Hornblum AM. They were cheap and available: prisoners as research subjects in twentieth century America. *BMJ* 1997;315:1437–1441.
4. Hornblum AM. Ethical lapses in dermatologic "research." *Arch Dermatol* 1999;135:383–385.
5. Gostin LO. Biomedical research involving prisoners: ethical values and legal regulation. *JAMA* 2007;297:737–740.
6. Gesch CB, Hammond SM, Hampson SE, Eves A, Crowder MJ. Influence of supplementary vitamins, minerals and essential fatty acids on the antisocial behaviour of young adult prisoners: randomised, placebo-controlled trial. *Br J Psychiatry* 2002;181:22–28.
7. Hibbeln JR, Ferguson TA, Blasbalg TL. Omega-3 fatty acid deficiencies in neurodevelopment, aggression and autonomic dysregulation: opportunities for intervention. *Int Rev Psychiatry* 2006;18:107–118.

Clinical Research in Resource-Poor Countries

Research is urgently needed on diseases such as malaria and HIV infection, which are ravaging resource-poor countries. Medical interventions commonly used in developed nations may not be feasible in settings that lack refrigeration, clean water, or medical infrastructure. In addition, pharmaceutical manufacturers are increasingly carrying out clinical trials in resource-poor countries, where costs are lower and a large number of patients have not received previous treatment. Clinical trials sponsored by pharmaceutical companies often involve drugs for diseases such as hypertension and diabetes, whose primary market will be in developed countries. As illustrated in Table 22.1, research in resource-poor countries raises numerous ethical concerns at each step of a project.

HOW IS RESEARCH IN RESOURCE-POOR COUNTRIES DIFFERENT?

In resource-poor countries, the two primary means of protecting participants—IRB review and informed consent—may be inadequate. IRBs in developing countries may lack training, experience, and resources. IRBs in the United States are unlikely to be familiar with conditions in the host country (1). Informed consent may be problematic in a country where people are poorly educated and lack health literacy, and where physicians in clinical practice usually do not tell patients their diagnosis, admit uncertainty, or obtain consent. Participants may not accept Western models of disease. Furthermore, participants might hear rumors and other misinformation about a research study.

In several highly publicized cases, researchers from developed countries have been harshly criticized for allegedly carrying out inappropriately risky studies in resource-poor countries without adequate consent (3). Allegations of exploitation are complicated by the history of colonialism and the vast economic discrepancies between the North and South. For these reasons, researchers conducting international studies need to be particularly sensitive to ethical concerns. Randomized trials to prevent mother-to-child transmission of HIV infection dramatized these ethical issues (4,5).

| STUDY 22.1 | Prevention of mother-to-child transmission of HIV infection. |

The vast majority of perinatal HIV infections occur in resource-poor countries. In 1994, a placebo-controlled randomized controlled trial (RCT) showed that zidovudine reduced the rate of transmission of HIV from infected pregnant women to their children from 25% to 7%. The treatment regimen was oral zidovudine starting in the second trimester plus intravenous zidovudine during labor plus oral administration to children for 6 weeks after birth. Although this treatment was quickly adopted in the United States and other developed countries, it

STUDY 22.1 **(Continued).**

was not feasible in resource-poor countries, where women often do not receive early prenatal care and intravenous therapy is not feasible.

To determine whether perinatal HIV infection could be prevented in developing countries, a much simpler regimen was tested: oral zidovudine starting at 36 weeks of gestation plus a more frequent oral dose during labor and delivery. The control group received placebo. Similar trials were carried out in Thailand and sub-Saharan Africa, including countries where breastfeeding is the cultural expectation.

DOES THE RESEARCH ADDRESS A HEALTH PRIORITY?

It would be an imprudent use of limited health care resources in a developing country to conduct human-participants research that does not address a health or public health priority in the host country. In light of the dire health care problems in resource-poor countries, there is little benefit from gaining knowledge about low-priority issues. Furthermore, research projects often pay higher salaries to health care workers than are available in clinical practice, eroding the medical and public health infrastructure. Because the ratio of benefits to burdens in such research would be inappropriate, the study would be unethical unless fair benefits could be negotiated with the communities in which the study is carried out. Since the results would not be relevant in the host country, the participants and their communities would bear the risks of research without the prospect of benefiting from the findings of the study. In particular, it is ethically problematic for researchers and sponsors from developed countries to carry out clinical trials to evaluate drugs that will be marketed exclusively or predominantly in developed countries.

ARE STUDY INTERVENTIONS APPROPRIATE?

Because of scarce resources and logistical constraints, medical interventions that are standard in developed countries may not be available or feasible in resource-poor countries where the trial is conducted. This creates an ethical tension between providing a benefit to research participants and obtaining generalizable scientific knowledge.

TABLE 22.1 **Questions About Clinical Trials in Resource-Poor Countries**

1. Does the research address a health or public health priority in the host country?
2. Are study interventions provided to participants appropriate?
   - Is a placebo control proposed?
   - Is background care for the condition under study appropriate?
   - Is ancillary care for other conditions appropriate?
   - If the control intervention would not be acceptable in the researchers' own country, special justification is needed.
3. Are there barriers to informed consent, and how can they be overcome?
4. Will participants and their communities receive fair benefits?
5. Is IRB review rigorous?
6. Are stakeholders in the host country partners in the study?

USE OF PLACEBOS IN CLINICAL TRIALS IN DEVELOPING COUNTRIES

As discussed in Chapter 26, although placebo controls enhance the scientific rigor of a clinical trial, they may also raise ethical concerns. It is unethical for researchers to withhold a therapy that is known to be effective for the condition being studied if the subjects will suffer significant harm as a result of their participation.

Critics sharply attacked the use of placebos in Study 22.1 because an effective drug regimen was available in developed countries. It would be unethical to carry out a placebo-controlled trial for this condition in the developed world, and critics argued that a double standard that allowed a placebo control in developing countries would also be unethical. One critic wrote, "Residents of impoverished, postcolonial countries, the majority of whom are people of color, must be protected from potential exploitation in research" (6). From this viewpoint, an appropriate study design would be an equivalency trial comparing the short-course regimen with the standard treatment offered in the United States. The deputy editor of the *New England Journal of Medicine* attacked these placebo-controlled studies because they "subordinate the subjects' welfare to the objectives of the study" (7). She compared these studies with the infamous Tuskegee study, which withheld effective treatment from poor, uneducated black research participants.

The 2000 revisions to the Declaration of Helsinki declared that new interventions "should be tested against . . . the best current prophylactic, diagnostic, and therapeutic methods" (8). Hence, the control group should receive the standard of care that is available in developed countries. In its deliberations, the World Medical Association rejected an alternative standard, that the control group should receive the "highest attainable and sustainable" level of care in the host country.

Others defended these mother-to-child transmission trials because placebo controls were necessary to address the health priorities of the host country (1). In a resource-poor country, the pertinent research, clinical, and public health question is whether short-course antiretroviral therapy (ART) would be more effective than what is currently available in the country, not how it compares with care that is unaffordable and impossible to implement. An equivalency trial would not address the former question. In this view, an equivalency trial would indeed be unethical because the results would not be relevant in the host country, and therefore the country would bear the risks of research without benefiting from its findings.

As a result of these debates, a "clarification" to the Helsinki Declaration was issued in 2002: "a placebo controlled trial may be ethically acceptable, even if proven therapy is available . . . [if] for compelling and scientifically sound methodological reasons its use is necessary to determine the efficacy or safety of a prophylactic, diagnostic or therapeutic method" (8). In 2007, the World Health Organization declared: "The use of a placebo control arm is ethically acceptable in a biomedical HIV prevention trial only when there is no HIV prevention modality of the type being studied that has been shown to be effective in comparable populations" (9). For example, if HIV prevention trials in the developed world are carried out with participants who are injection drug users or men having sex with other men, the results will not be applicable to populations in developing countries where HIV is predominantly transmitted through heterosexual intercourse.

The issue is commonly framed as the "standard of care" that must be provided to all study participants. However, in this chapter we avoid this term because it suggests that certain interventions are required or obligatory. It is contested whether researchers must provide to study participants all interventions that are "standard" in developed countries.

STUDY 22.1   (Continued).

Study 22.1 is permissible under current international ethical guidelines. Without a placebo-controlled trial, it would be impossible to address a pressing public health question in the host country.

> **STUDY 22.1   (Continued).**
>
> *In these perinatal HIV trials, the placebo group had a lower transmission rate compared to historical rates. Thus, an equivalency trial would have overestimated the absolute benefit of the short-course intervention.*
>
> *These clinical trials established proof of principle that antiretrovirals are feasible in developing countries. Subsequently, billions of dollars were made available through United Nations Joint Programme on HIV/AIDS (UNAIDS), the President's Emergency Plan for AIDS Relief (PEPFAR), and the Gates Foundation to provide antiretroviral therapy in resource-poor countries. Additional clinical trials were funded to test even simpler regimens and address transmission through breastfeeding. In these later trials, the control arm received the regimen that previous trials had shown to be the most effective in resource-poor settings.*

WHAT IS THE RESEARCHER'S OBLIGATION TO PROVIDE BACKGROUND CARE?

What obligations do researchers have to provide to participants in a clinical trial interventions in addition to the study intervention? As the following case illustrates, there are two distinct questions: what background care researchers should provide for the condition being studied, and what ancillary care should they provide for other conditions they identify? This section deals with the former question, and the latter question is analyzed in the next section.

> **STUDY 22.2   HIV prevention trial.**
>
> *Researchers are carrying out a randomized controlled trial of a new microbicide for HIV prevention. Participants will return for follow-up evaluations 1 month after receiving the study or control intervention and every 6 months thereafter for 2 years. What obligations do researchers have to provide other HIV prevention measures, such as counseling and condoms?*

According to the ethical obligation to minimize harm to participants, researchers should provide interventions that are known to be effective and feasible to prevent or treat the condition addressed in the clinical trial. In HIV prevention studies, researchers have a strong obligation to provide counseling for risk reduction and condoms (9). As discussed in Chapter 6, participants in clinical trials commonly have a therapeutic misconception; for example, in Study 22.2 they might mistakenly believe that they will receive an intervention that effectively prevents HIV infections. If researchers do not recommend and provide condoms, participants might mistakenly believe that they no longer need to use them. They might even increase risky behaviors as a result of this misunderstanding. Thus, to prevent harm to participants, HIV prevention researchers should provide standard, proven prevention measures (9). Such background care must be provided even though it will tend to reduce the number of study endpoints and thus lower the power of the trial. To avoid conflicts of interest, researchers could train persons who are independent of the study to provide high-quality counseling.

Specifying what interventions are standard or proven in resource-poor countries is often controversial. The general rule is that researchers should do what a reasonable physician in the host country would do under the circumstances. However, the interpretation of this general maxim depends on the specific circumstance. Condoms and counseling are affordable, feasible, and included in international guidelines for HIV prevention. A more controversial issue is whether researchers are obligated to provide all "state of the art" prevention services regardless of cost and sustainability. If the sponsor provides as background care intravenous medicines that are not feasible outside a research setting for the foreseeable future because of a lack of clean water and electricity, the results of the trial will not be applicable in the host country. Similarly, in a HIV prevention trial in injection drug users, it would make little sense for researchers to provide preventive measures that would not otherwise be permitted or available in the host country. For example, if methadone and needle exchange for injection drug users are illegal in the host country, researchers should respect such prohibitions. Furthermore, even if the researchers could persuade government officials to allow these measures for the duration of the trial, providing them to study participants would make the results of the trial inapplicable to other persons in the host country. Participants in the host country would therefore undergo risks and inconvenience to gain knowledge that would not benefit their countrymen. Arguably, the ratio of benefits to risks would then be unacceptable.

WHAT IS THE RESEARCHER'S OBLIGATION TO PROVIDE ANCILLARY CARE?

During a clinical trial, researchers might discover that participants have other illnesses or conditions that can be readily treated. What ancillary care should investigators provide during the study for these other conditions?

STUDY 22.2   (Continued).

During a trial of a new microbicide to prevent HIV infection in high-risk seronegative women in a sub-Saharan country, researchers identify some participants with the following conditions:

- *Sexually transmitted infections, which could be treated with a short course of antibiotics.*
- *Pulmonary tuberculosis (TB), which would require an extended course of several months.*
- *New HIV infection in participants who were seronegative upon entry to the study.*
- *Children of participants are at risk for malaria, which could be prevented by mosquito nets.*

What responsibility do the investigators have for providing care to prevent or treat these other medical conditions during the study?

By ancillary care, we mean interventions for other conditions that are not required to make a clinical trial scientifically rigorous or minimize risks caused by study procedures. Some claim that researchers have no responsibility to provide ancillary care during a clinical trial because the role of the researcher differs from that of the treating physician. In this view, the only interventions that researchers must provide are those needed to carry out the study in a safe and scientifically valid manner. Researchers cannot be expected to address all the medical problems that participants have or develop. An open-ended obligation to provide ancillary care in a resource-poor setting with limited basic health care might keep researchers from fulfilling their primary and unique goal of obtaining generalizable knowledge. However, this position has been criticized as treating participants merely as a means to achieve the ends of research. To critics, it seems inhumane for researchers not to alleviate suffering if they can readily do so at little burden to themselves.

One approach to ancillary care is based on reciprocity (10). In this view, participants in a clinical trial give permission for researchers to collect personal health information and carry out interventions. As a matter of reciprocity, researchers have limited obligations to respond to aspects of the participant's health that are related to those interventions or to the information they need to conduct the trial. An alternative view of ancillary care is that participants entrust certain aspects of their health to the researcher (11,12). Such partial entrustment creates certain reciprocal obligations for researchers to respond to those aspects of health that were entrusted to them. However, it is questionable whether the researcher-participant relationship can be properly characterized as entrustment.

The extent of the researcher's obligation to provide ancillary care during a clinical trial therefore will depend on several factors (10). There must be some limit to a researcher's obligation to provide ancillary care, to ensure that there will be adequate resources to carry out the study protocol.

The Connection Between the Participant's Condition and the Research Topic and Interventions

The more closely the condition is related to the research question and study design, the greater is the researcher's responsibility to provide ancillary care.

STUDY 22.2   (Continued).

It is expected that some participants will develop HIV infection in the course of the trial; indeed, this is the primary endpoint of the study. Thus, identifying women with new infections is integral to the study design and researchers have a strong obligation to provide ancillary care, such as ART.

In Study 22.2, during follow-up evaluations, some participants can be expected to have sexually transmitted diseases (STDs). Researchers should be testing for STDs as part of the protocol because STDs may be a confounder or an adverse effect of the study intervention. Treatment for STDs is simple, and it would be convenient for the study participants to receive it from the researchers rather than a local source of medical care. It also would strengthen the validity of the study to document exactly what treatment was given.

In contrast, although TB and malaria are common in the host country, they are not as tightly linked to the study topic. Hence the obligation of researchers to provide care is weaker for the latter conditions.

The intensity and duration of the researcher-participant relationship

The stronger the researcher-participant relationship, arguably the stronger is the researcher's responsibility to participants. And the more that a participant has done for a study, the stronger is the reciprocal obligation of the researchers to provide ancillary care.

STUDY 22.2   (Continued).

Researchers will have a strong relationship with participants. They will spend considerable time educating women about the proper use of the microbicide and answering their questions about this intimate intervention. This close relationship creates greater responsibilities to provide ancillary care.

The relative cost of ancillary care relative to the study budget

Researchers should try to write into their budget the costs of justified ancillary care. However, it would be unreasonable to expect researchers to spend so much time and study resources on ancillary care that they compromise the goal of obtaining generalizable knowledge.

STUDY 22.2   (Continued).

Treating STDs does not require follow-up visits or high costs. Although some study sponsors (such as the NIH) do not allow funds to be used for clinical care, a strong argument can be made that treating STDs is justified for research purposes as well as clinical purposes. In contrast, treating a chronic illness such as TB is more complicated and costly, requiring many follow-up visits.

The Extent of Ancillary Care Obligations

Researchers should first inform participants of other conditions they discover, explain what further care would be desirable, and arrange for additional care. In general, it is desirable to have participants receive ancillary care from providers outside the study site to prevent confusion over the researcher's role. If the host country has a functioning health care system for the problem, referral would be sufficient. Dilemmas arise when, as often occurs in resource-poor countries, this is not the case. One option is for researchers to collaborate with a local hospital, for example, by establishing a research or demonstration project for conditions that would be unfeasible to treat at the research site, such as TB. Alternatively, the investigators could volunteer to serve as physicians or teachers at the hospital or clinic to improve the quality of care there.

Providing ancillary care only to trial participants but not to others in the community where the trial is conducted will widen health disparities in the resource-poor host country. Exacerbating health disparities violates the principles of justice (13). Thus, researchers who provide ancillary care should do so in a way that ameliorates rather than worsens health disparities within the host country (13).

STUDY 22.2 **(Continued).**

Researchers should provide ART to trial participants who develop incident HIV infection in a manner that would ameliorate health disparities. If researchers provide ART to participants at the research site, women in the trial who seroconvert will have much better care than women in the community who also develop HIV infection. Instead, it would be preferable for researchers to arrange to have research participants receive care through the country's national HIV program and provide funds to do so if necessary. If the country does not need additional funding, researchers should provide an amount equivalent to the cost of antiretrovirals to improve the quality of care, for example, by reducing waiting times or improving transportation to national clinics.

Even in situations where researchers have no ethical obligation to provide ancillary care, it is praiseworthy for them to do so. Many researchers carrying out studies in resource-poor countries have devoted considerable time and energy to raising the standard of clinical care in the community where they conduct their research; this is to be commended and encouraged.

STUDY 22.2 **(Continued).**

Although a researcher has only weak obligations to persons who are not study participants, there are humanitarian reasons to prevent serious disease in children, which would be more severe in the context of concomitant HIV infection acquired through mother-to-child transmission. Researchers could partner with charitable agencies that provide children with insecticide-treated mosquito nets to prevent malaria.

WILL PARTICIPANTS AND COMMUNITIES RECEIVE FAIR BENEFITS?

Because participants in a research study help researchers, sponsors, and society at large, they should receive some benefit in return as a matter of reciprocity. Advocates contend that researchers and sponsors must avoid taking unfair advantage of participants and their communities by providing those who bear the risks of research appropriate benefits, in addition to the long-term benefit of generalizable knowledge.

AVAILABILITY OF THE STUDY INTERVENTION AFTER THE TRIAL

Researchers and sponsors need to consider whether the study intervention will be available in the host country if it is shown to be effective and safe.

| STUDY 22.3 | **Recombinant surfactant in infants wth respiratory distress syndrome (RDS).** |

In 2001, the manufacturer of a new recombinant surfactant proposed a randomized placebo-controlled trial in infants with RDS, a common life-threatening condition in premature infants. The study would be conducted in Latin America. In a three-arm trial, the other groups would receive placebo and an approved surfactant drug. In the developed world, natural surfactants are the standard of care for this condition, and a placebo-controlled trial would be considered unethical. Critics condemned the study as "exploitative" and charged that developing countries would not be able to afford the drug after the trial.

The sponsor responded that the premature babies in the placebo arm would receive much better care than they would outside the trial in a country with few neonatal intensive care units (ICUs). Thus, participants in the control group would be much better off than if the trial were not carried out. The placebo design would shorten the trial by about 2 years, saving many lives in the long run if the recombinant drug were proven effective. If the study drug proved successful, the sponsor promised to supply the drug at a little above cost for 10 years and also to provide training and equipment.

Study 22.3 raised several ethical concerns. Similarly to Study 22.1, the placebo arm of the trial was sharply attacked. Critics argued that better prenatal and obstetrical care is a much higher priority in resource-poor countries than neonatal intensive care. Thus, the placebo arm could not be justified (unlike Study 22.1) on the grounds that it was required to address a pressing public health priority in the host country.

An additional concern was access to the study intervention after the trial if it proved to be effective. The costs of the recombinant surfactant and ICUs would be prohibitive except for wealthy persons. Furthermore, the market for the drug would be much larger in developed countries than in the poor country where the trial was carried out. Thus, although the participants in Latin America would bear the risks of the trial, wealthier nations would obtain most of the benefits of the knowledge gained. This discrepancy violates the principle of justice.

To avoid such unfairness, some have proposed that if a trial shows that the study intervention is effective and safe, it should be made reasonably available in the host country (14). In this view, because the participants helped the researchers, sponsor, and society at large, they should receive some benefit in return. One proposed standard is *reasonable access* after the conclusion of the trial to treatments proven to be effective in the host country.

A number of practical and conceptual issues need to be worked out regarding reasonable availability or fair benefits.

When is an Intervention Proven to be Effective?

Usually the results of a single clinical trial do not change clinical practice. In general, favorable results from a clinical trial need to be replicated or confirmed in other research. Thus, it may be premature to introduce an intervention as a new standard of care on the basis of a single clinical trial.

To Whom Should an Effective Intervention be Made Accessible?

For participants in the active arm of a trial, the case for continued access would be particularly strong if the drug improved clinical symptoms in a chronic illness; it would be callous to withdraw the drug and allow relapse to occur. However, approval of a new drug in the host country is beyond the sponsor's control and may require additional clinical trials. Thus sponsors are not in a position to guarantee post-trial access—they can only make good-faith efforts to provide it.

Participants in the control group, who have provided crucial outcomes data for the trial, have a strong reason to receive the investigational agent after the termination of the trial if it is medically appropriate. The argument again is based on reciprocity: all participants in a clinical trial deserve some personal benefit in return for their contributions. In Study 22.3, however, infants in the control group would not be eligible for surfactant at the conclusion of the trial.

Other persons in the community where a trial is carried out, who did not participate in the trial, have weaker claims to access to the investigational agent. Their contributions were substantially less than those of the participants. Furthermore, it would require a much greater commitment of resources to provide the study agent to such a large number of people.

What Constitutes Reasonable Access to the Study Intervention?

The term "reasonable access" is ambiguous. Must the new drug be free to host country citizens, or may the sponsor make it available at its cost? In Study 22.3, the cost to the manufacturer for the recombinant surfactant would still be prohibitive in an impoverished country. In addition, the cost of ICU equipment and staffing is considerable. Yet another question to be addressed is, how long after the conclusion of the trial should the researcher and sponsor make the intervention accessible?

Many discussions regarding reasonable access fail to take into account that rigorous evidence of the efficacy and safety of an intervention often set in motion forces that result in lower prices and new resources to provide the intervention. The hepatitis B vaccine and ART to prevent mother-to-child transmission of HIV infection are widely available today in developing countries because costs dropped sharply after pivotal trials were published and more resources became available to purchase them, not because they were guaranteed at the onset of the trial.

Who is Responsible for Ensuring Reasonable Access?

No single stakeholder has both the means and the resources to guarantee reasonable access (13). Although researchers are the public face of the trial, they do not have the long-term financial resources to guarantee access. Some sponsors, particularly large multinational drug companies, may be able to afford to pay for access to the intervention. However, small biotechnology startup companies may not be able to do so. The NIH cannot ensure post-trial access because it is forbidden by law to pay for the costs of clinical care. Finally, the host-country government plays a crucial role because only it has the authority to approve a new drug and provide the medical infrastructure to deliver it. In some cases, an argument could be made that the government's responsibility to basic provide health care to its population should include covering a new drug in its national health program or trying to obtain external funds to cover it.

Overly high expectations to ensure reasonable availability of the study drug during the planning of a clinical trial will be counterproductive if they delay well-designed and ethically responsible clinical trials to evaluate a promising intervention.

In summary, none of these questions regarding post-trial access to a study drug have a definitive answer. Reasonable arguments can be made on both sides. The appropriate resolution will depend on the specifics of the situation and will need to be negotiated by the stakeholders.

FAIR BENEFITS

Some ethics experts point out that providing reasonable access to study interventions after a trial may be an inadequate reciprocation for participation in research. First, it is too limited and weak an obligation. If the study is something other than a pivotal clinical trial (for example, an epidemiological study), no additional benefits will be required. Even if the study is a clinical trial, it might be a negative study. Second, other benefits might be more useful to participants or their communities than the trial drug. For example, they might benefit more from better primary care or better education for host country health care workers. Third, the appropriate target group for benefits may be all persons in the community where the study is carried out, not just trial participants. Providing benefits only to trial participants will widen health disparities in the resource-poor host country and therefore raise concerns about causing injustice (13). Thus, providing benefits to the host country should be done in a way that ameliorates rather than worsens health disparities.

For these reasons, some writers argue that researchers and sponsors from the developed world should provide fair benefits to the research participants and their communities in reciprocity for what they contribute to the research (14). Otherwise, researchers and sponsors would be taking unfair advantage of them. "Fair benefits" is a broader and more flexible concept than reasonable access to the study intervention. Researchers could provide benefits to research participants in a number of ways, such as by providing health education or some basic health services; training local health care workers, researchers, and IRBs; donating equipment at the end of the study; and giving local investigators a key role in analyzing data and writing papers. Such contributions ensure that the community where the research is carried out will receive benefits in reciprocity for participating in the research. By building infrastructure, researchers can help provide sustainable improvements that will help to narrow health disparities between rich and poor nations.

The type and amount of such collateral benefits to participants and communities should be negotiated among the sponsor, investigators, and host-country stakeholders before the study is launched. To overcome disparities in negotiating power, agreements should be made public so that other communities and countries will know what benefits might be achieved.

STUDY 22.3 **(Continued).**

Because of concerns about fairness, this trial was not carried out as proposed. Instead, an international multicenter RCT was conducted at sites in developed as well as developing nations. The control group in all countries received a currently approved form of surfactant.

Conducting the trial in both developed and developing countries resolved concerns about exploitation of vulnerable participants and communities, because participants in developed countries that would benefit from the intervention also assumed the risks of the clinical trial.

Under a framework of fair benefits rather than reasonable access, investigators could provide benefits to the communities where the trial was conducted by building pediatric ICUs and clinical laboratories, improving prenatal care, and training health care workers. Arguably, these measures will provide a broader-based and more durable benefit to the community than promising access to the study drug.

ARE THERE BARRIERS TO INFORMED CONSENT?

Investigators in developing countries can overcome the challenges of obtaining informed consent, as the following study illustrates (2,15).

STUDY 22.4 **Prevention of postpartum hemorrhage.**

Worldwide, more than 150,000 women die each year from postpartum hemorrhage. The majority of these deaths occur in developing countries, almost exclusively in women who give birth outside of hospitals. An RCT was conducted to compare oral misoprostol, a prostaglandin analogue, with placebo in postpartum hemorrhage in women in rural India. In this setting, most pregnant women have no access to physicians and hospital facilities. Auxiliary nurse midwives perform deliveries at home or at village centers, but are not permitted to give injections. Oxytocin, the standard of care in the developed world for postpartum hemorrhage, requires refrigeration and injection, and therefore is not feasible in resource-poor countries. Previous clinical trials in developed countries showed that misoprostol is safe and effective, though somewhat less effective than injectable oxytocin. Because the drug costs about $1 a dose and does not require refrigeration, it can be used in resource-poor countries.

STUDY 22.4   **(Continued)**

Several ethical concerns were raised about this trial. First, was a placebo ethically appropriate in light of the known effectiveness of oxytocin? Second, were the risks to participants acceptable? All participants with severe hemorrhage were provided access to a hospital, where transfusion, surgical procedures, and ICUs were available. Third, could informed consent be obtained in this setting from illiterate women who traditionally defer to their husbands and mothers-in-law? The study was approved by the Ministry of Health in India and the ethics board of a local medical school.

In this clinical trial, the use of placebo in a resource-poor country was ethically justified even though an effective treatment was available in developed countries. A comparison between oxytocin and misoprostol was not relevant to the clinical and public health question posed in this study: Is an oral drug more effective than no treatment at all (the currently available level of care in this setting)?

Study 22.4 illustrates the challenges of obtaining informed consent in resource-poor countries (15). A purely individual approach to informed consent is not appropriate in many cultures. In some cultures, people regard themselves primarily as members of a family or community, rather than as autonomous individuals. People might not make important decisions by themselves, and instead consult with others or defer to their opinion. In such cultures, participants should be offered the options of consulting with others about the decision to participate in research or allowing others to make the decision. In Study 22.4, researchers needed the approval of village elders and leaders to carry out the study. Furthermore, in rural India, women traditionally defer to their husband or mother-in-law and do not make decisions independently of their families. Researchers should allow participants to choose whether to involve these family members in the consent process. Ultimately, however, a woman must have the right to refuse to participate in research, even if others want her to participate (1). Researchers should devise a consent process that protects participants from undue influence or coercion and protects women who disagree with their family against reprisal. In some cases, a woman might want to participate in research despite the objection of others. Researchers need to ascertain that she understands the psychosocial risks in this situation and take steps to minimize those risks, for example, by heightening confidentiality protections. However, as with any informed adult, she should be allowed to enroll in the study if she wishes.

STUDY 22.4   **(Continued).**

Women were allowed to consult with relatives about participating in the trial. If she wished, a woman was permitted to obtain her husband's approval to participate. However, no one was entered into the study without her individual consent. Consent discussions were carried out in the local language. To protect illiterate women, a relative had to witness the consent procedure.

Detailed consent forms might serve little purpose in low-literacy populations. Although careful translation and back-translation of consent forms are necessary, they are not sufficient to ensure that the consent process is culturally appropriate. Moreover, insisting on signatures or thumbprints may alarm some participants, who fear that the document could be used against them later (for example, if there is a change in the government) (1). Participants may also suspect that they are giving away something. Instead of requiring a signature or fingerprint, researchers could have persons who are independent of the study witness the consent process.

Steps can be taken to enhance informed consent from poorly educated persons in resource-poor countries (16). Stakeholders in the host country, such as community-based organizations, can identify common misconceptions and concerns about the trial and offer suggestions for improving the consent process and explaining difficult terms. For instance, to explain randomization, investigators have used the analogy of testing fertilizers or new seeds on randomized plots.

Innovative means of communicating information, such as street theater and group meetings where people can ask questions, can precede and supplement individual discussions with potential participants (1).

Researchers should administer a questionnaire to participants to ascertain whether they understand key features of the study (16). Although disclosing information about a research study is necessary, the key ethical issue is whether the participants comprehend the disclosed information. If potential participants fail to show adequate comprehension, researchers should hold additional discussions with them until they achieve an acceptable level of understanding.

STUDY 22.4   (Continued).

This trial showed that misoprostol was effective at reducing the incidence of postpartum hemorrhage (from 12.0% to 6.4%) (2). One case was prevented for every 18 women treated.

IS THE IRB REVIEW RIGOROUS?

In some clinical trials in resource-poor countries, the IRB review and approval process may fail to achieve the goal of protecting participants.

STUDY 22.5   Oral antibiotic for meningococcal meningitis.

During a 1996 epidemic of meningococcal meningitis in Nigeria, an RCT was conducted to compare a new oral antibiotic, trovafloxacin, with injections of ceftriaxone, a standard therapy for children with this life-threatening infection. At the time of the study, trovafloxacin was not approved by the FDA and had been given orally to only one child. The study drug was to be given to half the participants as either an oral solution or an intravenous formulation. Due to a shortage of nurses, the control antibiotic was usually given intramuscularly rather than intravenously. Because these intramuscular shots were very painful, children commonly received lower than standard dosages. The protocol did not include a second lumbar puncture to assess response after the antibiotic was started.

Many parents were illiterate. Allegedly, they were told that it was a new medicine and that they could say no, but were not told that the antibiotic was investigational and that standard care was available nearby at a medical camp run by a humanitarian organization.

One 10-year-old girl died after receiving the oral form of the experimental antibiotic. The day after receiving the drug, she developed weakness and cranial nerve palsies. Her treatment was not changed after her symptoms worsened. She died on the third day after starting the intervention. Overall mortality rates in the control and intervention arms were both around 6%, comparable to outcomes in U.S. hospitals and at the local medical facility.

U.S. employees of the pharmaceutical manufacturer who sponsored the study flew into the country to carry out the study and left after 3 weeks, when the treatment phase was concluded. They returned 4–6 weeks later for follow-up visits. Although the company said it was trying to respond quickly to the epidemic, critics said that during the epidemic the country needed more resources for standard care, not a hastily planned research study.

The study files contained a letter of approval from an ethics committee at a local teaching hospital. However, the hospital later said it had no ethics committee at the time the trial was carried out.

An oral antibiotic that is effective against meningococcal meningitis would greatly benefit resource-poor countries, where outbreaks occur but intravenous medications generally are not feasible. Although an oral antibiotic would not be used in the United States to treat meningitis, data from the trial could support FDA approval of the oral form of drug in children with other infections.

Ethical concerns about Study 22.5 included not only the previously discussed issues of unacceptable risks and inadequate informed consent, but also lax oversight and a one-sided relationship between the sponsor and in-country stakeholders.

STUDY 22.5   (Continued).

In this trial, the risks were unacceptable because of the lack of pharmacokinetic data in children, the lack of follow-up lumbar punctures to identify children who were not responding, and, most seriously, the absence of a plan to switch nonresponders to another antibiotic. The fact that overall mortality levels were good in both arms does not excuse these shortcomings in the study design.

With regard to informed consent, it is inappropriate to characterize an investigational agent as a "new medicine." Potential participants should have been informed that its safety and effectiveness were unknown and that standard care was available nearby through a humanitarian agency.

CHALLENGES IN IRB REVIEW

Review by a panel that is independent of the investigators is a fundamental protection for participants. Careful scientific and ethical reviews should identify problems with risks and consent. However, studies designed by pharmaceutical companies may be reviewed only in house, not by independent experts. FDA reviews for new drugs and new indications for licensed drugs typically focus on design issues rather than ethical concerns.

A U.S. IRB may not understand conditions in the host country and thus may not appreciate the relevance of the study there, problems with the administration of study medications, the clinical alternatives available at the study site, or the need for a salvage regimen.

IRB review in the host country is intended to address some of these shortcomings of IRB review in the United States. However, in many resource-poor countries, IRBs often lack training in research ethics, experience in reviewing complicated protocols, and resources to carry out their work. For example, photocopying documents or sending them electronically to committee members may not be feasible.

STUDY 22.5   (Continued).

For this trial, there evidently was no local IRB. Forging IRB approval would be a grave violation of ethical and legal standards.

FACILITATING IRB REVIEW

Researchers can facilitate IRB review of international studies if they take the initiative to provide the U.S. IRB with background information they will need to conduct their review. The U.S. IRB needs to understand how the research context in the host country differs from that in the U.S. The IRB must then consider how those differences will affect its judgments about the informed consent process and the risks and benefits of the research. Investigators might provide the following specific information:

1. What are the options for medical care for the condition being studied in the country where the research will be carried out?
2. What increased psychosocial risks do participants in the host country face, compared with risks participants in the U.S. would face if the study were carried out there? For example, risks might be greater because of weaker confidentiality protections or greater stigma. How will the investigators minimize these additional risks?
3. What are barriers to informed and free consent in the host country that are not present in the U.S.? Potential issues include low literacy, non-Western beliefs about illness and health care, atti-

tudes toward written contracts and signatures, and the role of third parties, such as spouses or village elders, in decision-making. There may be sources of undue influence or coercion that would not be present in the U.S. How will the investigators minimize these barriers?

4. If subjects will be paid for participating in the study, what does the amount means in terms of an average or living wage in the host country? An amount that would not be an undue influence in the U.S. may be so in the host country.

ARE STAKEHOLDERS IN THE HOST COUNTRY PARTNERS?

Research in resource-poor settings is best viewed as a partnership between investigators and sponsors from the developed world and stakeholders in the host country. This would include scientists, clinicians, public and patient representatives, community groups, and government officials (17–19). Ideally, these stakeholders would be involved in the research, beginning with the planning phase. WHO and UNAIDS urge communities to be involved "in an early and sustained manner in the design, development, implementation, and distribution of results" of a trial (9,20). This should be "an open, iterative, collaborative process that involves a wide variety of participants," and generally will require "outreach and engagement measures to support participation." Various terms have been used to refer to this cluster of related ideas, such as community engagement, community participation, and community involvement (18,19,21). Similarly, different models of collaboration have been used, including community advisory boards and working with existing civil society organizations.

Host-country partners can help U.S. researchers understand the needs of the host country, risks associated with conditions in the country that may not be apparent to persons from developed nations, concerns that potential participants might have about the study, and barriers to recruitment, informed consent, and follow-up. In addition, stakeholders might suggest how to overcome these challenges, improve the study design, and help design an ethically appropriate recruitment and consent process.

STUDY 22.5   (Continued).

The researchers were accused of exploiting third-world persons. The protocol was developed in the U.S. and presented to Nigerian authorities for their approval as a finished product. Local physicians said they had no opportunity to suggest changes to address the ethical problems in the protocol.

Research team meetings should be conducted in ways that promote partnerships (17). In many countries, people receive deference based on age, experience, social status, and gender; this might frustrate efforts to elicit feedback and discussion. Those who chair meetings might need to explicitly invite people from developing countries to give their views, ask junior people to speak before more senior people have stated their position, or ask participants about their views in private as well as in group meetings.

STUDY 22.5   (Continued).

Two years after the trial was conducted, a multisite international clinical trial of trovafloxacin for meningitis was conducted in the U.S. as well as at sites in Latin America, South Africa, and Hungary. All the above ethical problems were corrected. An intravenous formulation was used. The protocol included follow-up lumbar punctures, and nonresponders were switched to another antibiotic. Trovafloxacin was, for a time, widely prescribed in the U.S. However, because it was found to cause fatal liver toxicity, its use was later limited to severe infections caused by multiresistant bacteria.

TAKE HOME POINTS

1. Vast discrepancies in wealth between developed and developing countries raise concerns about research carried out in resource-poor countries by investigators and sponsors from developed countries.

2. To ensure that such trials are ethically sound, researchers must carefully consider the use of placebos, the provision of background and ancillary care, informed consent, access to the study intervention after the trial, and collaboration with host-country stakeholders.

ANNOTATED BIBLIOGRAPHY

Lo B, Bayer R. Establishing ethical trials for treatment and prevention of AIDS in developing countries. *BMJ* 2003;327:337–339.
  Argues that stakeholders in the host country should be involved in the project from the early planning stages.
Miller FG, Mello MM, Joffe S. Incidental findings in human subjects research: what do investigators owe research participants? *J Law Med Ethics* 2008;36:271–279.
  Analyzes the arguments supporting different theories about what investigators owe research participants as a matter of fairness.
UNAIDS. Good participatory practice guidelines for biomedical HIV prevention trials. 2007. Available at: http:// data.unaids.org/pub/Manual/2007/jc1364_good_participatory_guidelines_en.pdf. Accessed May 9, 2008.
  Detailed guidelines for involving community groups in prevention trials.
Woodsong C, Karim QA. A model designed to enhance informed consent: experiences from the HIV prevention trials network. *Am J Public Health* 2005;95:412–419.
  Researchers should administer a questionnaire to ensure that participants understand the key features of a study.

REFERENCES

1. National Bioethics Advisory Commission. *Ethical and Policy Issues in International Research*. Rockville, MD: National Bioethics Advisory Commission; 2001.
2. Derman RJ, Kodkany BS, Goudar SS, et al. Oral misoprostol in preventing postpartum haemorrhage in resource-poor communities: a randomised controlled trial. *Lancet* 2006;368:1248–1253.
3. Page-Shafer K, Saphonn V, Sun L, Vun M, Cooper D, Kaldor J. HIV prevention research in a resource-limited setting: the experience of planning a trial in Cambodia. *Lancet* 2005;366:1499–1503.
4. Shaffer N, Chuachoowong R, Mock PA, et al. Short-course zidovudine for perinatal HIV-1 transmission in Bangkok, Thailand: a randomised controlled trial. Bangkok Collaborative Perinatal HIV Transmission Study Group. *Lancet* 1999;353:773–780.
5. Wiktor SZ, Ekpini E, Karon JM, et al. Short-course oral zidovudine for prevention of mother-to-child transmission of HIV-1 in Abidjan, Côte d'Ivoire: a randomised trial. *Lancet* 1999;353:781–785.
6. Lurie P, Wolfe SM. Unethical trials of interventions to reduce perinatal transmission of the human immunodeficiency virus in developing countries. *N Engl J Med* 1997;853–856.
7. Angell M. The ethics of clinical research in the third world. *N Engl J Med* 1997;337:847–849.
8. World Medical Association. Declaration of Helsinki. 2004. Available at: http://www.wma.net/e/ethicsunit/helsinki.htm. Accessed August 30, 2008.
9. UNAIDS/WHO. Ethical considerations in biomedical HIV prevention trials. 2007. Available at: http://search.unaids.org/Preview.aspx?d=en&u=pub/Report/2007/jc1399-ethicalconsiderations_en.pdf&p=%2fcgi-bin%2fMsmGo.exe%3fgrab_id%3d0%26page_id%3d10082%26query%3dhiv%2520prevention%2520trials%26hiword%3dhiv%2520prevention%2520trials%2520%26PV%3d1. Accessed May 9, 2008.
10. Miller FG, Mello MM, Joffe S. Incidental findings in human subjects research: what do investigators owe research participants? *J Law Med Ethics* 2008;36:271–279.
11. Richardson HS. Gradations of researchers' obligation to provide ancillary care for HIV/AIDS in developing countries. *Am J Public Health* 2007;97:1956–1961.
12. Belsky L, Richardson HS. Medical researchers' ancillary clinical care responsibilities. *BMJ* 2004;328:1494–1496.
13. Lo B, Padian N, Barnes M. The obligation to provide antiretroviral treatment in HIV prevention trials. *AIDS* 2007;21:1229–1231.
14. Emanuel EJ. Benefits to host countries. In: Emanuel EJ, Grady C, Crouch RA, Lie RK, Miller FG, Wendler D, eds. *The Oxford Textbook of Clinical Research Ethics*. New York: Oxford University Press; 2008:719–728.
15. Geller SE, Adams MG, Kelly PJ, Kodkany BS, Derman RJ. Postpartum hemorrhage in resource-poor settings. *Int J Gynaecol Obstet* 2006;92:202–211.

16. Woodsong C, Karim QA. A model designed to enhance informed consent: experiences from the HIV prevention trials network. *Am J Public Health* 2005;95:412–419.
17. Lo B, Bayer R. Establishing ethical trials for treatment and prevention of AIDS in developing countries. *BMJ* 2003;327:337–339.
18. Bhan A, Singh JA, Upshur RE, Singer PA, Daar AS. Grand challenges in global health: engaging civil society organizations in biomedical research in developing countries. *PLoS Med* 2007;4:e272.
19. Tindana PO, Singh JA, Tracy CS, et al. Grand challenges in global health: community engagement in research in developing countries. *PLoS Med* 2007;4:e273.
20. UNAIDS. Good participatory practice guidelines for biomedical HIV prevention trials. 2007. Available at: http://data.unaids.org/pub/Manual/2007/jc1364_good_participatory_guidelines_en.pdf. Accessed May 9, 2008.
21. Morin SF, Maiorana A, Koester KA, Sheon NM, Richards TA. Community consultation in HIV prevention research: a study of community advisory boards at 6 research sites. *J Acquir Immune Defic Syndr* 2003;33:513–520.

Ethical Issues in Specific Types of Research

23

Research With Existing Data and Biological Materials

Using existing health data and biological materials allows researchers to address important research questions more efficiently than if they were to carry out primary data collection. Research using existing data and specimens has helped to establish associations between smoking and lung cancer, between *Helicobacter pylori* and gastric cancer, and between human papilloma virus and cervical cancer (1,2). Secondary data analyses also allow trainees and junior faculty to perform studies quickly and gain valuable research experience. Although such research causes no physical risks, it still raises ethical issues regarding consent and confidentiality.

RESEARCH USING EXISTING DATA

STUDY 23.1	**Review of electronic medical records.**

Researchers wished to study whether patients taking the selective cyclo-oxygenase-2 (COX-2) inhibitors rofecoxib or celecoxib were at greater risk for serious coronary artery disease than patients who were taking the nonselective NSAID naproxen or had discontinued these drugs. The researchers planned to study the computerized medical records of a large health maintenance organization (HMO), which included inpatient and outpatient care and prescriptions. Over a 2-year period, more than 1.3 million patients had filled prescriptions for these medicines. More than 23,000 persons were included in the study. It would be impossible to obtain permission from each person to access their records.

When this study was planned, the evidence regarding the cardiovascular adverse effects of selective and nonselective COX-2 inhibitors was uncertain. A randomized controlled trial (RCT) had shown that rofecoxib increased the risk of myocardial infarction compared to naproxen. However, it was unclear whether COX-2 inhibitors increased cardiac risk or whether naproxen had a protective effect. It would take several years to carry out an RCT to resolve this issue. With the use of existing records, however, it would be possible to address it in a matter of months (3).

Because so many participants were required to answer the research questions in Study 23.1, it was impossible to obtain consent to access their medical records. The justification for conducting such studies without individual informed consent is that the value of the research to society greatly outweighs the disrespect to persons whose data are used without their knowledge or permission.

In research using existing data and materials, the risks can be made very small. The primary risk is a breach of confidentiality, which may lead in turn to psychosocial harms, including stigma and discrimination. These risks are usually smaller than those of observational or interventional studies, which involve time, inconvenience, and, in many cases, physical risks.

STUDY 23.1   **(Continued).**

In this study, rofecoxib increased the relative risk of serious coronary disease by 1.59 compared to celecoxib. Naproxen did not protect against coronary disease compared to past use of NSAIDs. Study 23.1 had a major impact on the nation's health by supporting the withdrawal of rofecoxib from the market.

WHEN IS INFORMED CONSENT NOT REQUIRED?

If the study involves only existing data or specimens that were collected for a purpose other than the specific research project, consent may not be needed in certain situations. In Chapter 6 we discussed the federal regulations regarding informed consent, including the exceptions to consent. Because these regulations are complicated, in this chapter we present a practical series of questions researchers can ask to determine whether consent is needed in a study involving only existing data or specimens (see Fig. 23.1).

ARE THE DATA OR SPECIMENS PUBLICLY AVAILABLE?

For research with existing data and specimens, the risks are invasion of privacy and breach of confidentiality. If the data and specimens are publicly available, the research is exempt from the Common Rule because it poses no additional risks to the privacy or confidentiality of participants. For example, the federal government makes certain information from the census and various national health surveys publicly available. These data sets are constructed in a manner that ensures that participants cannot be identified.

ARE THE DATA OR SPECIMENS IDENTIFIABLE?

A project is not considered human subjects research if researchers cannot link existing data or specimens to identifiable individuals, either directly through overt identifiers (such as name or Social Security number) or indirectly through codes. Therefore, the Common Rule and HIPAA do not apply, and consent is not required. Data and specimens may not be identifiable in several situations.

Data and Specimens Were Collected Anonymously

If the data or specimens were collected anonymously without any identifiers, the federal regulations consider them not identifiable and therefore not human subjects research.

Data are Recorded so That Participants Cannot be Identified

Although investigators may have access to identifiable information, they can record the research data in such a manner that the participants cannot be identified. For instance, a researcher may review medical records but record the data for subjects 001, 002, etc., with no link whatsoever between these numbers for subjects and their identities. In other words, there is no key to determine who subject 001 is.

Data and Specimens are De-identified

The data or specimens may have been collected without identifiers, but the identifiers were removed before the researcher receives them. Historically, the removal of explicit identifiers, such as name, address, telephone number, Social Security number, and medical record number, has sufficed to de-identify data or specimens. The HIPAA privacy regulations set stricter standards: a de-identified health data set may not contain 18 specified identifiers, not even the last two digits of zip codes and dates more specific than the year.

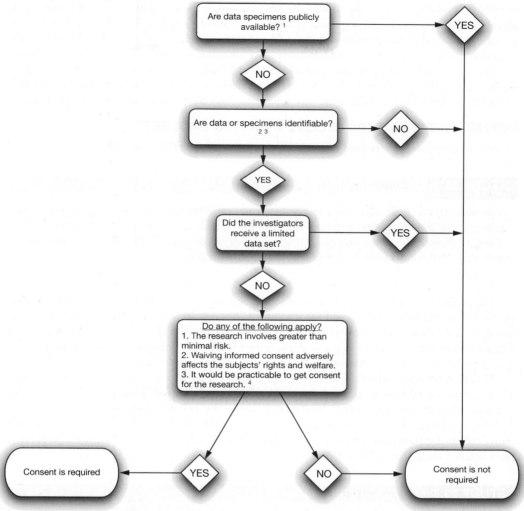

FIGURE 23.1. Is informed consent required for research involving only existing data and specimens?

[1] If yes, the activity is exempt from federal regulations on human subjects research
[2] If no, activity is not human subjects research
[3] If using coded data or specimens, this may be accomplished if:
a.) The key to deciphering the code is destroyed before the research begins
b.) The investigator and the key-holder agree to prohibit the release of the key to the investigator
c.) There are institutional, legal and/or IRB-approved policies prohibiting the release of the key to researchers
[4] If none of the criteria apply to the research project, it qualifies for a waiver of informed consent.

Data and Specimens are Coded, but Investigators Have no Access to a Link to Decipher the Code

Electronic medical records systems, repositories, and biobanks, which store identified specimens or data, may provide researchers with nonidentifiable coded materials and data without explicit consent from the persons whose data or specimens are released. There are three ways to render the data and specimens nonidentifiable. First, the repository may destroy the key to decipher the code before the research begins. Second, the researcher and the repository may negotiate an agreement prohibiting release of the code to the investigators. Third, the repository may have written policies, approved by the IRB, to prohibit release of the code to the investigators, or there may be other legal requirements prohibiting release. An exception is made to allow the release of identifying information after the subjects die (because deceased persons are not considered human subjects). The issue for IRBs is how the researcher receives data and specimens, not how they are stored in the medical record or repository.

The terms "unlinked" and "anonymized" are used loosely to refer to data or specimens whose identifiers have been removed. Rather than use such ambiguous terms, researchers should specify precisely which identifiers have been removed and whether they have access to a key to decipher codes.

DID THE INVESTIGATORS RECEIVE A LIMITED DATA SET?

In some projects, researchers need information that is one of the HIPAA identifiers.

STUDY 23.1   (Continued).

The researchers must have the exact dates when patients received medications from the pharmacy and experienced coronary endpoints. A de-identified data set would not allow them to answer their research questions. However, researchers may obtain a limited data set without obtaining explicit permission from the participants.

The project may still be carried out without explicit authorization from the persons whose data are used if the researchers obtain and use a so-called "limited data set." Limited data sets may contain dates and full zip codes (but not the other 16 HIPAA-specified identifiers). To obtain a limited data set, researchers must agree to use or disclose the information only for a specific purpose, to use appropriate confidentiality safeguards, and to not identify or contact the participants.

The disadvantage of a limited data set is that it can only be used for a specific research purpose. The researchers would not be permitted to use the data set to study a different research question, for example, whether selective COX-2 inhibitors decrease the risk of developing colorectal cancer. Prohibiting additional analyses of the data set can reduce the efficiency of research without significantly enhancing protection of the persons whose data are being analyzed. Chapter 7 contains a more detailed discussion of limited data sets.

STUDY 23.1   (Continued).

The data manager for the HMO may give the investigators a data set that identifies individuals as 001, 002, etc., and destroy the code linking these study numbers to the participants' identities. In this study, the investigators need exact dates of hospitalization and prescriptions to calculate the time between receiving a prescription and having a clinical event. Thus the researchers need to sign an agreement to obtain a limited data set.

DOES THE RESEARCH QUALIFY FOR A WAIVER OF INFORMED CONSENT?

In some research studies, researchers need to have identifiable information about participants. Although the previous exceptions to informed consent do not apply, it may be permissible to carry out the research without informed consent for other reasons.

STUDY 23.2   Retaining identifiers to link to the National Death Registry.

In Study 23.1, the researchers want to link information about participants from the HMO to information in the National Death Registry to identify persons who died outside the HMO. To do so, they need explicit identifiers such as name and Social Security number.

TABLE 23.1	Waiver of Informed Consent

Informed consent may be waived or modified if all of the following criteria are met:

1. The research involves no more than minimal risk to the subjects.
2. The waiver or alteration will not adversely affect the rights and welfare of the subjects.
3. The research cannot practicably be carried out without the waiver or alteration.
4. Whenever appropriate, the subjects will be provided with additional pertinent information after participation.

May this study be carried out without permission from the thousands of patients whose records are being studied? The researchers need identifiers to combine information from different data sets. The study cannot be conducted if consent from all of these persons is required. Another common example is retaining identifiers to link Medicare databases to state databases of hospital discharge summaries, which contain discharge diagnoses. When identifiers are retained, the risk of a breach of confidentiality is increased.

Under the Common Rule, human subjects research may qualify for a waiver or modification of informed consent if all of the four criteria in Table 23.1 are satisfied. Figure 23.1 simplifies this regulatory language.

The fourth criterion in Table 23.1 is intended for research that involves deception of participants, and does not apply to research with existing data or specimens.

The HIPAA privacy regulations have somewhat different requirements for a waiver or modification of consent:

1. The use or disclosure of the protected health information presents minimal risk to the privacy of individuals.
2. The research cannot practicably be conducted without the waiver or alteration of authorization.
3. The research cannot practicably be conducted without access to and use of the protected health information.

In practice, provided that researchers use appropriate security protections, the HIPAA requirements are met when the Common Rule criteria are satisfied (4). One difference is that under the HIPAA regulations, coded information is not considered identifiable if the code was generated from identifying information. For example, the code may not contain the last four digits of a participant's Social Security number.

STUDY 23.2	(Continued).

This study meets the regulatory criteria for waiving consent. The risk of the study is a breach of confidentiality, and this risk is minimal (i.e., no greater than the risks of daily life and routine medical tests) provided that adequate confidentiality protections are taken. Protections should include training research staff, establishing careful and explicit procedures for combining data sets, and, in some studies, obtaining a federal certificate of confidentiality. The rights and welfare of the patients whose computerized records are studied will be respected if no identifiers are given to researchers and if the IRB or privacy board approves the study. It would be impractical to try to obtain consent from the large number of participants needed to achieve adequate power to answer the research question. Moreover, attempts to obtain consent are likely to introduce bias into the study. Finally, the research cannot be carried out without access to this information.

CONCERNS ABOUT RESEARCH WITH EXISTING MATERIALS

The use of existing biological materials allows investigators to study important research questions efficiently without harming or wronging the donors of the materials.

STUDY 23.3	Use of existing pathological specimens.

In women with breast cancer, amplification of the human epidermoid growth factor receptor type 2 (HER2) is associated with a poor clinical prognosis. Trastuzumab (Herceptin) is a monoclonal antibody directed against a region of the HER2 protein product. Clinical trials showed a benefit of Trastuzumab in women with advanced breast cancers that overexpress the HER2 protein. The test used in these trials is a research test that is not feasible to use in clinical practice. Researchers wish to test the accuracy of a simpler test for HER2 using 600 tumor tissue specimens from pathology archives. The specimens will be de-identified so that researchers will receive no identifying information about the women.

Many women had not specifically consented to have their tumor tissue used for research, although they had signed admission papers allowing the hospital to use tissue left over after clinical tests were carried out for teaching or research. The surgical consent form also contained a sentence allowing materials removed at surgery but not needed for clinical care to be used for teaching and research.

Trastuzumab therapy is typically considered when women develop metastases. Because biopsies are usually not performed on metastatic lesions, HER2 testing generally must be done on archived specimens from the primary tumor. Because the specimens for Study 23.3 have already been obtained and will be irreversibly de-identified, the risks are extremely low and far less than the potential benefits of the research.

Although the women had signed forms to be admitted to the hospital or to have surgery that mentioned the use of removed tissue for research, it would be disingenuous to claim that women had provided informed consent for research such as Study 23.3. Patients typically do not read such consent forms carefully, because they need medical care and tend to regard the consent form as a mere formality. Moreover, patients are not told what might be involved if their tissue is used for research, what kinds of studies might be done, or what the risks might be. Without such information, a patient's decision to donate her tissue will not be truly informed. Furthermore, patients may not appreciate that they can obtain medical care without allowing their specimens to be used for research.

RATIONALE FOR USING DATA AND SPECIMENS WITHOUT CONSENT

There are several ethical justifications for allowing researchers to use de-identified data and materials without consent if participants cannot be identified. First, there can be no breach of confidentiality. Thus the risks of research are very small, and the benefits of research should not be foregone simply because it is impractical to get consent from participants. The benefits of the research to society are judged to outweigh the small risk of a breach of confidentiality and the dignitary harm of using a person's medical information without her consent. Second, it is assumed that almost all people would allow their de-identified data or biological materials to be used in such a manner. Indeed, empirical studies have shown support for such research using existing data and specimens (5). However, it is not known how well respondents understand what kinds of research might be done (6). Furthermore, respondents have not been specifically asked whether they would object to having their specimens used in research that is controversial or, to some persons, objectionable. Third, citizens have a moral obligation to allow their de-identified data or materials to be used in such low-risk research (7). In this view, because everyone benefits from research carried out with existing data and specimens from previous patients, it is only fair for people to allow their data and specimens to be used to benefit others.

However, these rationales may not hold in several circumstances. If the research project includes whole genome sequencing, which is expected to become feasible soon, it might be possible to re-identify the specimens (see Chapter 27). Another concern is that some participants might object to certain uses of their biological materials or clinical data, even if they are de-identified.

Although researchers need to understand and comply with regulatory requirements, they must also appreciate that the regulations do not resolve some important ethical issues regarding consent. In certain situations, an investigator's ethical responsibilities regarding consent may go beyond her legal duties, as in the following project involving de-identified existing specimens.

STUDY 23.4	Derivation of stem cell lines from discarded oocytes.

A researcher is deriving stem cell lines using somatic cell nuclear transfer. The researcher plans to obtain discarded oocytes that failed to fertilize in vitro from an infertility practice. The researcher plans to remove all identifying information from the specimens. Under the Common Rule, this project is not considered human subjects research, and therefore informed consent is not required.

Stem cell research is controversial. Around one-third of Americans oppose embryonic stem cell research because they believe embryos have the moral status of persons. One study reported that about 22% of infertility patients with frozen embryos intended to discard them rather than donate them for stem cell research (8). Furthermore, oocytes may have special significance compared to, for example, cancer tissue removed at surgery. Another study found that about 25% of women who provide oocytes to patients in infertility clinics would not want their oocytes to be used for research (9). Using a person's reproductive materials for purposes to which she would strongly object violates the ethical principle of respect for persons. De-identifying the materials would not overcome her objections. Hence an IRB might decide to not exempt Study 23.4 from the informed consent requirement, even though no identifiable materials would be involved and thus, strictly speaking, it would not be considered human subjects research. This example shows that cutting-edge research that is technically in compliance with the Common Rule may still be ethically problematic.

More generally, some persons may object if existing blood or tissue specimens left over from their clinical care were to be used in research projects they consider offensive (1,10,11). Anonymizing the specimens would not overcome their objections. Other examples of potentially offensive research using de-identified biological materials might include studies on contraception, ovulation, the genetic determinants of violence or criminal behavior, and research on human evolution. In such research, waiving requirements for informed consent would be disrespectful to persons who strongly object for deeply held moral reasons.

STUDY 23.5	Use of samples from a previous study.

Extra tubes of blood from a prospective study of cardiovascular risk in young men have been stored for future research studies. There is also extensive clinical data on the participants, including data on marital status, use of alcohol and illicit drugs, employment, and incarceration. There is oversampling from African-American and Latino men. The participants agreed to allow their samples to be used for future research on heart disease and "other serious medical illnesses affecting young men, such as diabetes or cancer." Now researchers want to use the stored samples and data to identify genes that are associated with substance abuse or criminal behavior, which they operationalize as incarceration.

Study 23.5 raises additional ethical concerns because the topic of study is controversial and the information on participants is highly sensitive. A breach of confidentiality would be more damaging than, for example, a breach of the information on COX-2 inhibitors and heart disease in Study 23.1.

Is it ethically acceptable to carry out Study 23.4 using de-identified existing biological materials without obtaining specific consent? The consent under which the material was originally obtained does not cover the proposed study because criminal behavior is not a medical disease. However, the Common Rule allows research using existing coded samples and data to be carried out without consent provided that the researcher cannot readily identify the participants, for example, if the coordinating center destroys the link between the code and the identities of the participants. Anonymizing the data and materials eliminates the risk of breach of confidentiality.

Even if samples are irreversibly de-identified, in some situations there may still be ethical concerns (see also the Appendix to Chapter 6). Although they cannot be identified as donors, some people may not want the samples and information they provided to be used for a study they consider objectionable or offensive (1,10,11). Some might consider research on genetic predisposition to incarceration a much lower priority than research on the economic and social roots of criminal behavior. Furthermore, people of color might fear that the study will reinforce the stereotype that certain ethnic groups are more likely to engage in crime. They might contend that they would not have given permission for Study 23.5 had they been asked. They certainly did not have such a study in mind when they enrolled in the original study. Nor were they informed during the consent process for donating materials that their data and materials might be used in controversial projects. Still other donors may not want their biological materials to be used in research that might undermine personal responsibility for antisocial behaviors. They may fear that if Study 23.5 found a genetic basis for criminal behavior, society might conclude that people cannot be held responsible or punished for crimes. Furthermore, some people may not want their materials used in studies of human evolution. Hence people with a wide variety of political views might object to using anonymized biological materials for sensitive and controversial studies without specific consent. Because of these objections, it would be ethically preferable to carry out Study 23.5 only on samples from persons who had given specific consent for that type of study.

A rule of thumb for identifying sensitive and controversial research is to consider how donors would respond if they were told explicitly about the project. Might a significant minority of donors—say over 10%—feel wronged or offended that their materials were used for this project? If so, researchers and IRBs should question the use of existing samples without explicit consent. An advisory group representing the communities where the original donors were enrolled could help researchers and the IRB understand objections that might be raised.

HOW TO COLLECT BIOLOGICAL MATERIALS FOR FUTURE RESEARCH

Clinical data and biological materials collected for a research project are a valuable resource for future research. Hence when collecting new data and materials for a study, researchers should consider how to facilitate their use in future projects. The NIH requires applicants to discuss what arrangements will be made to share data and materials with other investigators.

There are several options regarding consent for future studies. It is not practical for participants to provide specific consent for each future research project when it is carried out. Furthermore, some participants may not want to receive multiple requests for consent and may regard repeated contact as an invasion of privacy or an annoyance, even if they do not object to the research. Thus, researchers collecting biological materials should obtain permission to use them in a variety of future projects.

NO CONSENT REQUIRED

As discussed above, no consent is required to use materials that were originally obtained for clinical care but are not needed for that purpose, provided that the participants cannot be identified. Examples include tissue removed at surgery, biopsy materials, and extra tubes of blood (12). These diagnostic or pathologic materials will be removed from the patient whether research is conducted or not, and de-identification eliminates breaches of confidentiality. Furthermore, clinicians performing routine care cannot be expected to set up consent protocols for storing tissues for future research projects.

Under the Common Rule, researchers may use leftover materials that were collected for another research project after de-identifying them, without further permission from the donors. However, when collecting specimens for one research project, investigators should already be considering collecting additional specimens for future studies. To fulfill their ethical requirement to treat research participants with respect, investigators should seek permission for future studies when collecting the original specimens.

GENERAL CONSENT

Participants may give permission for their data and biological materials to be used in any future research studies. In surveys, most individuals (more than 80% in most studies) say they are willing to provide samples for future unspecified research (5). Most are willing to donate materials for research on other diseases, for genetic research, and for research carried out by for-profit organizations (5). General consent makes sense for future projects that almost no one would object to; more elaborate consent procedures would be cumbersome but provide little protection. Such one-time general consent is also consistent with current federal regulations.

However, general consent raises both conceptual and practical concerns. Critics argue that it is not informed consent because donors have little idea of what kinds of research might be done in the future. Researchers cannot specify all future research projects that might be done with biological materials. Donors cannot understand the nature, benefits, or risks of unspecified future projects. As noted above, some people would not want their materials to be used in certain sensitive research, such as Study 23.4 on the genetic basis of criminal behavior, research on embryonic stem cells (see Chapter 6), whole genome sequencing (see Chapter 27), or human evolution (1,10,11). However, donors may not appreciate that such sensitive research could be carried out with materials they provide, or may not have considered this possibility when they gave general consent for research.

Although it is hard to define the term "sensitive research" precisely, one rule of thumb is that a substantial minority of people, say 10%, would object to it. When donors give general consent for future use of their materials, they implicitly trust that IRBs will not allow their tissue to be used in offensive or objectionable research. IRBs are more likely to be aware that some donors might regard a research project as objectionable if they include articulate members from the communities where donors were recruited.

Blanket or general consent is complicated because HIPAA regulations require separate authorization for each use or disclosure of identifiable health information or biological materials (13). To fulfill this requirement, biobanks have several options. One option is to provide researchers with de-identified data sets or limited data sets; however, researchers may need identifying information to carry out their research. Alternatively, biobanks may provide researchers with identifiable data and materials under a waiver of consent or authorization from the IRB or privacy board. Although most institutions will grant such waivers routinely if confidentiality is adequately protected, each research project still requires a separate application.

OPTING OUT

Researchers who are using existing specimens to study sensitive or controversial topics may allow donors to opt out; that is, the research team will try to contact donors to notify them of the research and give them the opportunity to decline to participate. If no objection is voiced, the sample will be used. This process provides a measure of respect to donors of materials beyond what the regulations require. As discussed above, de-identified existing materials may be used for research without consent. Although this process is sometimes called "passive consent," this is a misnomer because no consent is actually given.

TIERED CONSENT

When donating materials for research, participants may select from a range of options. One option is to give permission for only the current research study. Additional options would be to (14):

- Consent to future studies addressing the same general topic, such as cancer or heart disease.
- Give general consent to all future research.
- Give specific permission for various types of highly sensitive studies, such as research on embryonic stem cells or whole genome sequencing. For such research, it would be important to explain the nature of the research and its risks and benefits.
- Give permission to be contacted by researchers in the future about additional research studies. This would allow researchers in the future to describe sensitive studies that were not considered at the time of donation and obtain consent to use previously collected materials for such research.

The challenges in tiered consent are to know what categories of studies are meaningful to participants and to provide enough information so that participants will understand the types of sensitive research that might be conducted.

The Office of Human Research Protections (OHRP) provides guidance on setting up repositories of stored tissues on its website at http://www.hhs.gov/ohrp/humansubjects/guidance/reposit.htm.

OHRP strongly recommends that investigators who receive specimens from the repository not receive the identities of the donors of the materials or information by which they might ascertain their identities.

MAY DONORS WITHDRAW SPECIMENS FROM RESEARCH PROJECTS?

Research participants have the right to withdraw from a research project. Specimens that are still identifiable should then be discarded and no additional research on them should be carried out. If the samples have already been anonymized, they cannot be discarded. The right to withdraw from research should not be interpreted as requiring researchers to destroy work already performed under the original consent. It is unfair to nullify work researchers have done when they were justifiably relying on the original consent.

A recent case in which a researcher moved to a new university illustrates the issues involved when donors change their minds about donated materials (15).

STUDY 23.6   **Control over stored specimens.**

A professor of urology and his colleagues collected a large repository of prostate tissue from patients for use in research. The university provided space, funding, and staff for the repository. When the professor moved to another university, he sought to take the samples to his new institution to continue his research. At his request, over 6000 donors asked the original university to withdraw their specimens and allow the professor to take them to the new university. However, the first university claimed that it had sole right of ownership of the specimens and refused to relinquish them.

Researchers who have invested great effort in collecting materials for biobanks understandably want to control the research uses of those materials. Donors of materials for research may want to have a voice in how those materials are used. However, research institutions that have devoted resources to maintaining a biobank may want to have it available for other faculty members to use.

These different priorities need to be reconciled. Ideally, expectations should be worked out and made clear to donors when they when agree to provide specimens.

STUDY 23.6   **(Continued).**

The federal district court ruled in favor of the university, ruling that the university now owned the materials the donors had given. Although they retained to right to withdraw from research (for example, to have their still-identified specimens destroyed), the donors had no right to transfer the donated materials to another institution. The case is still under appeal.

In its reasoning, the court conceptualized the use of human biological materials as property: having given away their tissue, donors have no right to transfer ownership and control over the materials to another individual (16). However, donors could withdraw from research by revoking the donation. Although regarding human biological materials as property may seem impersonal, the lesson of Study 23.6 is that materials may be withdrawn from research (if still identifiable) but may not be transferred to another institution. These arrangements should be clarified in the consent form for the original donation.

TAKE HOME POINTS

1. Research with existing data or specimens may be carried out without consent under certain circumstances.
2. When researchers collect specimens for one study, they should make plans to use the stored materials for future studies.
3. Researchers and IRBs need to appreciate that some research topics are so sensitive that they should obtain explicit consent to use specimens collected for another purpose.

ANNOTATED BIBLIOGRAPHY

Hansson MG, Dillner J, Bartram CR, Carlson JA, Helgesson G. Should donors be allowed to give broad consent to future biobank research? *Lancet Oncol* 2006;7:266–269.
 Analysis of broad versus specific consent for future research.

REFERENCES

1. National Bioethics Advisory Commission. *Research on Human Stored Biologic Materials*. Rockville, MD: National Bioethics Advisory Commission; 1999.
2. Hansson MG, Dillner J, Bartram CR, Carlson JA, Helgesson G. Should donors be allowed to give broad consent to future biobank research? *Lancet Oncol* 2006;7:266–269.
3. Graham DJ, Campen D, Hui R, et al. Risk of acute myocardial infarction and sudden cardiac death in patients treated with cyclo-oxygenase 2 selective and non-selective non-steroidal anti-inflammatory drugs: nested case-control study. *Lancet* 2005;365:475–481.
4. Office for Human Research Protections. Guidance on research involving coded private information or biological specimens. 2008. Available at: http://www.hhs.gov/ohrp/humansubjects/guidance/cdebiol.htm. Accessed November 11, 2008.
5. Wendler D. One-time general consent for research on biological samples. *BMJ* 2006;332:544–547.
6. Laurie G. Evidence of support for biobanking practices. *BMJ* 2008;337:a337.
7. Knoppers BM, Chadwick R. Human genetic research: emerging trends in ethics. *Nat Rev Genet* 2005;6:75–79.
8. Lyerly AD, Faden RR. Embryonic stem cells. Willingness to donate frozen embryos for stem cell research. *Science* 2007;317:46–47.
9. Kalfoglou AL, Geller G. A follow-up study with oocyte donors exploring their experiences, knowledge, and attitudes about the use of their oocytes and the outcome of the donation. *Fertil Steril* 2000;74:660–667.
10. Nuffield Council on Bioethics. *Genetics and Human Behavior: the Ethical Concerns*. London: Nuffield Council on Bioethics; 2002.

11. Greely HT. The uneasy ethical and legal underpinnings of large-scale genomic biobanks. *Annu Rev Genomics Hum Genet* 2007;8:343–364.

12. van Diest PJ. No consent should be needed for using leftover body material for scientific purposes. *BMJ* 2002;325:648–651.

13. Rothstein MA. Expanding the ethical analysis of biobanks. *J Law Med Ethics* 2005;33:89–101.

14. National Cancer Institute. The National Cancer Institute Tiered Consent Form. Available at: http://prostate nbnpilot.nci.nih.gov/blue_app_i.asp. Accessed December 18, 2008.

15. Glantz L, Roche P, Annas GJ. Rules for donations to tissue banks—what next? *N Engl J Med* 2008;358:298–303.

16. Hakimian R, Korn D. Ownership and use of tissue specimens for research. *JAMA* 2004;292:2500–2505.

24

Observational Studies

I n observational studies, researchers observe participants or make measurements on them without intervening with them or their environment. Because interactions with participants usually consist of interviews, questionnaires, and simple clinical tests, such studies pose fewer risks than interventional studies. This chapter describes the ethical issues that arise particularly in observational studies. Some specific ethical issues involving cross-sectional studies and prospective cohort studies were covered in detail in previous chapters; we summarize those issues here to give the reader a sense of how several issues can work out in a particular type of study. Research conducted in the home raises several unique issues, which we analyze in depth in this chapter.

CROSS-SECTIONAL STUDIES

In cross-sectional studies, researchers take measurements at a single point in time. This design allows researchers to describe variables, their distributions, and their associations.

STUDY 24.1	Survey to patients.

Researchers are studying access to primary care in patients who present for care at the emergency department (ED) or urgent care clinic. They plan a cross-sectional questionnaire to determine what barriers the patients faced in obtaining primary care and what needs were not addressed during the ED or urgent care visit. The questionnaire contains items about mental illness, substance abuse, and alcoholism, which are important health problems that may not be effectively discussed or treated in these settings. Participants will have the option of completing the survey by themselves on a laptop computer in a private area of the waiting room, or having the questionnaire read to them by research staff. Participants will receive $25 for completing the survey. A list of the names and Social Security numbers of the participants is required for accounting purposes.

WHAT ARE THE ETHICAL CONCERNS ABOUT CROSS-SECTIONAL STUDIES?

Psychosocial Risks

Although observational studies generally entail low physical risks, they might present serious psychosocial risks. As in Study 24.1, investigators might ask participants sensitive questions that cause them embarrassment, shame, or stress, or make them unwilling to continue with the study. In addition, breaches of confidentiality might result in tangible harms. Disclosure of information about mental illness or alcoholism may lead to stigmatization, disruption of social relationships, or discrimination in employment. Disclosure of information about substance abuse may also lead to legal liability. As discussed in Chapter 5, investigators have a duty to minimize the harms that their interventions might cause participants, which includes protecting confidentiality.

Informed Consent

Informed consent is usually required and generally presents no insurmountable ethical problems. Chapter 6 discusses issues regarding how eligible participants are contacted and when an exception to consent is appropriate. Note that because the questionnaire in Study 24.1 asks about illegal and stigmatizing behaviors, it does not qualify for an exemption to informed consent.

HOW SHOULD RESEARCHERS RESPOND TO ETHICAL ISSUES IN CROSS-SECTIONAL STUDIES?

As in any study, researchers need take adequate safeguards to protect confidentiality (see Chapter 7) and minimize risks (see Chapter 5) in cross-sectional studies.

STUDY 24.1	(Continued).

It is possible to carry out the research using de-identified data. The investigators have no need to link responses to the identities of the participants. If records of payments must include Social Security numbers, there should be no link to the participants' responses.

PROSPECTIVE COHORT STUDIES

In prospective cohort studies, researchers follow a group of participants over time. The investigators measure baseline characteristics and then determine whether the outcomes of interest occur or not. This design allows investigators to describe the incidence of outcomes over time and to analyze the associations between predictor variables and outcomes. Prospective cohort studies allow researchers to measure predictor variables (also called independent variables) more accurately and more completely than they could in retrospective studies. Cohort studies can also be carried out in a retrospective manner with data that have already been collected at two different times. Thus retrospective cohort studies involve a type of secondary analysis using data and specimens that have already been collected. In addition to the issues previously discussed for cross-sectional studies, researchers in cohort studies face additional ethical issues, as the following study illustrates. In this section, we briefly summarize these issues, referring to detailed discussions of specific issues in other chapters.

STUDY 24.2	Epidemiology of hepatitis C.

After the hepatitis C virus was identified, researchers proposed a prospective cohort study of risk factors and incidence. Persons at high risk for blood-borne infections, such as injection drug users and persons with multiple sexual partners, will be eligible. Participants will be evaluated every 6 months. Blood samples will be collected for liver function tests, viral hepatitis serologies, and HIV testing, as well as a new test for detecting hepatitis C infection and viral load. Participants also will be asked about risk factors for liver disease and blood-borne infections, including alcohol use, injection drug use, and sexual behaviors. Participants will receive counseling about substance abuse and HIV prevention, with referrals to agencies that provide such services as needed. The study will be sponsored by the National Institutes of Health (NIH).

WHAT IS ETHICALLY SPECIAL ABOUT PROSPECTIVE COHORT STUDIES?
Ongoing Relationship With Participants

Researchers who follow a cohort prospectively have continued contact with the participants. Furthermore, investigators try to develop a good rapport with participants to obtain a high follow-up rate and ensure the scientific validity of the study. Because of this ongoing relationship, researchers have reciprocal obligations to participants. Researchers need to encourage participants to attend follow-up visits. Although incentives for participation should be strong enough to make the continuation rate acceptable, they must not be so strong that they create an undue influence.

Confidentiality of Contact Information

Prospective cohort studies pose heightened risks to confidentiality. Researchers need to contact participants to arrange follow-up visits. Furthermore, it would be useful for participants to provide the name of a contact person in case they move or change telephone numbers. Thus researchers need to have considerable personal information about participants. In addition, after each follow-up visit, researchers need to link the new data with the previously collected data about each participant. Investigators therefore need to retain codes that link new data with identifying information about participants. In Study 24.2, researchers will collect sensitive data about highly private or illegal activities. If confidentiality is breached, the participants might suffer significant harms.

Observation of Risks

In the course of their research, investigators may become aware of risks that the participants already face, whether or not they participate in the research, that are not caused by the research interventions. These risks differ from those caused by research interventions because they

- exist whether or not the study is carried out,
- may not be related the topic of research, and
- may not be identified through procedures in the study protocol.

Although researchers in any observational study might become aware of such risks, it is more likely to occur in prospective cohort studies because researchers develop a close relationship with the participants.

STUDY 24.2	(Continued).

During a follow-up interview, one of the participants begins to tear up and reveals to the interviewer, "I haven't told anyone else about this, but I don't think I can bear it any more. My boyfriend keeps beating me if I don't do what he tells me. Sometimes I can't go out of the house for days because I don't want people asking me about the bruises. There are times when I want to get a gun and shoot him, it's so bad."

This participant reveals sensitive information about domestic violence to the interviewer, with whom she has previously discussed intimate issues. After building a relationship with participants and encouraging them to discuss private topics such as sex and injection drug use, researchers should not be surprised if they also reveal other personal information that is not related to the study questions.

Researchers may consider these risks outside their scope of responsibility. However, as Chapter 10 discusses in detail, researchers may be in a unique position to prevent or ameliorate serious harms because they have expertise or a unique opportunity to intervene. The ethical issue is how serious and how likely the danger must be to require intervention by the researcher.

STUDY 24.2	(Continued).

The participant may be at serious and imminent risk, and there is also a risk of violence to the partner. Furthermore, most states have domestic violence reporting laws that require designated health care workers to report domestic violence to public safety officials. Thus, there are strong reasons for the research team to provide emotional support and urgent referrals to social service agencies, as well as to comply with the state reporting laws.

Results of Research Tests

Because participants in a cohort study undergo repeated measurements over time, many subjects may want to know their individual results. As Chapter 11 discusses in detail, it is important to distinguish established clinical tests that are carried out as part of the research protocol from research tests that are being developed or validated during a study. In Study 24.2, liver function tests are established clinical tests, whereas a new assay to quantify the load of hepatitis C is a research test.

HOW SHOULD RESEARCHERS RESPOND TO ETHICAL ISSUES IN PROSPECTIVE COHORT STUDIES?

Researchers need to anticipate these ethical issues and discuss in the protocol how they will respond to them.

Provide Incentives to Continue to Participate, Without Undue Inducement

Acceptable measures to encourage ongoing participation include education about health issues, building a relationship through newsletters and token gifts such as mugs and t-shirts, and offering to participants (and their primary physicians) individual results of tests done as part of the study that are routinely available in clinical practice. However, some incentives would be unacceptable, such as paying subjects for the time they spend on the research project only if they complete all visits, rather than prorating the payments.

Maintain Confidentiality

In their zeal to maintain high follow-up rates, researchers must be careful not to compromise confidentiality. In addition to the measures to protect confidentiality presented in Chapter 7, researchers also need to pay attention to how they recontact participants.

STUDY 24.2   **(Continued).**

When leaving phone messages for the participants, researchers should not reveal the reason for the call or the nature of the study. It is best just to leave their name and phone number. Participants may be stigmatized if someone in their household finds out that they are at risk for hepatitis. Similarly, when talking to a participant's contact person, it would be prudent not to mention the nature of the study.

Offer Results of Research Tests Whose Validity has Been Established

As discussed in Chapter 11, researchers generally should offer the results of common clinical tests carried out as part of the study. For tests that are being developed for research purposes, several factors determine whether results should be offered, including the analytic and clinical utility of the test, and the clinical and personal significance of the results for participants. Researchers may also have ethical obligations to inform participants of test results that have important clinical implications.

STUDY 24.2   **(Continued).**

Participants should be offered results of the liver function tests, tests for HIV and hepatitis B, and standard tests for hepatitis C. These tests are commonly ordered in clinical practice, and their clinical utility is established. Indeed, as a condition of receiving NIH funding, researchers are required to notify participants if their HIV tests show that they are infected. Infected persons may also need to be reported to public health officials, depending on local public health regulations. Participants need to be told of these requirements during the informed consent process. Participants who are told they have HIV infection or hepatitis B or C also need counseling and referral for follow-up care.

RESEARCH IN THE PARTICIPANT'S HOME

Conducting research in the participant's home allows researchers to measure variables that cannot be measured in the clinic or research office. Research in the home raises additional ethical issues, as in the following case.

| STUDY 24.3 | Causes of asthma in children. |

Asthma is disproportionately common in inner-city areas that have low incomes, poor housing, and predominantly minority populations. To identify factors associated with asthma and asthma-related symptoms and disability, researchers are planning a cross-sectional study in which they will collect dust samples from participants' homes, test the samples for cockroach and dust mite antigens, and inspect the home for mold. They will also administer questionnaires regarding respiratory symptoms and their impact on activities and school attendance, and other triggers of asthma, such as cigarette smoke and pets. While making these home visits, the research assistant notices:

- *A gun case in the living room.*
- *A hole in the floor, larger than a child, with a drop-off to the floor below.*
- *A child who is not a participant in study is disciplined by a blow to the head with a broomstick. His arms have multiple visible bruises of different colors.*
- *Visible mold on the walls.*

WHAT IS ETHICALLY DIFFERENT ABOUT RESEARCH IN PARTICIPANTS' HOMES?

Loss of Privacy

Home visits involve a loss of privacy because the researcher cannot help observing information beyond what is needed for research purposes (1). Such loss of privacy may lead to embarrassment or shame, such as when researchers notice poverty or messy housekeeping. Guests in a home are expected to be polite and respectful. Researchers who are invited into the home for research purposes do not have *carte blanche* to comment on or intervene in other activities there.

Impact on Persons who are not Research Participants

Research conducted in the home also intrudes on the privacy of other residents in the household who are not research participants, even if researchers do not interact with them or collect identifiable information about them. Other household residents may experience embarrassment or shame if they are observed to be living in substandard conditions. Moreover, residents may face legal liability—for example, if the researcher notices illegal behaviors such as injection drug use.

Observation of Risks

During home visits, researchers may become aware of risks that are not caused by research interventions or related to the research topic, and would not be apparent in clinical or office settings. Some argue that researchers who observe children in poor housing environments should "rescue" them and provide better living conditions (2). Although it is a natural humanitarian impulse to help children in need, it is unreasonable to expect researchers to rescue subjects; this is almost always beyond the researchers' power and resources, and beyond the relationship the parents have agreed to. Furthermore, interventions intended to reduce risks may be meddlesome, ineffective, or even counterproductive. Researchers' attempts to help may have unintended adverse consequences. If tenants complain about a hole in the floor, for example, the landlord might retaliate by raising rents, enforcing lease violations more strictly, or reporting illegal immigrants. Moreover, parents' views about childrearing and firearms may differ from those of the researchers; they deserve respect except when the child is endangered. Investigators have an obligation to do what is reasonable under the circumstances. The appropriate course of action will depend on the specific situation, including the type of risk identified, who is at risk, the nature of the research project, and the availability of community resources, as we next discuss.

RECOMMENDATIONS

Inform Other Household Residents of the Study and the Time of Home Visits

When designing a study in the participant's home, researchers need to anticipate how the study might affect other residents in the household even if they are not research participants under the Common Rule definition (1). Other residents may want to be absent during research visits to protect their privacy, or they may want to be present during educational portions of the visit. The researchers can ask study participants to inform other residents and provide information sheets for doing so.

Respond Directly to Imminent and Serious Risks

Investigators should first assess whether a risk is imminent and serious. As Chapter 10 discusses in detail, researchers have an ethical obligation to intervene to prevent or mitigate imminent, serious harms. In several situations, such as child abuse, they have a legal duty as well.

Have a Plan for Responding to Risks That are not Imminent and Serious

Researchers have less responsibility to respond to risks that are not imminent and serious. They need to balance the likelihood of preventing serious harm against the harm caused by a breach of confidentiality. Generally, a respectful discussion with the participant or parent on how to mitigate the risk will suffice. The researcher may also refer the parents to community organizations. For instance, legal services organizations can help families enforce their rights as tenants or protect them from retaliatory evictions.

STUDY 24.3 **(Continued).**

In the situation involving the gun case, researchers should discuss with the study parent whether the case contains a loaded and unlocked gun. If it does, the parent should be urged to unload, lock, and remove the gun from the child's access. If the parent does so, no other action need be taken other than offering additional information or referrals on gun safety. If the parent is unwilling or unable to make the situation safe, the researcher has an ethical (and in most states a legal) obligation to notify child protective services.

If a child is struck on the head and has multiple bruises, the probability of child abuse is sufficiently high that the investigator should report the situation to child protective services. If the situation is covered by state child abuse and neglect laws and the researcher is a mandated reporter, reporting is required rather than optional. Investigators should be sensitive to possible retaliation by the perpetrator. For example, if someone other than the parent is perpetrating the abuse, the researcher or the child abuse team needs to discuss with the parent the possibility of retaliation by the perpetrator on the family.

In the situation involving the hole in the floor, the ages of the children and the steps the parents have taken to protect them are relevant. The parents may have instituted effective measures to mitigate the hazard, such as continuous supervision of younger children. In contrast, if the parents refuse to acknowledge that the risk is imminent and serious to young children, the investigators may be obligated to report the situation to child protective services.

With regard to mold, although it may cause or exacerbate asthma, it is not a serious and imminent threat. It suffices for the researchers to provide information and referrals to community organizations, such as tenants' groups or legal aid services, that can offer assistance.

Chapter 10 discusses in detail how researchers should respond to incidentally discovered risks.

Inform Participants of Potential Interventions During the Consent Process

During the consent process, researchers need to explain how the study might affect other residents and what kinds of risks might require intervention, including, in some cases, reporting to legal authorities. Parents or participants need such information to make an informed decision about whether to participate in a study.

TAKE HOME POINT

1. Prospective cohort studies and research in the participant's home may raise difficult ethical issues regarding privacy and confidentiality, and observation of risks not related to the study. Researchers need to anticipate such issues and describe in the protocol and during the consent process how they will address them.

REFERENCES

1. Lo B, O'Connell ME, eds. *Ethical Considerations for Research on Housing-Related Health Hazards Involving Children*. Washington, DC: National Academies Press; 2005.
2. Sharav VH. Children in clinical research: a conflict of moral values. *Am J Bioeth* 2003;3:W-IF 2.

25

Translational Research

T 1 translational research, also known as bench-to-bedside research, has been defined as "the transfer of new understandings of disease mechanisms gained in the laboratory into the development of new methods for diagnosis, therapy, and prevention and their first testing in humans" (1). Its goal is to develop a new test or treatment that can be brought to market. T1 translational research is essential to show proof of principle in humans and to define the pharmacodynamics (PD) and pharmacokinetics (PK) of new agents. PK describes the relation between the dose of a drug and its plasma or tissue concentration over time. PD describes how the plasma concentration of a drug is related to its effect on the body. It depends on the drug's mechanisms of action.

T1 translational research raises ethical concerns because some first-in-human trials can cause unanticipated serious adverse events. There is an unavoidable tension between protecting participants in such trials and the interest of study sponsors in making the drug discovery process more efficient and maintaining a competitive advantage. Furthermore, obtaining informed and voluntary consent may be particularly challenging.

The term "translational research" is also applied to so-called T2 translational research, which aims to translate the results of research studies into clinical practice in the community (1). In this book we use the term "translational research" to refer only to T1 research.

ETHICAL CONCERNS ABOUT FIRST-IN-HUMAN TRIALS

A recent first-in-human trial vividly illustrates how research participants might suffer unexpected life-threatening adverse events.

STUDY 25.1   **Monoclonal antibody stimulating the immune system.**

In 2006, investigators conducted a Phase I first-in-human trial of TGN1412, a monoclonal antibody that directly activates the CD28 receptor on T-lymphocytes, stimulating the production and activation of T lymphocytes (2,3). The first six participants received the investigational drug on the same day, one after the other, as per the protocol. They all suffered immediate life-threatening vascular collapse, requiring emergency hospitalization and intensive care. All survived, but 3 months after the study they had memory loss, headaches, and poor concentration. One had dry gangrene of the fingers and toes (2).

Participants in the trial alleged that the possibility of serious adverse events was not disclosed, and the payment of £2000 (U.S. $3500) to participants may have been an undue inducement (4). The drug manufacturer went bankrupt shortly after these events occurred.

STUDY 25.1   (Continued).

Studies revealed that the investigational agent had triggered a "cytokine storm." This had not occurred in animal studies of TGN1412. However, because the structure of the CD28 receptor varies across species, the biological effects of TGN1412 in mice and monkeys may not predict the effects in humans (5). Some scientists suggested in retrospect that the possibility of serious adverse events should have been anticipated in light of adverse events caused by another monoclonal antibody that also activates T cells without a second signal (4).

Most examples of drug toxicity are "side effects" that are not related to the drug's intended mechanism of action (3). However, in Study 25.1, life-threatening toxicity was caused by the action of the drug on its intended biological target (3). Until a novel target is manipulated for the first time in humans, toxic effects cannot be reliably predicted. Because of differences between human and animal physiology, safety data in animal studies may not accurately predict safety in humans. The possibility of unexpected serious adverse events is a particular concern when there are no good animal models for studying the mechanism of the investigational drug, as is the case with highly specific monoclonal antibodies directed against the human immune system (6).

In addition to scientific concerns, Study 25.1 raises ethical concerns. Study sponsors wish to proceed as efficiently as possible through the preclinical and clinical studies needed to obtain regulatory approval for a new therapy. However, some steps that reduce the time and expense of the approval process may increase risk to participants in an unacceptable manner (3,6).

WHAT ARE THE RISKS TO PARTICIPANTS?

Regulators and scientists alike questioned whether the serious toxicity in Study 25.1 should have been anticipated. Because of the increased risk of unexpected serious adverse events, some experts suggest that stricter oversight and more careful peer review are needed for monoclonal antibody trials that employ a new mechanism of action, address a target that lacks appropriate animal models, and have a new type of engineered structure (6). Heightened review might provide greater protection to research participants, but would also add to the time and expense of the drug approval process for sponsors.

In Study 25.1, the number of serious adverse events was increased because the protocol called for six participants to receive the investigational drug on the same day, one after another. This arrangement reduces costs and time for the study sponsor. However, had there been an observation period after the study intervention was administered to each participant, the study would have been halted after the first participant suffered this life-threatening reaction, and the remaining five participants would not have been harmed (3,6).

In addition to studies of monoclonal antibodies that are immune modulators, other types of research raise particular concerns about risk in first-in-human trials. Nanomedicine deals with materials that are about the size of DNA or a virus and smaller than a red blood cell. They are potentially useful as drug delivery devices and to image lymph nodes and tumors (7). However, nanomaterials raise special ethical concerns regarding risk (7). Their size, shape, and properties depend on the microenvironment and may change when they enter an organism. Changes in size and shape may dramatically alter their toxicity. Nanomaterials may enter the blood stream and be transported to other organs, where their effects are not known. Some nanomaterials can trigger inflammatory and immune responses. They also may accumulate in the body and cause long-term toxicity. Thus in vitro and preclinical studies in nonhuman animals may not accurately predict toxicity in humans. Finally, early-phase clinical trials are unlikely to detect long-term risks and rare adverse events.

HOW ARE SUBJECTS SELECTED?

The selection of subjects in first-in-human clinical trials presents clinical and ethical dilemmas. Researchers often select healthy volunteers because their results are more reproducible than those in sick persons. The PK and PD of the drug in sick patients may be highly variable because of the effects the disease or other treatments (6). Thus investigators and sponsors may prefer healthy volunteers for these studies because the data will be more precise. Furthermore, healthy volunteers may be less susceptible to adverse events than sick patients. However, the use of healthy subjects may be inappropriate for some biologics, such as new monoclonal antibodies, because their biological effects on the immune system of healthy persons may differ radically from the effects in patients who will receive the therapy, whose immune system is altered by the disease or other medications.

HOW IS INFORMED CONSENT OBTAINED?

In retrospect, there were concerns that the consent of the volunteers in Study 25.1 may not have been informed and voluntary. Critics charged that the level of payment may have been an undue inducement and that the participants may not have appreciated the fact that serious risks can occur in such first-in-human trials.

In other Phase I clinical trials, concerns have been raised about enrolling poor people and paying them high fees (8). Some participants view enrolling in such trials as a job that is more lucrative than a minimum-wage job. They may be reluctant to drop out of trials that are risky and unpleasant, particularly if they paid money to travel to the site and obtain housing, and to complain to sponsors about poor conditions. Moreover, they often receive no coverage for medical injuries resulting from the trial. In response, defenders of these arrangements point out that participants have agreed to enter the trial, that they are better off financially than they would be if they did not participate, and that it is more respectful and beneficial to give participants higher payments than lower ones.

PHASE 0 CLINICAL TRIALS

Less than 10% of investigational therapies that begin with human trials are ultimately submitted to the FDA for approval. It would benefit companies that develop drugs, as well as the public, to identify more efficiently which candidate therapies should not proceed to further development. To reduce the time and resources expended on candidate products that are unlikely to succeed, the FDA has issued guidance on exploratory investigational new drug (IND) studies (9), also known as Phase 0 trials. Because such studies are thought to present substantially less risk than traditional Phase I studies, preclinical testing may be less extensive.

TRADITIONAL PHASE I STUDIES

Researchers are required to conduct preclinical studies in nonhuman animals to select a safe starting dose for humans, evaluate toxicity, estimate the margin of safety between a clinical and a toxic dose, and estimate PK and PD parameters in humans. These extensive preclinical tests require significant investments in product synthesis, animal use, laboratory analyses, and time. Many resources are invested in candidate products that subsequently are found to be unacceptable for humans.

DESIGN OF PHASE 0 STUDIES

Exploratory IND studies are conducted before traditional Phase I studies in humans. The new FDA guidance allows them to proceed with fewer animal toxicology studies than is required for traditional Phase I trials. Exploratory IND studies usually involve very limited human exposure in terms of dose, duration of administration, and number of participants. Such studies can serve a number of useful goals. For example, an exploratory IND study can help investigators (9):

- determine whether a mechanism of action observed in animal models can also be observed in humans (e.g., a binding property or inhibition of an enzyme);

- describe PK and PD in humans;
- select the most promising candidate designed to interact with a particular therapeutic target in humans; and
- explore a product's biodistribution using imaging techniques.

Phase 0 studies represent a paradigm shift in clinical trials because their goal is to inform drug development, not to assess safety and dosage (10).

ETHICAL ISSUES IN PHASE 0 STUDIES
What are the Risks to Participants?

Peer reviewers of a Phase 0 study need to critically examine the assumption that such trials present very low risk because of the very low dosages used and the short duration of administration. For some innovative interventions, serious unanticipated adverse events may still occur at very low doses, such as through activation of effector pathways, positive feedback loops, or replication of cells. Reviewers also need to question the assumption that the knowledge gained in Phase 0 studies is generalizable to higher doses that will have a pharmacological effect. PK data from microdose studies may poorly predict the PK at therapeutic doses if molecules have nonlinear PK or high-affinity binding to their targets (11).

In light of the absence of any direct benefit to participants (10,12,13), the risk of any invasive study procedure needs to be carefully justified. For example, investigators may wish to carry out serial biopsies to validate biomarkers that can be used in later phase trials to assess the effects of the study agent (11). Although the risks of serial biopsies may be justified in clinical care, they may not be justified in research when carried out with no possibility of benefiting a research participant.

How is Informed Consent Obtained?

Because the design of a Phase 0 trial is so novel, participants might misunderstand the goals and risks of the study and how it differs from other clinical trials, including classic Phase I trials. In classic Phase I studies, there is a possibility of direct benefit to participants, albeit a low one (see Chapter 5). Furthermore, cancer specialists often tell patients that the best cancer therapy can be obtained in a clinical trial because of the collateral benefits of more careful follow-up and individualized attention. However, in Phase 0 studies there is no possibility of benefit.

Other misunderstandings may arise if participants in Phase 0 studies are asked to undergo serial tumor biopsies to validate biomarkers for the study agent (11). Because biopsies are a standard part of clinical care, participants might infer that they will benefit from the biopsy. However, in Phase 0 studies the biopsy is being carried out solely for research purposes and will not provide any clinically meaningful information to participants.

Finally, participants in a Phase 0 study may not realize that participation in a Phase 0 study may exclude them from other clinical trials that might offer them the prospect of personal benefit, or delay their participation (13). Although some writers advocate the inclusion of Phase 0 participants in subsequent phase trials of an agent, patients may not appreciate the fact that few agents studied in Phase 0 are expected to proceed further in drug development, and that clinical trials of other agents may exclude persons who participated in previous trials.

RECOMMENDATIONS TO ADDRESS ETHICAL ISSUES

In innovative T1 research, there is a tension between the protection of participants and the interests of the sponsor in developing drugs efficiently. In recent years, several healthy or highly functioning participants have died or suffered life-threatening complications in clinical research. In addition to the cases described in this chapter, 18-year-old Jesse Gelsinger died from liver failure as a result of a Phase I gene transfer trial in 1999, and 24-year-old Ellen Roche died as a result of a study on the pathophysiology of asthma in 2001 (see Chapter 1). In light of these tragedies, it is important for researchers, review panels, and study sponsors to meet their obligation to minimize risks to participants, as required by the Common Rule (see Chapter 3). The protection of participants should take priority over the efficient conduct of clinical research.

WHAT ARE THE RISKS TO PARTICIPANTS?

Several features of these cases suggest additional steps to minimize risks to participants, as listed in Table 25.1.

Review Higher-Risk Protocols With Particular Care

Study 25.1 alerted scientists that preclinical safety studies might poorly predict human toxicity for certain types of highly innovative agents. The regulators who approved Study 25.1 suggested that heightened reviews should be carried out when good animal models for the mechanism of the study agent do not exist (6). In any first-in-human study, reviewers should ask whether there are particular concerns that the preclinical evidence might poorly predict toxicity in humans—for example, because the study involves an immune-modifying monoclonal antibody or nanoparticles. IRBs must ensure that a rigorous scientific review has been carried out.

Such stringent reviews are possible only if reviewers and regulatory agencies have access to all pertinent data regarding the safety of the novel agents. Drug and biotechnology companies commonly consider data on the safety of compounds that will not proceed to further development to be trade secrets. Hence, a new investigator or sponsor may not be aware that previous attempts to manipulate the selected target or to administer structurally similar compounds resulted in unacceptable toxicity (10). When such safety data are kept confidential, participants may suffer serious harm. There are several approaches that can be used to protect participants while also respecting the interests of previous sponsors.

First, if a participant in a Phase I clinical trial is hospitalized for an illness that is possibly or probably related to the study agent, the treating physicians in the hospital should file an adverse event report to the FDA. Second, study sponsors can file with the FDA confidential reports of serious unexpected adverse events in Phase 0 and Phase I trials that are possibly, probably, or definitely related to the study agent. The FDA should retain such reports in a searchable manner so that they can be examined when the FDA is approached about related investigational agents. In this situation, the protection of participants should take priority over the competitive advantage of study sponsors. It is not in the public interest for companies to pursue therapeutic approaches that are already known to have unacceptable risk.

Administer the Study Agent Only After Clinical Evaluation and Review of Laboratory Tests

In the Gelsinger case, the investigational agent was administered before laboratory results drawn that day were checked. Jesse Gelsinger had abnormal liver function tests that day, and the liver toxicity was one of the expected adverse effects of the study agent. During a first-in-humans trial, researchers

TABLE 25.1	Minimizing Risks to Participants in T1 Research
Review higher-risk protocols with particular care.	
Administer the study agent only after clinical evaluation and review of laboratory tests.	
Evaluate symptoms rigorously.	
Provide free care for adverse events.	

should administer investigational agents only after they have carried out a clinical evaluation and checked laboratory tests. Again, the precautions taken in administering investigational agents should be at least as rigorous as those taken before administering cytotoxic cancer chemotherapy; patients should be evaluated for fever and symptoms of infection, and their blood counts checked before the drug is administered.

Evaluate Symptoms Rigorously

When participants in the above-mentioned cases developed common symptoms, such as cough, fever, and vomiting, investigators and physicians assumed they were self-limited illnesses, rather than possible adverse events due to the administered agent. A more conservative approach would be to assume that any symptoms related to the target organ system of the administered agent are related to the agent, until proven otherwise. Furthermore, if the investigational agent is an immune modulator, it would be prudent to assume that any unexplained febrile symptoms might be an opportunistic infection. Finally, research staff should have the necessary qualifications and experience to respond immediately to unexpected serious complication. Precautions should be at least as careful as those applied during anesthesia. Although the vast majority of anesthesia procedures are performed without complications, the anesthesiologist needs to be prepared to identify and manage rare but catastrophic complications, such as malignant hyperthermia.

Provide Free Care for Adverse Events

If participants require medical care for adverse medical events that are caused by the study agent, it seems fair for the study sponsor to pay for such care, not the participant (14). Although such care is desirable for any research injury, it is particularly important in T1 research, where the risks are uncertain. Financial liability can be limited by restricting coverage to "direct and proximate" complications (15).

HOW SHOULD INFORMED CONSENT BE OBTAINED?

Informed consent is a particular concern in T1 research. No matter what information is in the consent form, participants may not appreciate several key features of such studies:

- Researchers do not know whether the study agent is safe or effective.
- The study differs from ordinary clinical care that is expected to benefit the participants personally.
- There is no direct therapeutic benefit to participants in Phase 0 studies.
- Serious, life-threatening, or fatal adverse events may occur. In studies that have no good animal models, this possibility is even greater.

For particularly innovative studies in which preclinical studies may poorly predict toxicity in humans, it would be prudent to have investigators administer a questionnaire to ascertain that participants understand these key points before enrolling them in the study.

CONFLICTS OF INTEREST IN EARLY-PHASE CLINICAL TRIALS

In translational research, conflicts of interest can arise when a scientist has financial and intellectual interests in the outcomes of early-phase clinical trials. The following case and analysis are from a comprehensive report by the American Association of Medical Colleges (AAMC) and Association of American Universities (AAU) (16). Chapter 15 provides a more detailed discussion of conflicts of interest, including the requirements for investigators to disclose to their universities or research institutions their financial relationships with industry. This chapter applies that framework to early-phase clinical trials.

STUDY 25.2   Financial relationships with a startup company.

Dr. S discovers a protein in ovarian cancer cells and shows that a monoclonal antibody to it can reduce the progression of cancer in a mouse model. Dr. S patents her discovery and starts a biotech company to develop a clinical therapy. The university licenses the monoclonal antibody technology to her startup company. The company proposes a Phase I clinical trial to administer the monoclonal antibody to human subjects with ovarian cancer and evaluate its effect on the progression of the cancer. Dr. S is proposed as the principal investigator because she is most familiar with the experimental intervention.

Dr. S owns 100,000 shares of founders stock and options. She is not an officer or a member of the board of directors of the company. However, she is a member of its scientific advisory board and she receives an annual payment of $30,000 for her service on it. The university and Dr. S will both receive licensing payments.

ANALYSIS OF CONFLICTS OF INTEREST

Dr. S's significant financial and intellectual interests in this clinical trial may influence her judgment in the conduct of the trial and the subsequent evaluation of the resulting data. The following questions can help investigators, sponsors, and IRBs analyze conflicts of interest in early-phase clinical trials.

What are the Risks to Participants?

There is a risk that Dr. S's financial interests could influence her judgment in the selection, recruitment, and consent process. She might, for example, select and recruit participants and assign them to experimental groups in ways that would enhance her financial interests but would not be in the best interests of the participants. She might obtain their consent without fully disclosing the risks or her personal financial interests.

Other concerns arise if Dr. S provides care to patients with ovarian cancer. If she invites her own patients to enroll in the study, they might find it difficult to say no to their treating physician, even if they do not wish to participate.

What is the Risk to Data Integrity?

As the principal investigator, Dr. S would be in a position to influence the outcome of the trial in ways that would favor her company's financial interests. She might select patients with a favorable prognosis for the study or interpret the data in ways that would favor the effectiveness of the monoclonal antibody.

What are the Benefits of Allowing an Investigator With a Conflict of Interest to Participate in the Research?

In some clinical trials, a scientist who has made crucial discoveries regarding the new therapy has unique expertise to develop the product or carry out the trial. For example, a scientist who discovers and patents a target for therapy may have unique expertise for designing the product, scaling it up for production, selecting the starting dosage, or selecting study endpoints. However, it should be possible to identify researchers with no relationship to the company who have the expertise to recruit participants, obtain informed consent, administer the monoclonal antibody, assess the progression of cancer, and analyze outcomes data.

Are There any Institutional Conflicts of Interest?

Because the university receives royalties from the patent, it has a financial interest in the success of the product. It might be questioned whether it can objectively oversee the research.

HOW TO ADDRESS CONFLICTS OF INTEREST IN T1 RESEARCH

As discussed in Chapter 15, the standard responses to conflicts of interest are disclosure, management, and prohibition. Dr. S's relationship with the company needs to be disclosed to the university, the institutional conflict of interest committee, the IRB, the participants in the clinical trial, and in all relevant publications and presentations. Consensus guidelines from the AAMC set a rebuttable presumption that researchers with a significant conflict of interest should not conduct human participants research. Exceptions are permitted if there are compelling circumstances related to design or participant safety (16).

We next present additional recommendations for managing or prohibiting conflicts of interest based on the following questions (Table 25.2)

What Steps Should be Taken to Ensure Integrity of Data?

The trial could be carried out with another principal investigator who has no financial interest in the company, is not a close friend or relative of Dr. S, and does not report to her professionally. Dr. S could serve as a consultant or coinvestigator, but should not control the design of the study or the data analysis. She should play no role in the selection and enrollment of participants or the ascertainment of endpoints. These key aspects of the study require no expertise regarding the study intervention in this case. They should be carried out by persons who have no financial relationship to the company other than the research contract or grant for the clinical trial. If Dr. S's laboratory performs assays on the level of antibodies or pathophysiological effects, the samples should be blinded so that the laboratory does not know the dose administered or the timing of the dose.

Some common suggestions made regarding such circumstances are actually not feasible. Dr. S could divest her financial interest in the company to eliminate a financial conflict of interest, but she would still have an intellectual commitment to her discovery. Appointing a monitor to oversee the study is not practical, given the large number of steps in a clinical trial. It would be more efficient and effective simply to have someone without conflicts of interest serve as the principal investigator.

What Steps Should be Taken to Protect Research Participants?

Someone other than Dr. S should identify eligible participants and invite them to participate. If Dr. S cares for patients with ovarian cancer, it is particularly important for someone else to discuss the study with her patients.

What Steps Should be Taken to Protect Trainees?

The department chair should appoint another faculty member to ensure that trainees working with Dr. S's group participate in research projects that offer appropriate opportunities for intellectual creativity and professional development.

What Steps Should be Taken to Address Institutional Conflicts of Interest?

The university should address its institutional conflict of interest, for example, by eliminating its holdings in the company or having the trial carried out at another institution.

TABLE 25.2 Approaching Conflicts of Interest in T1 Research
What steps should be taken to ensure integrity of data?
What steps should be taken to protect research participants?
What steps should be taken to protect trainees?
What steps should be taken to address institutional conflicts of interest?

TAKE HOME POINTS

1. In early-phase clinical trials, there may be an ethical tension between protecting research participants and carrying out the research in an efficient manner.
2. Trials of highly innovative interventions may result in serious unexpected adverse events. It may be appropriate to require heightened scientific and ethical review, and to ensure that participants appreciate the key features of the study.
3. T1 research often raises conflict of interest issues that need to be addressed.

ANNOTATED BIBLIOGRPAHY

AAMC-AAU Advisory Committee on Financial Conflicts of Interest in Clinical Research. *Protecting Patients, Preserving Integrity, Advancing Health: Accelerating the Implementation of COI Policies in Human Subjects Research.* Washington, DC: American Association of Medical Colleges; 2008.
> Available at http://www.aamc.org/research/coi/start.htm.
> Consensus report on conflicts on interest in research; several detailed case studies regarding translational research are presented.

Kummar S, Kinders R, Rubinstein L, et al. Compressing drug development timelines in oncology using phase '0' trials. *Nat Rev Cancer* 2007;7:131–139.
> Overview of the science and ethics of Phase 0 trials.

Schneider CK, Kalinke U, Lower J. TGN1412—a regulator's perspective. *Nat Biotechnol* 2006;24:493–496.
> Review of the TGN1412 trial, with suggestions for heightened review of Phase I trials in which preclinical safety data may be misleading.

REFERENCES

1. Woolf SH. The meaning of translational research and why it matters. *JAMA* 2008;299:211–213.
2. Dowsing T, Kendall MJ. The Northwick Park tragedy—protecting healthy volunteers in future first-in-man trials. *J Clin Pharm Ther* 2007;32:203–207.
3. Wood AJ, Darbyshire J. Injury to research volunteers—the clinical-research nightmare. *N Engl J Med* 2006; 354:1869–1871.
4. Wadman M. London's disastrous drug trial has serious side effects for research. *Nature* 2006;440:388–389.
5. Goodyear M. Learning from the TGN1412 trial. *BMJ* 2006;332:677–678.
6. Schneider CK, Kalinke U, Lower J. TGN1412—a regulator's perspective. *Nat Biotechnol* 2006;24:493–496.
7. Resnik DB, Tinkle SS. Ethical issues in clinical trials involving nanomedicine. *Contemp Clin Trials* 2007;28: 433–441.
8. Elliott C, Abadie R. Exploiting a research underclass in phase 1 clinical trials. *N Engl J Med* 2008;358:2316–2317.
9. Center for Drug Evaluation and Research, FDA. Exploratory IND studies. Available at: http://www.fda.gov/cder/guidance/7086fnl.htm. Accessed August 3, 2008.
10. Kimmelman J. Ethics at phase 0: clarifying the issues. *J Law Med Ethics* 2007;35:514, 727–733.
11. Marchetti S, Schellens JH. The impact of FDA and EMEA guidelines on drug development in relation to phase 0 trials. *Br J Cancer* 2007;97:577–581.
12. Kummar S, Kinders R, Rubinstein L, et al. Compressing drug development timelines in oncology using phase '0' trials. *Nat Rev Cancer* 2007;7:131–139.
13. Kinders R, Parchment RE, Ji J, et al. Phase 0 clinical trials in cancer drug development: from FDA guidance to clinical practice. *Mol Interv* 2007;7:325–334.
14. National Bioethics Advisory Commission. *Ethical and Policy Issues in Research Involving Human Participants.* Rockville, MD: National Bioethics Advisory Commission; 2001.
15. Lomax GP, Hall ZH, Lo B. Responsible oversight of human stem cell research: the California Institute for Regenerative Medicine's medical and ethical standards. *PLoS Med* 2007;4:e114.
16. AAMC-AAU Advisory Committee on Financial Conflicts of Interest in Clinical Research. *Protecting Patients, Preserving Integrity, Advancing Health: Accelerating the Implementation of COI Policies in Human Subjects Research.* Washington, DC: American Association of Medical Colleges; 2008.

Clinical Trials

Clinical trials are essential to establish the effectiveness and safety of interventions. In a clinical trial, researchers intervene with participants by administering a study drug and thereby exposing them to risk. Researchers must ensure that the experimental intervention does not put participants at unacceptable risk. The goal of a clinical trial, which is to obtain valid information about the effectiveness and safety of an intervention, may conflict with the best interests of an individual participant. In a clinical trial, many aspects of the participants' care are determined by the protocol, not by a personal physician (1). The intervention may be assigned by randomization. Study personnel and participants may be blinded to what intervention is provided. Some participants may receive a placebo rather than an active drug. Adjustments in drug dosage may be determined by the protocol, not by individualized decisions tailored to the participant's condition. Additional therapies may be limited or prohibited. Although these provisions allow the research question to be answered more rigorously, they may not be best for individual participants. For example, a participant might benefit from concurrent medications forbidden by the protocol, or from an individualized adjustment in the dose of the study drug. In such circumstances, the participant would be better off not participating in the trial. However, participants often do not appreciate how a clinical trial differs from usual clinical care, and their decisions to participate in clinical trials may not be truly informed.

The following example illustrates how each step in the design of a clinical trial may involve ethical issues. The same design features that make clinical trials rigorous may also raise ethical concerns.

STUDY 26.1   **Prevention of nephropathy in patients with Type II diabetes.**

A randomized controlled trial (RCT) was conducted to determine whether an angiotensin II receptor blocker (ARB) can prevent the progression of renal disease in patients with diabetes who have microalbuminuria. The control group received a placebo. All participants received the usual care for diabetes from their primary physicians.

At the time the study was proposed, randomized trials had already shown that angiotensin-converting enzyme (ACE) inhibitors slowed the progression of nephropathy in persons with Type I diabetes. Some smaller studies had suggested benefits in patients with Type II diabetes as well. Many physicians in clinical practice had extrapolated these findings from published studies and were already prescribing ACE inhibitors to patients with Type II diabetes.

In Study 26.1 (2), some physicians contended that it was unethical to randomize participants to a placebo because the benefits of ACE inhibitors were already accepted. Others argued that it would be preferable to study ACE inhibitors rather than ARBs. Still others were concerned that investigators had a conflict of interest regarding background care for diabetes. Tighter control of glucose would reduce the endpoint of diabetic complications, but it would also reduce the power of the study to detect a difference between the two arms, and thus researchers, wanting the clinical trial to succeed, might be less vigorous about controlling blood glucose levels.

RANDOMIZATION

WHY IS RANDOMIZATION USEFUL?

RCTs, as in Study 26.1, are the most rigorous design for evaluating interventions because randomization is the best way to make the baseline characteristics of the intervention and control groups similar. Any differences at the onset of the study could lead to a difference in outcomes between the control and active groups.

WHAT ARE THE ETHICAL CONCERNS ABOUT RANDOMIZATION?

RCTs raise particular ethical concerns because the intervention that a participant receives is determined by chance rather than by a personal physician making an individualized judgment about what is best for that participant. Furthermore, there are concerns that randomization may harm participants if they receive a less effective or riskier intervention. Recent metaanalyses have shown that the outcomes of participants in an RCT are generally comparable to those of patients who are eligible to participate but receive conventional care (3,4). These data are controversial because people who volunteer for clinical trials may be healthier or more compliant than eligible patients who do not enroll.

WHEN IS RANDOMIZATION JUSTIFIED?

Researchers and ethics experts agree that it is appropriate to randomize participants in clinical trials in certain circumstances, but they cannot agree on why that is the case.

The Concept of Equipoise

One ethical justification for assigning treatment by randomization is that the arms of the protocol are in equipoise. Equipoise is a concept that intuitively seems clear but is hard to define precisely. The general idea is that there is genuine uncertainty or controversy over which arm of the trial is superior. Intuitively, the concept of equipoise makes sense: if there is no convincing evidence that one arm is superior, the relative benefit/risk ratios of the study arms will be comparable, and participants will not be harmed if they agree to allow their care to be determined by randomization rather than by an individualized decision by their personal physician. However, philosophers debate over how to define equipoise and whether randomization is most convincingly justified by equipoise, the researcher's duty to act in the best interests of individual participant, or the duty of nonexploitation (5).

Equipoise is sometimes taken literally to mean an exact balance between the two arms, but this is almost never the case. Sponsors and investigators would be unlikely to propose a trial for a new drug if they did not have some evidence that it was superior to current therapy. Also, as data accumulate in a clinical trial, trends emerge and the arms of the trial will no longer be in balance. In addition, results from other trials may be pertinent. It is illogical to say that equipoise must be exactly 50-50 or that a researcher may never compromise a patient's personal best interests to any degree; from this perspective, a randomized clinical trial could never be completed. If randomization may be acceptable despite some evidence favoring one arm, the crucial questions are: How much imbalance between the arms is acceptable, and who decides what is acceptable? Metaphorically, the balance arm need not be exactly level, but the weight of evidence may not tip completely to one side. The concept of equipoise should be interpreted broadly to include interventions that may not be quite as effective as standard care but may be less complicated, less expensive, or have fewer side effects. Our intuition is that researchers in a clinical trial may compromise a participant's interests only for very good reasons and only to a limited extent. In Study 26.1, there was some evidence to support the effectiveness of ARB, but it was not definitive.

Levels of Equipoise

In practical terms, equipoise or uncertainty should exist on three different levels:

The community of scientific experts. One requirement for equipoise is that existing evidence on the research question is inconclusive; that is, experts who have critically reviewed the evidence disagree. Judgments about the superiority of one treatment or another should follow the convention that requires statistical significance at the level of $p < .05$. This determination of equipoise is made by peer reviewers, IRBs, and study sponsors when they approve an RCT.

The individual physician, acting as an investigator or a referring MD. This option is often criticized because individual physicians might base their judgments on intuition, custom, or ignorance rather than evidence-based deliberation. However, it would be ethically troubling to ask physicians to ignore their personal clinical judgment when making recommendations to potential research participants or when carrying out a research study. In clinical practice, physicians are expected to extrapolate from published evidence when making decisions regarding individual patients. Moreover, many patients rely on their physician's recommendations about entering a clinical trial. Physicians who believe that one arm of the trial is superior cannot refer patients to it without violating their ethical obligation to act in the best interests of their patients. Nor can such physicians in good faith serve as an investigator in the trial without violating their obligation as researchers to ensure that the risks of the research are minimized and acceptable in light of the benefits.

Individual research participants. Even if experts and individual physicians believe that equipoise holds, an individual patient may decline to be randomized because he strongly prefers one of the arms. In Study 26.1, patients who would benefit from ARB or ACE inhibitors because they have congestive heart failure should not accept randomization. As another example, if a trial compares surgical and medical approaches to a disease, some persons may find the short-term risk or the long-term complications from surgery to be unacceptable, while others may not be willing to take medication daily.

If few patients are willing to be randomized to receive either treatment, as a practical matter, the trial cannot be carried out. Hence even if the scientific peer reviewers and the IRB judge that a randomization is appropriate, the trial will fail if referring physicians or potential participants do not agree that equipoise exists.

CHOICE OF INTERVENTIONS

The choice of interventions in a clinical trial may give rise to ethical as well as scientific concerns.

ACTIVE INTERVENTIONS

In Study 26.1, the choice of the active intervention was controversial. Some experts contended that ACE inhibitors should have been studied rather than ARBs. Because several ACE inhibitors were available in generic format or were going off patent, the cost of long-term therapy would be much less for ACEs than for on-patent ARBs. Thus an RCT showing that ACE inhibitors are effective would provide greater benefit to society than an RCT of ARBs. However, drug manufacturers who sponsor trials like Study 26.1 have much more incentive to study ARBs, because sales of patented drugs generate greater profits.

CONTROL INTERVENTIONS

The choice of interventions for the control group may raise ethical concerns. In some clinical trials, the choice of interventions has been criticized as biased because the control intervention was known to be ineffective for the condition studied, or was administered at suboptimal doses in the clinical trial (6). Such use of control interventions is unethical both because it puts participants at unacceptable risk and because it leads to overestimates of the benefits of investigational agent. Rigorous scientific peer review of protocols is the best safeguard against such design bias.

TABLE 26.1	Acceptable Use of Placebo Controls
No effective treatment exists for the condition.	
Participants have failed to respond to established treatment.	
Participants have refused established treatment.	
No serious or irreversible risks will occur.	
Alternative study designs will not produce valid conclusions.	

USE OF PLACEBO CONTROLS

Placebos are substances that are inactive for the condition being studied. Their use strengthens the rigor of a clinical trial, but it also raises ethical concerns. Administering a placebo rather than no intervention at all in the control group controls for the possibility that outcomes are due to the participant's belief that the intervention will work, rather than a biological effect. However, if effective treatment is available, participants might be harmed if they receive a placebo rather than the active treatment. Placebos are ethically acceptable under several circumstances (Table 26.1).

No effective treatment exists for the condition under study. Placebos are appropriate if there is no effective treatment, provided that participants understand that they might receive an inert pill and consent to this possibility. However, if an effective treatment exists for the condition being studied and is feasible to administer, intentionally withholding effective therapies would violate the ethical principle of "do no harm." A more ethically acceptable design is an "add on" design: all participants receive the current standard of care plus either the investigational agent or a placebo.

Participants have failed to respond to established treatment. A placebo would not harm persons who fail to respond to the standard treatment or cannot tolerate it, because they would not benefit from the treatment they have foregone.

There are no serious or irreversible risks to participants. In mild, self-limited conditions, such as allergic rhinitis, insomnia, mild hypertension, and pain from a dental extraction, participants would not suffer significant harm if they received a placebo. Indeed, many patients with these conditions decide not take medications. Potential participants need to be informed that effective interventions are available outside the research study.

Informed refusal of standard therapy. Participants may be entered into a placebo-controlled trial if they have made an informed refusal of standard and effective therapy (7). The criteria for judging whether they are informed should be strict. For example, participants should be administered a questionnaire to ascertain that they understand the availability of effective treatment and the risks that might occur if they forego it. The more serious the condition and the potential harm from omitting standard therapy, the stricter the criteria should be. Also, such participants should be offered the opportunity to change their minds, withdraw from the clinical trial at any time, and receive standard treatment.

STUDY 26.2	Placebo-controlled trial of acellular pertussis vaccine.

In Italy in 1992, a pertussis vaccine was not required for children, and the national vaccination rate was about 40%. A major reason for this low rate of vaccination was the perception that the whole-cell pertussis vaccine had an unacceptable rate of complications. A randomized clinical trial in Italy compared two acellular vaccines with the whole cell vaccine currently used in the United States and with a placebo. The two acellular vaccines were found to be immunogenic, effective, and safe, whereas the effectiveness of the whole-cell vaccine was unexpectedly low. Adverse events (AEs) occurred much more frequently with the whole-cell vaccine.

In Study 26.2, relatively few children in Italy received pertussis vaccine, because of parental concerns about side effects. Parents who strongly preferred their children to receive an active vaccine could choose to receive the licensed whole-cell vaccine outside the trial. Thus, the trial was carried out in children whose parents were willing to forego an active vaccine.

More controversially, placebos may be acceptable under the following circumstances:

Alternative study designs will not produce valid conclusions. In some situations, if placebo controls are not used, the research question cannot be answered in a rigorous manner. One such situation is when the difference in outcomes between standard treatment and placebo for the condition varies greatly from one clinical trial to another.

It has been reported that participants in about one-third of well-designed and well-conducted clinical trials involving major depression failed to distinguish a drug that was known to be effective from a placebo (8). The percentage of people who respond to antidepressants also varies greatly from trial to trial. This is due to a number of reasons, including great variability in response from person to person, spontaneous remissions, refractory cases, and modest efficacy.

STUDY 26.3	Variable outcomes in clinical trials for depression.

A placebo-controlled RCT is proposed for a new antidepressant. The participants will be persons with major depression. They will be informed that standard therapies for depression are available outside of the trial.

In Study 26.3, if a new intervention is compared only with standard therapy (an active control design), the study results will be difficult to interpret if no significant difference is found between the two arms. Without a placebo comparison arm, the FDA has determined that it would be impossible to determine whether both drugs are effective in this trial or whether both are no better than placebo. Hence without placebo controls, the study might not yield valid knowledge, and therefore any risk to participants would be unethical.

Strict measures need to be taken to ensure that risks to participants are acceptable and minimized in such placebo-controlled trials (9). Serious or life-threatening outcomes may occur if an exacerbation of depression is not treated promptly. In Study 26.3, participants need to be monitored closely for the development of suicidality. Because severely depressed persons may not take the initiative to seek care, it would be prudent to enroll only persons who have someone who can help monitor their condition and help them seek medical care if needed. The participant (as well as a relative, partner, or close friend) should be educated on the importance of reporting symptoms of worsening depression or suicidality immediately to the investigators. Investigators need to be available at all times to respond to such serious AEs. Appropriate plans must be made to remove suicidal patients promptly from the study and provide individualized treatment, which might include off-study medications and voluntary or involuntary hospitalization. When participants are removed from the trial because they are suicidal, they should be counted as a treatment failure.

Placebo-controlled trials are also appropriate, even though effective treatments are available, for conditions that have a waxing-waning course or spontaneous remissions, or whose therapies are only partially effective and have serious adverse effects (9).

It may not be acceptable to carry out a placebo-controlled trial in resource-poor countries that would be considered unethical in the United States. For instance, such trials are not appropriate simply because people in the host country cannot afford therapies used in the United States. As discussed in Chapter 22, such trials need to address a health care priority in the country, and alternative study designs that do not use a placebo would not produce valid conclusions.

BLINDING

Blinding of investigators and participants, which helps prevent bias, can raise ethical problems. Blinding eliminates bias in the ascertainment of endpoints. It also minimizes the clinical impact of a participant's belief that she is receiving an effective intervention (the so-called placebo effect). However, blinding can be detrimental if the patient suffers a serious AE that may be related to the study intervention. Thus, there must be a procedure to override blinding when necessary to provide needed medical care to a participant. Blinding is often imperfect because participants can determine by the adverse effects what intervention they are receiving.

STUDY 26.1   (Continued).

If a participant in Study 1 develops life-threatening hyperkalemia, the blind should be broken. If the participant was on ARB, it would be reasonable to monitor the potassium level carefully after stopping the study medication to ensure that the potassium returns to normal. If the participant was on placebo, a workup for other causes of hyperkalemia would be indicated.

BACKGROUND CARE

Background care or concurrent care is the care participants receive for the condition being studied in addition to the study or control intervention. Protocols commonly specify what background care will be permitted; this standardization enhances the internal validity of the study. Ethical concerns arise if the quality of background care is substandard. In Study 26.1, background care for diabetes includes counselling on diet and exercise and home glucose monitoring. These interventions are known to improve glucose control and thereby reduce the progression of nephropathy. However, they also reduce the power of the study to detect a difference between the two arms. Thus study staff might unconsciously underemphasize lifestyle changes and self-management. Further dilemmas arise if a study adopts "usual care" for background care but the quality of care available to participants is known to be substandard. Even though the researchers are not personally providing a substandard level of care, they have some responsibility for the care participants receive for the condition they are studying. If investigators allow substandard care to continue without comment, participants may infer that the experts approve it. Researchers can address concerns about background care by providing treating physicians with results of clinical tests carried out as part of the research project and offering suggestions to the referring physicians. For example, in Study 26.1, investigators should provide results of hemoglobin A1c and cholesterol tests, and suggest prescribing statins or increasing the dose to meet target goals for cholesterol management. Alternatively, to avoid a conflict of interest, the investigators could arrange for independent diabetes experts to monitor these tests and make recommendations. For persistently suboptimal glucose control, the researchers could offer treating physicians the opportunity to refer participants to free counseling for diet and exercise that is provided by clinicians who are independent of the study and blinded to the intervention the participant receives. In addition, investigators should also provide care for conditions that might affect the endpoint of the trial; for example, untreated hypertension could cause progression of renal insufficiency.

A related issue is ancillary care—care for other conditions that are not the object of study. In countries with a well-functioning health care system, participants can be referred to their usual source of medical care. Chapter 22 discusses the issue of ancillary care in resource-poor settings, where access to basic health care is compromised.

STANDARDIZATION OF INTERVENTIONS

Protocols commonly specify the doses of medications and the circumstances in which the doses may be changed. Such standardization increases the internal validity of the study. However, it can be problematic if participants do not appreciate that decisions about their medications are determined by the protocol, and not by individualized decisions about what is in their best interests. The ethical tension between scientific rigor and acting in the best interests of individual participants can be alleviated if the study is designed as a "large simple trial," in which participants are allowed to receive a broad spectrum of background care in addition to the study intervention (5). Furthermore, participants may be recruited from diverse populations and practice settings (10). Such pragmatic trials also have the advantage of greater external validity because they are directly applicable to decision-making in clinical practice.

CHOICE OF ENDPOINTS

Clinical endpoints, such as death, myocardial infarction, functional status, or disease-related quality of life, are meaningful to patients. Rigorous evidence that an intervention can improve such clinical endpoints provides a strong basis for a change in medical practice. However, demonstrating an impact on clinical endpoints may require a large number of participants or a prolonged trial.

To make trials smaller and shorter, intermediate markers, such as laboratory measurements or physical signs, may be considered instead of a clinical endpoint. Intermediate markers are commonly used in Phase I studies, which are too small and short to reveal changes in clinical endpoints. For example, in a Phase I cancer trial, improvement in tumor markers, such as prostate specific antigen (PSA), or stabilization or reduction in tumor size may justify moving to a Phase II study.

Intermediate markers, however, should be used with great caution. In a number of clinical trials, the interventions had a beneficial effect on intermediate markers but a detrimental or no effect on clinical endpoints. Examples of such discrepancies include the following (11,12):

- Flecainide, encainide, and moricizine suppress ventricular arrhythmias after a heart attack but increase mortality.
- Milrinone and flosequinan improve cardiac output and exercise tolerance but increase mortality in congestive heart failure.
- Chemotherapy with 5-fluorouracil (5FU) improves complete and partial response rate of patients with advanced colon cancer but has no impact on overall survival.
- Fluoride increases bone mass but also increases vertebral fractures in patients with osteoporosis.
- Topical antibiotics reduce the incidence of nasal cultures of *Staph aureus* in surgical patients but do not reduce infection at surgical sites.

Intermediate markers were misleading surrogates for clinical outcomes in these studies. Inferring that the study intervention is effective solely on the basis of intermediate markers would have led to serious errors. Had clinical practice changed on the basis of these findings, many patients would have been seriously harmed. Thus in Phase III studies, intermediate markers, no matter how plausible, should be used as surrogates for clinical outcomes only if they have been formally validated as predicting clinical outcomes.

In summary, the choice of interventions, subjects, and endpoints can only be addressed in the context of a specific clinical trial. Integrated scientific and ethical review helps ensure that these issues will be addressed appropriately. First, the study should undergo rigorous scientific peer review by experts independent of the study. These experts can determine whether the existing evidence already indicates that one arm of the study is superior to the other(s), whether the endpoints are meaningful, what the medical risks are, and which participants might be at increased risk of AEs. Second, an IRB reviewing a clinical trial should have access to the scientific reviewers' recommendations on these issues and take them into account during its deliberations. The IRB should include members or consultants with scientific and clinical expertise pertinent to the study.

SELECTION OF SUBJECTS

The inclusion and exclusion criteria for a clinical trial may raise ethical concerns. Investigators need to decide, for example, whether to study the early or late stages of a disease or condition. Enrolling persons who are in the late stages of a disease and have a poor prognosis may limit the potential loss of quality-adjusted life years if serious AEs occur. However, depending on the disease and the condition, an intervention may fail to benefit patients with advanced disease but still benefit persons in the early stages of the disease.

Researchers should exclude persons who are at greatly increased risk of harm from the investigational or control intervention in the study. For example, persons should be excluded if they already have significant impairment in an organ system in which the investigational agent causes AEs.

Persons should also be excluded if they need to take the investigational agent and will be harmed if they do not receive it.

STUDY 26.1   **(Continued).**

Enrolling patients with impaired glomerular filtration would increase the number of clinical endpoints and shorten the length of the study. However, persons who already have significant renal failure might not respond to an intervention that would be effective in persons with early-stage nephropathy. Hyperkalemia is one adverse effect of ARBs. Thus the study might exclude persons who have a history of hyperkalemia or who need to take other medicines that can cause hyperkalemia. Finally, participants with congestive heart failure in addition to diabetes could be significantly harmed if they receive a placebo rather than ARB, and therefore should be excluded from the trial.

INFORMED CONSENT

Although investigators and IRBs pay great attention to consent forms, many participants—the majority in some studies—have fundamental misunderstandings about the purpose and nature of clinical trials (13–17). Participants often do not understand how clinical trials differ from standard treatment; this is often called "therapeutic misconception" (18). Furthermore, they commonly do not understand that they may be in a control group rather than the intervention group, and that being in a clinical trial may restrict their therapeutic options (18). Thus, investigators should try to improve the comprehension of the participants, such as by spending more time talking with them.

Obtaining consent may be particularly problematic in certain clinical trials (19):

- Phase 1 clinical trials whose aim is to determine the maximum tolerated dose of a new investigational agent.
- Placebo-controlled trials in which treatment of proven efficacy is withheld.
- Trials in which invasive procedures, such as biopsies, are performed solely for research purposes.
- Trials of interventions for which participants have high hopes of success, such as stem cell transplantation (20). (Chapter 28 discusses ethical issues in stem cell clinical trials in more detail.)

In these circumstances, the balance of benefits and risks may not be as favorable as in standard care.

Although many researchers and IRBs focus on disclosure of information, it may be more important ethically for researchers to ask eligible participants questions to ascertain whether they comprehend key information about the trial. As noted in Chapter 6, clinical trial participants need to appreciate:

- how research differs from clinical care;
- that the effectiveness of the research intervention is unknown;
- that the research intervention has risk; and
- that the interventions are determined by chance and not by what a physician believes is best for the individual participant.

If participants do not understand these issues, the investigators need to spend more time talking with them until their misunderstandings are corrected.

Trials in which many participants have low literacy or poor access to health care present particular challenges. Chapter 6 discusses how to overcome such barriers to consent.

Consent must be voluntary as well as informed. If an investigator in a clinical trial enrolls her own patients as participants, it raises ethical concerns because patients may be reluctant to say no to a physician on whom they depend for ongoing care.

DATA MONITORING

As data are collected in a clinical trial, they should be monitored to address the questions in Table 26.2. Data monitoring and interim data analyses are needed to determine whether it is ethical to continue the trial as planned.

DATA MONITORING PROCEDURES

To address these questions, the protocol should contain a data monitoring plan to address the following procedural questions:

When Will Data be Monitored?

The protocol should specify when data will be monitored. In Phase I studies, data are typically analyzed after a few participants have completed the protocol. In a classic dose-escalation protocol, three participants receive each dose, and researchers examine data from each cohort before proceeding to the next dosage level. In some circumstances, such as first-in-human studies of highly innovative interventions, data from each participant should be evaluated before the next participant is enrolled.

In Phase III studies, investigators often plan three interim analyses, for example, when 25%, 50%, and 75% of the planned participants are enrolled, or when these percentages of endpoints are observed. However, data monitoring schedules should be individualized for each trial.

Who Will Monitor Data From the Trial?

The most rigorous way to carry out interim analyses of the data as they accrue is through a data and safety monitoring board (DSMB) that is independent of the investigators and the sponsor (21). The DSMB can be unblinded while the investigators remain blinded, so that the study can proceed without bias.

The DSMB also examines unblinded data on safety and efficacy, looking at differences between the active and control arms. These unblinded data are kept confidential from the investigators and sponsor to ensure that no bias will be introduced into the trial.

The protocol should specify what data will be examined at each data monitoring session and what findings will lead to changes in the protocol. The DSMB receives data from the statistical center at each planned interim analysis. The DSMB examines data on patient accrual, retention,

TABLE 26.2	Questions for Data Monitoring and Interim Data Analysis

Are the risks and benefits substantially different from expected?

Has one arm been proven to have more benefit?

Has one arm been proven to have more harm?

Will the trial fail to provide a valid answer to the research question?

If the answer to any question is yes, several additional questions need to be posed:

Should the trial be continued?

Should the protocol be modified?

Should the informed consent process be modified?

protocol violations, and missing data. These data, as well as aggregate data on AEs, are often shared with the study leadership and sponsor in an open session. The DSMB also examines AEs and outcomes data by treatment arm in a closed session that the investigators and sponsor do not attend; the DSMB may unblind the arms during the closed session if needed.

Investigators can obtain more information about DSMBs at a number of websites. The National Institutes of Health (NIH) has guidance on DSMBs on its website at http://grants.nih.gov/grants/guide/notice-files/not98-084.html. The National Cancer Institute (NCI) has detailed guidance regarding DSMBs, including examples of plans for DSMBs, at http://www.cancer.gov/clinicaltrials/conducting/dsm-guidelines/page1. In addition, research institutions often have model DSMB policies on their IRB website.

Because DSMBs are costly, they are used primarily in Phase II/III trials. The NIH requires their use in the Phase III trials that it funds. However, for other studies, alternative options for data monitoring may be appropriate (22). In Phase I studies, the principal investigator, a colleague of the principal investigator, or the study sponsor may monitor the data for unexpected harm. However, these alternative arrangements may raise concerns about conflicts of interest.

ARE THE RISKS AND BENEFITS SUBSTANTIALLY DIFFERENT FROM EXPECTED?

Serious unexpected AEs related to the study agents may alter the risk/benefit ratio to the point that it is unacceptable or the risks are no longer minimized. Unexpected AEs are those that are not mentioned in the protocol or are more frequent or serious than anticipated. The DSMB also reviews whether the serious unexpected AEs are related to the study or control agents. If they are, the balance of risks and benefits in the trial must be reassessed to determine whether the risks are still acceptable and minimized. The DSMB may recommend additional or more frequent measurements to ascertain the incidence, severity, or mechanism of the AEs.

In some cases, the DSMB might recommend or require protocol modifications, such as reducing the dose of the investigative agent or excluding participants who are at greatly increased risk for AEs.

HAS ONE ARM BEEN PROVEN TO HAVE MORE BENEFIT?

Interim data analyses raise complex ethical and statistical issues, as the following study illustrates (23–25).

STUDY 26.4   Stopping a trial early for benefit.

In the Anglo-Scandinavian Cardiac Outcomes Trial (ASCOT) trial, participants with hypertension and other cardiac risk factors were randomized to receive an atenolol-based regimen (a thiazide diuretic could be added after a maximal dose of atenolol) or an amlodipine-based regimen (an ACE inhibitor could be added after a maximal dose of amlodipine). The trial enrolled over 19,000 patients. After an average of 4.6 years of follow-up, the DSMB found on interim analysis a nonsignificant trend in the primary endpoint—heart attack plus cardiac death—in favor of amlodipine regimens. Moreover, there was a highly significant trend in one of the seven secondary endpoints—stroke—favoring the amlodipine arm ($p < 0.00004$). Even taking into account that there were seven secondary endpoints, this p-value exceeded the stopping rule at the first analysis. The DSMB recommended stopping the trial on the basis of this secondary endpoint. However, after discussions with the leadership and other experts, it was agreed that the trial should be continued. Because beta-blockers were widely prescribed for hypertension, it was judged that more compelling evidence was needed to change clinical practice. Furthermore, an independent endpoint committee was still adjudicating some endpoints.

STUDY 26.4   (Continued).

At a second interim analysis after 5.5 years of follow-up, there continued to be a non-significant trend in favor of amlodipine for the primary cardiovascular endpoint and a significant trend for stroke. In addition, there was a trend favoring amlodipine in total mortality (13.9/1000 participant years vs. 15.5, p = 0.0247, which did not meet the statistical stopping rule) and in new-onset diabetes (p < 0.001, which met the stopping rule). The DSMB again recommended stopping the trial, and the trial was halted.

From an ethical perspective, if interim data already prove that one arm is significantly more beneficial, continuing the study as planned would be ethically problematic because it would delay providing the more effective intervention to participants in the other arm and to patients outside the trial. From a statistical viewpoint, however, trends seen on early interim analysis may be misleading because they may be reversed as more endpoints accrue. There is considerable fluctuation in interim trial results over time due to random variation (26). Furthermore, multiple analyses of data increase the likelihood of finding a difference between the two arms by chance when in reality no difference exists (a Type I error).

Statistical stopping rules address these issues by requiring a more stringent level of statistical significance (alpha) at each interim analysis than at the end of the trial. Generally, the alpha level at the first interim analysis is very small, and the alpha level at the final analysis is close to the two-sided alpha level of 0.05 for the completed study. The choice of stopping rules should be specified in the protocol. Unfortunately, DSMBs often do not apply proper statistical stopping rules and may base stopping decisions on an inadequate number of endpoints (27). As a result, clinically improbable effect sizes are sometimes reported when clinical trials are stopped early (28). This may lead to bias in systematic reviews (27). Some critics assert that stopping trials early for benefit leads to systematic overestimation of the magnitude of benefit (27). It is to be expected on statistical grounds, however, that point estimates of effectiveness are higher in trials that are stopped at interim monitoring for efficacy than in similar trials that are completed as planned (29). Another important consideration is that stopping a trial at interim analysis precludes gathering information on important long-term endpoints, such as long-term survival or recurrence of disease (26).

There often is an ethical tension between ensuring the short-term well-being of participants in a trial and discovering important new knowledge (30). Stopping an inferior intervention may protect trial participants from short-term harm. However, both future patients and trial participants have an interest in having the trial answer important research questions (for example, regarding long-term outcomes) or continuing the trial to see whether trends on secondary endpoints become statistically significant. In some cases, stopping a study at interim analysis makes it very unlikely that additional important questions will ever be answered. Moreover, in some circumstances, stopping a trial prematurely may decrease its impact on clinical practice, because practicing physicians may not find conclusions based on interim analyses persuasive. For example, this may occur if a trial reveals that a widely used treatment is less effective or less safe than the experimental intervention. As a result, future patients may be harmed by continuing to receive the inferior intervention. This dilemma can only be resolved in the context of a specific trial and clinical condition, taking into account all the data available at the time of the interim analysis.

HAS ONE ARM BEEN PROVEN TO CAUSE MORE HARM?

If the interim data prove that one arm causes significantly more harm than the other, continuing the trial would subject participants in that arm to excessive harms.

STUDY 26.5 **Stopping a trial early because of harm.**

In the Cardiac Arrhythmia Suppression Trial (CAST), the antiarrhythmic drugs flecainide, encainide, and moricizine were compared with placebo in heart attack survivors with ventricular premature beats. When this study was carried out, antiarrhythmic drugs were widely used in clinical practice in patients with myocardial infarction because they were known to suppress ventricular arrhythmias. Only participants whose ventricular arrhythmias were suppressed by one of the study drugs were randomized into the trial. At interim analysis after 10 months of follow-up, flecainide and encainide had a higher mortality than the placebo group (7.7% vs. 3.0%) and higher cardiac mortality (4.5% vs. 1.2%). The DSMB recommended stopping the trial.

Interim data suggesting that an experimental intervention is harmful have been called an "agonizing negative trend" (31). It may be difficult for the DSMB to decide whether to stop a trial because of harm, because two types of errors may occur. One error is stopping a trial too soon. If the evidence of harm is weak, the rejected intervention might be shown to be beneficial if the trial is continued. Furthermore, stopping a trial too soon may fail to provide sufficient evidence to persuade physicians to abandon a harmful drug that is being used in clinical practice (32). The opposite error is continuing a harmful trial longer than necessary and causing more participants to be harmed by a risky intervention.

STUDY 26.1 **(Continued).**

The DSMB allowed the trial to continue after it was already extremely unlikely that these drugs would be shown to improve mortality. Because antiarrhythmic drugs were widely used in clinical practice, the DSMB believed that it was important to show that these drugs increased mortality, rather than simply having no benefit. Study 26.5 produced the counterintuitive finding that these drugs increased mortality even though they had a beneficial effect on the surrogate endpoint. These results had a dramatic impact on clinical practice.

In some trials, there may be evidence of an increase in a serious but nonfatal AE that is statistically significant but relatively infrequent. Under these circumstances, a DSMB might decide to continue a trial but institute protective measures, such as scheduling more frequent interim analyses, excluding participants at high risk of developing the harm, and informing participants of the risk (33).

WILL THE TRIAL FAIL TO PROVIDE A VALID ANSWER TO THE RESEARCH QUESTION?

The power of a trial may become unacceptably low if there is very low enrollment or far fewer than expected outcome events. Furthermore, the validity of a trial may be compromised by frequent protocol violations or high dropout rates. If these problems occur, the DSMB may request that the investigators develop an action plan to correct the problems. For example, if enrollment falls well below projections, the investigators may add more sites, seek IRB approval to change the method of recruitment, provide additional training or support for study staff, or extend the duration of the study.

If steps to correct these problems are unsuccessful, the prospect of gaining valid and generalizable knowledge will be diminished. Thus it would be unethical to continue to expose participants to any risk and inconvenience.

ACTIONS AFTER INTERIM DATA ANALYSIS

In some situations, interim results and analyses may make it unethical to continue a clinical trial. In a Phase I trial, early data may already show unacceptable toxicity; for example, they may point to unexpected deaths that are definitely or probably associated with the investigational agent. The following examples from Phase III studies also raise the issue of terminating the trial.

Should the Trial be Continued?

If interim data show conclusively that one arm has more risk or is more effective, or that the trial will not provide a valid answer to the research question, it would be unethical to continue the study. Under these circumstances, continuing the trial would expose participants to the risks and inconvenience of participating in a clinical trial with the prospect of gaining little or no additional scientific knowledge. Compelling evidence of harm or benefit may be found in interim data or in the results of other clinical trials.

Should the Protocol be Modified?

Changes to the protocol may be required to reduce risk to participants, enhance the power of the study, or increase the validity of the data.

Should the Informed Consent Process be Modified?

In some situations, interim findings need to be discussed with participants because they would alter the willingness of persons to enroll in the trial or continue to participate in it. For instance, there may be evidence of unanticipated AEs or results from another clinical trial on the same condition that might be pertinent to a person's willingness to enroll in or continue in the trial. Providing such data to participants does not necessarily lead to a large number of participants dropping out of the trial (26).

After answering these questions, the DSMB sends a report to the study sponsor and leadership. It makes recommendations as to whether to continue or stop the trial, and describes any changes that should be made to the consent process or protocol. The study sponsor and leadership decide whether to accept the recommendations and communicate any protocol changes to site investigators, who pass it on to their local IRB. IRBs need to approve any protocol modifications.

CONTRACT RESEARCH ORGANIZATIONS

Contract research organizations (CROs) contract with clinical trial sponsors to carry out such activities as recruiting participants, collecting data, analyzing data, and writing articles (34,35). CROs are now participating in the majority of clinical trials. Many are for-profit companies, although a few are associated with academic health centers. CROs offer the advantages of greater efficiency and lower cost, often because they carry out research in low-cost countries. However, critics have alleged that because CROs depend on continued contracts from sponsors, they distort the science and place participants at risk to please sponsors. Both for-profit and academic-affiliated CROs have been criticized for alleged bias, incomplete disclosure of financial conflicts of interest, cases of serious injury to participants, and inexperienced and less educated staff (34,35).

RESPONSIBILITIES OF AUTHORS

As discussed in Chapter 13, authors of scientific publications have an ethical responsibility to vouch for the integrity and completeness of their findings. Authors should have access to all data from the trial and full control over data analysis and the writing and submission of the manuscript. Two serious ethical concerns about publication of clinical trials have recently been raised. First, some articles have been written by employees of drug companies that sponsored a trial for a university-based researcher who served as the lead author, but these ghostwriters were not named as authors or acknowledged in the paper (36,37). As shown in Chapter 13, this practice is dishonest, fails to give credit where it is deserved, and masks conflicts of interest. Second, negative findings from some clinical trials have not been published, or their publication has been markedly delayed (see Table 1.1 in

Chapter 1). Failure to publish clinically significant negative results is unethical and may cause serious harms to patients. To prevent such misconduct, all clinical trials must be registered at the onset in an acceptable public clinical trials registry (38). New requirements are being established to require timely reporting of results in a clinical trials registry as well.

TAKE HOME POINTS

1. Each step of an RCT—randomization, selection of interventions, and choice of endpoints, eligibility, and exclusion criteria—raises ethical issues that need to be addressed in conjunction with scientific and design issues.
2. Randomization is ethically appropriate if the arms of the trial are in equipoise.
3. Placebo controls are justified in certain circumstances.
4. Persons who are at greatly increased risk of harm should be excluded from the trial.
5. The protocol should include a sound plan for data monitoring and interim data analyses.

ANNOTATED BIBLIOGRAPHY

DeMets DL, Furberg CD, Friedman LM, eds. *Data Monitoring in Clinical Trials: A Case Studies Approach*. New York: Springer; 2006.
>   Excellent monograph on all aspects of data monitoring, including many thoughtful case studies of DSMB decisions that could not be made simply on the basis of statistical stopping rules.

Emanuel EJ, Miller FG. The ethics of placebo-controlled trials—a middle ground. *N Engl J Med* 2001;345:915–919.
>   Analysis of ethical and scientific issues regarding placebo controls.

Fleming TR, Sharples K, McCall J, Moore A, Rodgers A, Stewart R. Maintaining confidentiality of interim data to enhance trial integrity and credibility. *Clin Trials* 2008;5:157–167.
>   Discussion of the problems that occur if interim data analyses are inappropriately disseminated.

Pocock SJ. When (not) to stop a clinical trial for benefit. *JAMA* 2005;294:2228–2230.
>   Analysis of stopping clinical trials at interim analysis because of evidence of benefit.

REFERENCES

1. Appelbaum PS, Lidz CW. The therapeutic misconception. In: Emanuel EJ, Grady C, Crouch RA, Lie RK, Miller FG, Wendler D, eds. *The Oxford Textbook of Clinical Research Ethics*. New York: Oxford University Press; 2008:633–644.
2. Kurtzman NA. Drug companies should not have the final say in the design of clinical trials. *Am J Kidney Dis* 2001;38:1113–1114.
3. Vist GE, Hagen KB, Devereaux PJ, et al. Systematic review to determine whether participation in a trial influences outcome. *BMJ* 2005;330:1175.
4. Gross CP, Krumholz HM, Van Wye G, et al. Does random treatment assignment cause harm to research participants? *PLoS Med* 2006;3:e188.
5. Joffe S, Truog RD. Equipoise and randomization. In: Emanuel EJ, Grady C, Crouch RA, et al, eds. *The Oxford Textbook of Clinical Research Ethics*. New York: Oxford University Press; 2008:245–260.
6. Hampson LA, Bekelman JE, Gross CP. Empirical data on conflicts of interest. In: Emanuel E, ed. *Oxford Textbook of Research Ethics*. New York: Oxford University Press; 2008:767–779.
7. Lublin FD, Reingold SC. Placebo-controlled clinical trials in multiple sclerosis: ethical considerations. National Multiple Sclerosis Society (USA) Task Force on Placebo-Controlled Clinical Trials in MS. *Ann Neurol* 2001;49:677–681.
8. Temple R, Ellenberg SS. Placebo-controlled trials and active-control trials in the evaluation of new treatments. Part 1: Ethical and scientific issues. *Ann Intern Med* 2000;133:455–463.
9. Emanuel EJ, Miller FG. The ethics of placebo-controlled trials—a middle ground. *N Engl J Med* 2001;345:915–919.
10. Tunis SR, Stryer DB, Clancy CM. Practical clinical trials: increasing the value of clinical research for decision making in clinical and health policy. *JAMA* 2003;290:1624–1632.
11. Fleming TR. Surrogate endpoints and FDA's accelerated approval process. *Health Aff (Millwood)* 2005;24:67–78.
12. Fleming TR, DeMets DL. Surrogate end points in clinical trials: are we being misled? *Ann Intern Med* 1996;125:605–613.

13. Institute of Medicine. *Responsible Research: A Systems Approach to Protecting Research Participants.* Washington, DC: National Academies Press; 2003.

14. National Bioethics Advisory Commission. *Ethical and Policy Issues in Research Involving Human Participants.* Rockville, MD: National Bioethics Advisory Commission; 2001.

15. Advisory Committee on Human Radiation Experiments. *Final Report.* New York: Oxford University Press; 1998.

16. Wendler D, Emanuel EJ, Lie RK. The standard of care debate: can research in developing countries be both ethical and responsive to those countries' health needs? *Am J Public Health* 2004;94:923–928.

17. Lo B, O'Connell ME, eds. *Ethical Considerations for Research on Housing-Related Health Hazards Involving Children.* Washington, DC: National Academies Press; 2005.

18. Lidz CW, Appelbaum PS. The therapeutic misconception: problems and solutions. *Med Care* 2002;40:V55–V63.

19. Miller FG, Joffe S. Evaluating the therapeutic misconception. *Kennedy Inst Ethics J* 2006;16:353–366.

20. Lo B, Kriegstein A, Grady D. Clinical trials in stem cell transplantation: guidelines for scientific and ethical review. *Clin Trials* 2008;5:517–522.

21. Slutsky AS, Lavery JV. Data safety and monitoring boards. *N Engl J Med* 2004;350:1143–1147.

22. Amdur RJ. Provisions for data monitoring. In: Bankert EA, Amdur RJ, eds. *Institutional Review Board Management and Function.* 2nd ed. Sudbury, MA: Jones and Bartlett Publishers; 2006:160–165.

23. Dahlof B, Sever PS, Poulter NR, et al. Prevention of cardiovascular events with an antihypertensive regimen of amlodipine adding perindopril as required versus atenolol adding bendroflumethiazide as required, in the Anglo-Scandinavian Cardiac Outcomes Trial-Blood Pressure Lowering Arm (ASCOT-BPLA): a multicentre randomised controlled trial. *Lancet* 2005;366:895–906.

24. Pocock SJ. The simplest statistical test: how to check for a difference between treatments. *BMJ* 2006;332:1256–1258.

25. Pocock SJ. When (not) to stop a clinical trial for benefit. *JAMA* 2005;294:2228–2230.

26. Fleming TR, Sharples K, McCall J, et al. Maintaining confidentiality of interim data to enhance trial integrity and credibility. *Clin Trials* 2008;5:157–167.

27. Bassler D, Montori VM, Briel M, et al. Early stopping of randomized clinical trials for overt efficacy is problematic. *J Clin Epidemiol* 2008;61:241–246.

28. Montori VM, Devereaux PJ, Adhikari NK, et al. Randomized trials stopped early for benefit: a systematic review. *JAMA* 2005;294:2203–2209.

29. Goodman SN. Stopping at nothing? Some dilemmas of data monitoring in clinical trials. *Ann Intern Med* 2007;146:882–887.

30. Peppercorn J, Buss WG, Fost N, et al. The dilemma of data-safety monitoring: provision of significant new data to research participants. *Lancet* 2008;371:527–529.

31. DeMets DL, Pocock SJ, Julian DG. The agonising negative trend in monitoring of clinical trials. *Lancet* 1999;354:1983–1988.

32. DeMets DL, Friedman LM. The data monitoring experience in the Cardiac Arrhythmia Suppression Trial: the need to be prepared early. In: DeMets DL, Furberg CD, Friedman LM, eds. *Data Monitoring in Clinical Trials: A Case Studies Approach.* New York: Springer; 2006:198–208.

33. Hulley SB, Grady D, Vittinghoff E, et al. Consideration of early stopping and other challenges in monitoring the Heart and Estrogen/Progestin Replacement Study. In: DeMets DL, Furberg CD, Friedman LM, eds. *Data Monitoring in Clinical Trials: A Case Studies Approach.* New York: Springer; 2006:236–247.

34. Shuchman M. Commercializing clinical trials—risks and benefits of the CRO boom. *N Engl J Med* 2007;357:1365–1368.

35. Lenzer J. Truly independent research? *BMJ* 2008;337:a1332.

36. Moffatt B, Elliott C. Ghost marketing: pharmaceutical companies and ghostwritten journal articles. *Perspect Biol Med* 2007;50:18–31.

37. Mathews AW. Ghost story: at medical journals, writers paid by industry play big role. *Wall Street Journal (East Ed)* 2005 Dec 13:A1, A8.

38. De Angelis CD, Drazen JM, Frizelle FA, et al. Is this clinical trial fully registered?—a statement from the International Committee of Medical Journal Editors. *N Engl J Med* 2005;352:2436–2438.

CHAPTER 27

Genetics, Genomics, and Gene Transfer Research

Since the human genome was first sequenced in 2002, high-throughput technologies have lowered the cost of DNA sequencing. It is expected that it will soon be possible to sequence a person's entire DNA sequence for $1000. Research in many fields will increasingly incorporate genome-wide sequencing. Thus all researchers need to understand the particular ethical issues that genetics and genomics research raise.

Biobanks are repositories of biological materials that are linked with detailed clinical information about the donors, such as an individual's electronic medical records. Once samples are sequenced, researchers have both genotypic and phenotypic data on individuals. Sometimes the term "annotated sample" is used to refer to biological materials that are linked to extensive clinical information. Thus biobanks are more powerful research resources than tissue repositories that contain specimens associated with only limited clinical information. Sharing the information and materials in biobanks with other researchers can greatly facilitate research on inherited predispositions to diseases and responses to therapies. However, whole-genome sequencing of many specimens and the sharing of these data raise particular ethical concerns that researchers must address.

In this chapter, we first clarify how genetics and genomics research differs from other types of research. Second, we analyze the ethical issues that research with biobanks and genome-wide association research raise concerning consent and confidentiality. Third, we discuss the disclosure to study participants of individual results from genomic research tests. Finally, we analyze research involving pharmacogenomics and gene transfer.

STUDY 27.1   The deCODE project in Iceland (1,2).

In 1998, Iceland announced plans for a national biobank that would include information about virtually the entire population. The database would combine three sources of information. First, data from computerized health records would be entered on the basis of presumed consent. Citizens would be allowed to opt out or drop out of this part of the project, and about 7% did so. Second, genealogic data on all citizens would be obtained from existing public records. Third, individuals would provide blood samples, with explicit informed consent, for a specific project or for further research approved by a national panel. All data would be coded, and researchers would receive only de-identified data. The database thus would provide phenotypic, genealogical, and genotypic information.

In 2000, the for-profit company deCODE Genetics Inc. obtained an exclusive license to operate the database for 12 years. deCODE Genetics agreed to pay the government an annual payment plus 6% of any profits. The company ultimately worked with blood samples and clinical information provided by individuals. The company has published a number of studies to identify the genetic basis of common diseases, such as diabetes, coronary disease, asthma, and prostate cancer.

In addition to Iceland, several other countries, including the United Kingdom, Estonia, and Japan, are setting up large collections of biological materials for genomic analysis. These biobanks will contain between 50,000 and 500,000 specimens linked to clinical information. These large biobanks will enable research on the genetic basis of common multifactorial diseases and on gene–environment interactions (3,4). The NIH is encouraging the archiving of specimens from the research projects that it funds to be used in future studies. The NIH also is funding genome-wide association studies using archived specimens associated with clinical data. Furthermore, many hospitals, clinics, and for-profit companies are setting up biobanks. However, the concept of biobanks has also raised a number of ethical controversies, and a number of ambitious projects have floundered (4,5).

HOW IS GENETICS AND GENOMICS RESEARCH DIFFERENT?

Genetic or genomic information is commonly viewed as qualitatively different from other clinical information. We use the term "genomics" to refer to the DNA sequence of chromosomes, whereas "genetics" refers simply to the science of inheritance.

GENETICS PROVIDES INFORMATION ABOUT RELATIVES AND GROUPS

All genetic information, whether it is derived from a family history or a DNA test, provides information about relatives as well as the proband. This leads to a number of ethical issues. First, in many genetics studies, researchers collect information about the participant's relatives, which raises privacy concerns. Second, the results of genetics research may have clinical implications for relatives as well as the research participants. However, in some situations, a participant might refuse to share with relatives information that would enable them to take steps to prevent or treat a serious disease. Third, some genetics research may have implications for groups as well as individuals (see Chapter 20) (6,7). Certain groups may also be harmed if the research results contradict their spiritual traditions, historical narratives, or traditional beliefs. Groups also might be stigmatized—for example, if studies of the genetic basis of diseases such as alcoholism and schizophrenia are carried out on samples obtained from one ethnic group. Concerns about stigmatization are particularly salient for minority groups, such as African-Americans or Native Americans, who have suffered discrimination in the past.

GENES ARE VIEWED AS PREDICTIVE OF FUTURE HEALTH AND ILLNESS

The human genome has been termed a "blueprint" for life, or a "future diary" (8). These metaphors imply that a person's DNA sequence determines his or her future, which has been termed "genetic determinism." Genomic information is often considered to have greater predictive power than other medical information. To be sure, some severe diseases are caused by single-gene mutations that have complete penetrance, such as sickle cell disease or Huntington disease. However, the predictive value of genomics is commonly overestimated. Most genes have incomplete penetrance or variable expressivity, so their presence does not reliably predict the occurrence or severity of disease. Furthermore, most common conditions, such as diabetes and hypertension, are polygenic. Many laypersons mistakenly regard genetic influences as all-or-none, rather than probabilities. Furthermore, health and illness are matters of education and environmental factors such as diet, exercise, and exposure to viral illness, as well as heredity.

GENETIC INFORMATION MIGHT LEAD TO STIGMATIZATION AND DISCRIMINATION

Ideas about inheritance were used in the late 19th and early 20th centuries to support ideas of racial superiority and discriminatory social policies (9). Eugenics laws banned marriage or mandated the sterilization of people categorized as feebleminded, insane, or criminal. In addition, miscegenation laws and restrictive immigration policies were enacted. The science used to support such discriminatory policies was deeply flawed (9,10). Given this history, some people fear that genetic research today might be used to support discriminatory social policies. (11). The 2008 federal Genetic Information Nondiscrimination Act forbids discrimination in health insurance and employment, but does not cover disability, long-term care, and life insurance.

GENOMICS RESEARCH MIGHT UNDERMINE TRADITIONAL MORAL BELIEFS

Some critics fear that advances in genetic science might contradict moral and religious teachings and undermine human dignity (12). One concern is that if genes that predispose to alcoholism or drug addiction are identified, individuals with these conditions may no longer be held responsible for the consequences of their actions. Furthermore, genetics research might undermine traditional beliefs about human origins or the ancestry of specific groups. Some proponents of genomics research dismiss these harms as merely symbolic (13). However, the donors of materials for research might view such harms as very important (7).

SPECIAL ETHICAL ISSUES IN GENETICS AND GENOMICS RESEARCH

Genetics and genomics research raises novel ethical issues and requires innovative approaches to well-known ethical problems.

CONFIDENTIALITY

A major risk to participants in genetics and genomics research is a breach of confidentiality.

Confidentiality Concerns in Biobanks

Although no breaches of confidentiality with biobanks have been reported, the public might be concerned because of many reports of stolen or lost laptops containing large financial, research, or patient care databases with names and Social Security numbers. Although the overall probability of a breach of confidentiality can be minimized, the magnitude of harm following a breach would be great because a biobank contains a large amount of information on many persons. In several circumstances, concerns about confidentiality are heightened. First, identifying links must be maintained and used if clinical data in a biobank are updated periodically. Databases are vulnerable to breaches of confidentiality when they include data with identifiers. Second, commercial biobanks, like other startup ventures, might fail. If bankruptcy occurs, agreements between the biobank and the donors of materials, including confidentiality protections, may be voided during the bankruptcy proceedings (14).

Confidentiality Concerns With Genome-Wide Sequencing

After genome-wide sequencing, a "de-identified" sample may be converted into an identified one if the sequence data can be compared with a database that contains both sequence data and donor identities (15,16). For example, donors of biological materials found at a crime scene can be identified through DNA forensic databases maintained by the states and the Department of Justice (DOJ). As of August 2008, the DOJ had identified DNA profiles on over 6.2 million persons convicted of or accused of certain crimes. The DOJ database uses short tandem repeats (STRs) at 13 loci to identify individuals. The DOJ database thus cannot identify someone from information about single nucleotide polymorphisms (SNPs) in a research specimen. However, when full genomic sequencing in research subjects becomes feasible, STRs at the DOJ loci will be apparent, and donors of research samples will be identifiable if they are in the DOJ database.

Companies that offer genome-wide testing to the public via the Internet have databases that contain data on over 200,000 SNPs on each individual, together with identifiers. It is possible to identify a person on the basis of 80 independent SNPs (17). Hence, donors of research samples can be identified if their data are in one of these commercial biobanks.

The confidentiality of a research subject's sequencing data will therefore hinge on the security of databases that contain sequence data linked to identifiers. Re-identification will be even easier if the genomic sequence data are associated with demographic data such as date of birth and zip code; publicly available information such as voting registries allows identification of individuals based on such information (4). Both researchers and subjects will be uncertain about how secure such databases are. Internet companies offering genomic sequencing to the public may not be subject to HIPAA privacy regulations.

The probability of re-identifying participants from their genomic sequence is low. However, the adverse consequences to an individual might be great. As with other low-probability, high-magnitude research risks, reasonable measures must be taken to minimize the risk and reduce it to acceptable levels.

How Should Concerns About Confidentiality be Addressed?

First, strong security protections must be established, such as password protection, encryption, and prohibitions on transferring unencrypted identifiable data to laptop computers or portable storage devices such as CDs or memory sticks, which can be easily lost or stolen. Particular attention should be paid to protecting confidentiality when clinical data are updated. Only de-identified data and specimens should be provided to researchers when identifiable data are not necessary to carry out the research. Second, confidentiality should be discussed during the informed consent process, so that prospective participants will understand the risks and make informed decisions about participation. Participants need to understand that confidentiality cannot be guaranteed. Third, some have proposed techniques such as altering, masking, or binning genomic data to reduce identifiability. However, these measures compromise the scientific value of the data. Fourth, as we next discuss, the sharing of genome-wide sequencing data with other researchers should include strict protections.

WIDE SHARING OF SEQUENCING DATA

Collecting biological specimens and detailed clinical data is difficult, and whole-genome sequencing currently is expensive. Thus, international guidelines call for the results of genomic sequencing data to be widely shared to facilitate research by other investigators (18). For example, participants in one study might be used as controls in a study of another disease or condition. The NIH strongly encourages genome-wide association studies to deposit de-identified coded phenotype and genotype data in a central NIH data repository that will be available to other researchers (19). Principal investigators have a 12-month period of exclusivity for submitting analyses from the data set for publication. Although such sharing facilitates the progress of research, it complicates concerns about confidentiality and consent for future studies.

Approaches to Sharing Sequence Data

In one model for sharing, the National Center for Biotechnology Information has developed a database of Genotypes and Phenotypes (dbGaP), which allows authorized principal investigators to download individual-level genotype and phenotype data as de-identified data in encrypted files (20). Researchers must obtain approval from an NIH Data Access Committee and agree to data use restrictions and security measures. Another model for sharing provides access to a secure website. To access data, researchers must sign a data use agreement with strict confidentiality and security provisions. This arrangement would be most convenient for researchers, but it would be difficult to enforce the data use protections. Still another model is to give researchers only restricted access to sequence information to reduce the risk of misuse of genome-wide data. For example, researchers might be allowed access to data only at a central site where security will be strict or at an Intranet site controlled by the biobank (18). Finally, data analyses might be carried out by designated biostatistical centers with strict security, rather than by a biostatistician on the researcher's team. These options all involve trade-offs between confidentiality and efficiency of research.

How Should Data Sharing be Carried Out?

As noted in Chapters 3 and 23, research with de-identified existing biological materials is not considered human subjects research and does not require IRB oversight. However, because of the special ethical concerns raised by genomic research in biobanks, the biobank should establish an oversight committee and operating procedures (3,21,22).

A comprehensive policy for sharing genome-wide sequence data with researchers who want to carry out secondary analyses should include the requirements listed in Table 27.1 (3,18,22). The measures in Table 27.1 will enhance accountability and public trust. The biobank oversight body should review requests to obtain materials or access sequencing data. The biobank also should have a clear policy for identifying projects that are so sensitive that a substantial percentage of donors might find them objectionable, and should have a process for deciding whether to release data to such studies.

INFORMED CONSENT

Federal regulations allow existing biological materials and clinical data to be used for research without consent if no HIPAA identifiers are included in the data set (see Chapter 6). The underlying rationale is that there is no risk of breaching confidentiality and no one would object to the use of anonymized materials for research. However, the authors of these regulations did not anticipate that whole-genome sequencing might transform a de-identified sample into one whose donor could be identified with the use of other databases.

The underlying ethical rationale for allowing unidentifiable materials to be used without consent will no longer be tenable with whole-genome sequencing. Once the materials are identifiable, it will no longer be the case that the risks are minimal and virtually no one would object to the use of his or her data. Furthermore, whole-genome sequences will be widely shared with other researchers. Such sharing sharply limits a donor's control over future research uses of the data. Furthermore, some genomics research is sufficiently sensitive that it cannot be assumed that almost all persons would allow their materials to be used, as we next discuss. Thus there are strong reasons to require consent for whole-genome sequencing.

Withdrawal From Research

Research participants have the right to withdraw from a research project at any time. Thus, donors may ask the investigators or biobanks to which they gave specimens to destroy the specimens. However, if the specimens have been de-identified, it will not be possible to know which specimens are to be destroyed. Moreover, once genomic information has been widely disseminated to other researchers, it is not feasible to try to recover it or prevent it from being used in additional research projects. Participants should appreciate these limitations when they agree to enter genome-wide association studies.

Sensitive Future Studies

The rationale for establishing biobanks and sharing sequence data is to facilitate additional research by other investigators. However, no one can know what kinds of research might be done in the future with stored materials and data. When materials are collected in clinical settings, there may be

TABLE 27.1	Sharing Whole-Genome Sequences With Other Researchers

Researchers must be qualified, including training in data security and confidentiality.

The project must have scientific merit as determined by peer review.

Strong data security should be in place.

Researchers should agree to certain limitations on use; they may not try to re-identify participants, and may not give data to others.

little explanation of the types of research that might be done. For example, people might be asked to consent to "genetic analysis," with little explanation of what that involves or what the potential risks and benefits are. Few participants are likely to object to their genomic and clinical data being used in other research on serious diseases, for example, to serve as a control in a study of genetic susceptibility to cancer.

Participants may not realize, however, that their information might be used in research they would find objectionable. Some future research projects might be so sensitive that some donors would not want their specimens to be used (4,11,23). For example, researchers might study the genetics of antisocial behavior, operationalized as arrests or convictions by the criminal justice system. Some donors to biobanks might not want their materials used in such research because they believe that research should focus instead on the social and economic factors associated with crime. Alternatively, they might be concerned that such research could lead to racial profiling by police and discrimination against certain minority groups. As another example, researchers might study the genetics of addictive behavior, such as alcoholism or substance abuse. Some donors might not want their specimens used in such research because they fear that identifying genetic factors for such behaviors might lead lawmakers or judges to absolve individuals of responsibility for the consequences of their actions (12). Finally, some individuals might not want to participate in research on human evolution because they reject that theory on religious grounds (4). Thus, a range of cultural and political views may lead people to object to sensitive studies.

How Should Informed Consent for Genome-Wide Sequencing be Obtained?

Researchers who are prospectively collecting specimens for genomics research or biobanks should discuss with prospective donors during the informed consent process the critical characteristics of such research. Unless they understand the issues listed in Table 27.2, potential donors will not be able to make an informed decision about participation.

Researchers who are establishing biobanks should also clarify financial arrangements regarding patents, licensing fees, and royalties (see Chapter 14 for further discussion of patents). It is not feasible to offer to share income from patents with individual donors, since researchers will be working with de-identified materials and sequencing data. If a disease advocacy group helps recruit donors, access to tests or therapies developed from the research should be negotiated in the planning stages of the project, before specimens are obtained. After discoveries are made, researchers should make them freely available to other investigators carrying out noncommercial research, and grant narrow and nonexclusive licenses to develop products whenever possible (24).

There are several options for addressing concerns about future research projects that some donors might find objectionable. One option is to seek consent for all future research that is approved by an

TABLE 27.2	Informed Consent for Donating Materials to Biobanks

Investigators should explain to donors
- the possibility of re-identifying donors from whole genome data;
- the impracticality of withdrawing from research once materials or data have been anonymized or sequencing data have been disseminated; and
- the intention of researchers to patent discoveries;

Investigators should obtain consent for
- whole genome sequencing;
- dissemination of sequencing data; and
- use in future projects, some of which might be sensitive and objectionable to some donors.

IRB or oversight body at the biobank, with the understanding that they will review sensitive research projects very carefully. Another option is to require specific consent for highly sensitive research that can be anticipated, such as research on the genetics of antisocial behavior. Yet another option is to ask permission to recontact donors about particularly sensitive studies in the future.

There is a trade-off between carrying out future research efficiently and respecting the donors of biological materials. For consent to be informed, participants need to appreciate the consequences of their participation. Investigators collecting specimens have an affirmative obligation to explain the potential benefits and risks of donating specimens, and may not assume that the risks and benefits of genomic research are common knowledge. Furthermore, in research, as in clinical care, investigators should discuss unlikely but very serious risks. However, the more detailed the consent process, the greater will be the barriers to obtaining materials for biobanks. To obtain the advantages of biobanks, researchers may decide to include only donors who are willing to agree to whole-genome sequencing, wide sharing of genomic sequence data, and broad permission for future studies.

Consultation With Groups

As discussed in Chapter 20, when carrying out research with ethnic or minority communities that have authorized political leaders, are localized geographically, and have clear rules for group membership, researchers should obtain formal approval from those leaders (6,25). In other genetic studies, participants are recruited, in part, by their membership in an ethnic group that is geographically dispersed and culturally heterogeneous. In this situation, researchers ought to elicit feedback regarding the proposed research project from the communities where recruitment will occur, and should respond to concerns and suggestions that are raised. Researchers do not need to accept every suggestion, but they should explain why they choose not to accept them (26). Such consultations should be sought in addition to informed consent from individual participants. It is respectful and also is likely to increase participation in the study.

DISCLOSURE OF INDIVIDUAL FINDINGS TO PARTICIPANTS

Chapter 11 discusses the ethical issues involved in providing participants the individual results of research tests that are being developed as part of a research study. Genomic tests raise several special issues (27,28).

Offering genomic sequencing results is particularly complex for several reasons. First, genomic sequencing might lead to incidental findings that are not related to the research question and have adverse psychosocial or medical consequences. For instance, it might disclose that a child has been adopted or is not related to the putative father. Or it might reveal an allele that confers susceptibility to a serious but preventable disease, such as hereditary nonpolyposis colorectal cancer (29). Such incidental findings will occur more frequently because of the increasing availability of genome-wide analyses that provide sequencing data on loci other than the researcher's primary region of interest. Second, genomic sequence information will be widely shared among researchers performing secondary analyses on conditions other than the original focus of study. However, researchers carrying out secondary analyses usually use de-identified data sets, which makes it difficult for them to contact participants. Third, pleiotrophy (i.e., a single gene can have many different effects) is common. For example, testing for ApoE was originally developed to characterize the risk of coronary heart disease, but later was found to be associated with dementia as well. Thus, persons who agreed to receive information regarding their risk for heart disease subsequently were given information regarding their risk for dementia that they may not have wanted to know. Fourth, the clinical significance of genomic sequencing data will change over time as a result of other studies. A sequence that was not clinically significant when first discovered might become so after additional analyses are carried out or published by others. Fifth, genomics research is often conducted by investigators who have PhD degrees but no clinical training.

A researcher who performs research tests on participants should consider whether to disclose individual results to them. We use the term "research tests" to refer to innovative tests that are being developed as part of the research project and are not available in routine clinical care. Although this is an issue for all research tests (see Chapter 11), disclosure of genomic test results is particularly controversial because the clinical significance of the results might be uncertain, and the participants might be very likely to misunderstand the findings.

What are the Reasons for Providing Individual Results From Genomic Research Tests?

As discussed in Chapter 11, there are several reasons for offering individual results from research tests to participants, including showing respect for participants, giving them their due for participating in the study, and providing benefit to them. Even if the clinical significance of the results is unknown, they might be personally significant to participants.

When BRCA testing was first developed and used in research studies, many participants with a family history of breast cancer wanted to receive their individual results, even though at that time it was uncertain how their care should be changed by the test results. Some women who tested positive for a mutation associated with susceptibility to breast and ovarian cancer decided to undergo mammography more frequently or at an earlier age. Others considered bilateral prophylactic mastectomy or sought to enter prevention trials. Some changed plans for education, employment, or childbearing after learning that they were at increased risk. Still other women just wanted to know their probability of developing cancer.

What are the Concerns About Providing Individual Results From Genomic Research Tests?

Analytical validity is usually not a problem with well-established techniques of DNA sequencing. However, the clinical validity and significance of the research tests often is unclear. Associations between a polymorphism and the clinical phenotype need to be confirmed in an independent sample. Furthermore, optimal clinical management of persons with variant alleles is rarely certain.

As genomics research increasingly focuses on polygenic conditions such as diabetes, hypertension, heart attack, and stroke, additional issues need to be taken into account. The relative risk of a single predisposing gene for these conditions usually is small, less than 2.0. Clinically useful prediction would require the use of a panel of genomic tests, and the positive predictive value of the combined tests would need to be confirmed in an independent population. It may not be clear how much additional predictive power such genomic information would have compared to clinical information about risk factors, such as smoking and cholesterol levels as risk factors for heart attacks. Furthermore, until prevention trials are carried out with persons identified as being at high risk, it will not be clear whether to recommend interventions that go beyond advice on diet, exercise, and follow-up of established clinical risk factors, which would be recommended regardless of the results of genomic tests.

What Issues Might be Raised by Additional Genomic Research?

The clinical validity and significance of a genomic research test might increase over time after additional research is carried out. Often other researchers will perform secondary analyses with de-identified data. Do such researchers have an obligation to inform the participants of clinically significant findings? Even if the secondary researcher could obtain the participants' identifying information, the participants might regard it as an invasion of privacy to be contacted by someone they do not know about additional studies they did not realize were being carried out. However, the alternative of having the researchers who originally enrolled participants contact them may not be feasible. Researchers may change fields, retire, or lose funding. Hence, researchers who obtain biological materials and clinical data should not all be given long-term, open-ended responsibilities to keep up with additional research pertaining to their project or to stay in touch with the participants (28). The original researcher's responsibility will depend on the nature and strength of the research-participant relationship as well as the nature of the new findings. In ongoing cohort studies with the original participants, the research team does have an obligation to offer results that have become clinically significant.

How Should Individual Results From Genomic Research Tests be Disclosed?

Chapter 11 makes several suggestions regarding the disclosure of individual results from research tests. As with any research test results, genomics researchers should develop a plan regarding disclosure at the onset of the study and communicate the options clearly to participants. Several issues are particularly salient as regards genomics tests (27,28).

Weigh the benefits, risks, and burdens of disclosing results. The strongest case for offering to disclose genomic results is when the disease or condition is serious, the clinical validity of the genetic predisposition has been established, and the results have clinical significance and could alter clinical management (27).

Obtain informed consent to receive results. Even if participants indicate when enrolling in a study that they wish to receive individual genomic results, researchers should confirm they still want to receive the results before providing them.

Maximize the benefits and minimize the harms of offering results. Researchers need to educate participants about the significance and limitations of their test results. As with any test, the predictive value will depend on the prior probability of the disease or condition. Thus, the same allele might have a different clinical significance depending on the family history. Because of a mistaken belief that genes determine clinical outcomes, participants may overestimate the predictive value of genomics tests. The participant's primary physician may not understand genomic tests and therefore may be unable to provide counseling. Researchers may have to educate the participants' physicians and offer genetic counseling to participants.

Involve the IRB. The investigator and the IRB will need to take into account the seriousness of the condition, the effectiveness of interventions to prevent or ameliorate the condition, how the information would change clinical management, and what expectations participants have regarding recontact. If the results of the genomic test would lead some participants to alter their clinical care and obtain an effective intervention to prevent a potentially fatal condition, there are strong ethical reasons for offering participants their individual results from research tests.

PATENTING OF GENETIC DISCOVERIES

Chapter 14 discusses patents, including patenting of DNA sequences.

RESEARCH ON PHARMACOGENOMICS

The genomic revolution offers the promise of individualized therapy based on genetic susceptibility to disease and response to therapy. Pharmacogenomics is the study of how genetics influences a person's response to drugs (30). The hope is to develop more effective treatments with fewer side effects (30). Pharmacogenomics research may identify several subgroups of patients. Patients for whom the drug is not effective can be spared the risks and costs of the drug. Patients at increased risk for adverse effects can be given another drug or have the dosage modified to reduce risks. From a population perspective, identifying such patients might reduce the number and severity of adverse drug reactions. Yet another group might need higher doses than usual—for example, because of more rapid drug metabolism—to achieve therapeutic concentrations and clinical effectiveness. Finally, if the drug cannot be approved for general use, pharmacogenomics researchers might identify a subgroup for which it is effective and safe, allowing it to be licensed for that subgroup.

Pharmacogenomics may also change the process of drug development. Clinical trials may test a new drug together with a pharmacogenomic test to identify patients who are highly likely to respond. With this strategy, smaller and faster clinical trials may be possible. However, if a drug is approved only for a subgroup of patients who are predicted to respond to it, the potential market would be smaller. It is not clear whether pharmaceutical manufacturers will find it a sound business model to target a smaller market based on pharmacogenomic testing, even though that strategy might improve clinical outcomes for patients.

At this time, the potential of pharmacogenomics has yet to be fulfilled; only a few pharmacogenomics tests are used in clinical practice. The most contentious ethical issue raised by pharmacogenomics research is basing therapy on self-identified race, which is discussed in Chapter 20.

CLINICAL TRIALS OF GENE TRANSFER

New genomic knowledge may lead to innovative therapies, such as gene transfer. Although the scientific rationale is often strong for delivering a specific gene for therapeutic purposes, clinical trials of gene transfer raise a number of ethical concerns.

STUDY 27.2   Gene transfer causing severe adverse effects.

X-linked severe combined immunodeficiency (X-SCID), if untreated, is usually fatal in the first year of life. Treatment with antibiotics and intravenous immune globulin can reduce the incidence of infections. Bone marrow transplantation from a matched donor can reconstitute the immune system. In a clinical trial, gene transfer using a retrovirus vector was successful in nine of 11 children, allowing them to resume normal activities. However, three additional children who underwent gene transfer developed T-cell leukemia several years later (one subsequently died). These leukemias were shown to be related to mutagenesis caused by the insertion of the retrovirus near a protooncogene. As the cases of leukemia were announced, scientists and oversight boards struggled to decide whether the clinical trials should continue.

This experimental intervention apparently provided considerable clinical benefit as well as serious adverse effects. At one public meeting, a woman made a heartfelt plea to resume the X-SCID trial because her grandson, who had failed four bone marrow transplants, was on the waiting list for the gene transfer study.

Study 27.2 dramatizes several important ethical issues. First, outcomes in clinical trials are unknown. Although an intervention may have a strong scientific rationale and preclinical support, its effectiveness and safety in humans are not certain. As in Study 27.2, serious unanticipated adverse events may occur when an intervention is carried out in humans. Second, informed consent is challenging because many participants (or, in Study 27.2, their parents) have high hopes regarding experimental interventions.

As described below, a participant in another gene transfer trial died in 2007. Her death later was determined to be in all likelihood unrelated to the study drug—a "near miss" in terms of adverse consequences of the trial. However, a detailed investigation of the trial revealed several flaws in early-phase clinical trials and suggested several changes that might reduce risks to participants (31). In the spirit of quality improvement, researchers, sponsors, and IRBs should view these near misses as "accidents waiting to happen" that present opportunities to learn how to design better research systems and protocols (32).

> **STUDY 27.3** **Death of a participant in a gene transfer clinical trial.**
>
> *A company developed an intraarticular gene transfer intervention for persons with rheuma-toid arthritis and other types of severe inflammatory arthritis. The investigational agent is an adeno-associated virus (AAV) containing DNA encoding for recombinant human tumor necro-sis factor (TNF). It is the same DNA sequence used in the production of the drug etanercept, which is approved by the FDA for rheumatoid arthritis. The intended target population is per-sons with inflammatory arthritis who have a few joints that are not well controlled on sys-temic therapy, or who decline or cannot tolerate systemic therapy.*
>
> *A 36-year-old woman with a 15-year history of rheumatoid arthritis enrolled in the clinical trial. She had been treated with disease-modifying agents since the early 1990s and had been on TNF-antagonists since 2002. Since 2004 she had also been on methotrexate and low-dose prednisone. She was married, had a child, and worked full time. However, she had persistent disease in her right knee and had received several intraarticular steroid injections.*
>
> *She received the first injection of the investigational agent in February 2007, with little clinical improvement. Before the second dose, she had low-grade fevers and fatigue. The day after the second injection, she developed high fevers, chills, vomiting, and diarrhea, which worsened over the next week. She was hospitalized and developed hypotension, respiratory, liver and renal failure, and disseminated intravascular coagulation. Despite intensive care, in-cluding antifungal medication, she died. At autopsy she was found to have disseminated histoplasmosis. In retrospect, she was probably already ill with histoplasmosis on the day she received her second dose of the study drug.*
>
> *When a federal panel reviewed the case, the participant's husband asked, "Would my wife still be alive today if she had not participated in this study?" The committee considered whether the investigational agent contributed to her death through, for example, oversup-pression of the immune system or an immune response to AAV. It also considered whether replication-competent AAV could have contributed to the clinical course. The panel deter-mined that these possibilities were all very unlikely.*

Although the study agent in all likelihood did not contribute to this participant's death, the incident revealed several flaws in the way clinical trials of innovative agents are carried out. Future stud-ies need to consider how to correct these flaws so that the risk of serious adverse events is minimized.

ETHICAL CONCERNS ABOUT GENE TRANSFER TRIALS

What are the Risks to Participants?

When the participant in Study 27.3 developed nonspecific symptoms, her personal physician man-aged her care. Although continuity of care is desirable, researchers should have real-time involvement if patients develop unanticipated serious adverse events. In future studies of immune modulators, the possibility of opportunistic infections should be considered if patients develop unexplained new symptoms. When an investigational agent is an immune modifier, the suspicion of opportunistic in-fection should be even higher than when immune-modifying agents that are approved by the FDA are prescribed in clinical practice. The researchers may be able to raise awareness of the possibility of an opportunistic infection. Researchers might also suggest additional clinical studies, such as blood cultures for fungus infection or the collection of additional specimens for special studies that might clarify whether adverse events are related to the investigational agent. Such clinical involvement and archiving of specimens will add to the cost of the study.

How is Informed and Voluntary Consent Obtained?

In consent forms for gene transfer protocols, the benefits of the study intervention are often over-stated and the risks understated (33,34). This therapeutic misconception can be reinforced during the consent process. For example, the very term "gene therapy" implies an established treatment rather than an experimental intervention whose benefits and risks are unknown.

In Study 27.3, the participant was enrolled in the trial by her treating rheumatologist, who received payment from the study sponsor for enrolling participants. Enrolling participants through the offices of many community practitioners allows for more efficient enrollment than using only one or two sites. However, enrollment by treating physicians raises ethical concerns regarding undue influence and conflicts of interest. Patients may find it inconceivable that their personal physician would discuss a therapy, or prescribe or administer it, unless it would benefit them and the risks would be acceptable. These assumptions, which are appropriate in clinical practice, do not hold in clinical trials, where the safety and efficacy of the study agent are unknown. Even if the consent form states that the agent is unproven and that serious adverse effects might occur, patients might discount this information because of the role of their personal physician. In Study 27.3, the investigational agent also had strong scientific plausibility—the study agent gets into the patient's knee joint and makes the medicine that she takes by pill, raising the concentration of the drug where the arthritis is most severe. All of these factors might lead patients to have a therapeutic misconception, an unwarranted belief that the study agent will benefit them.

RECOMMENDATIONS FOR ADDRESSING ETHICAL CONCERNS

Strengthen Informed Consent

The website of the NIH Recombinant DNA Advisory Committee (RAC), which reviews gene transfer studies, suggests ways to describe gene transfer in terms a layperson can understand, and how to describe benefits and risks accurately. The website (at http://www4.od.nih.gov/oba/rac/ic/) gives examples of both problematical and useful language. The RAC discourages the use of terms such as "therapy" or "treatment." The discussion of possible clinical benefit should be realistic; in many Phase I studies, the goal is to determine safety and dosage for future studies, and it may be appropriate to state that no direct personal benefit is intended. The crucial ethical considerations usually can be framed without elaborate scientific detail. At a meeting of the RAC, one researcher explained how one parent summarized his decision: "You're telling me that this has a chance—a good chance—of letting my son lead a normal life, without all the intravenous treatments. But he also might get another fatal disease."

Optimize the Balance of Benefits and Risks

The RAC oversight committee commonly makes a number of recommendations to modify the design of gene transfer protocols to reduce risks to participants (35). The most frequent recommendations are to:

- Increase the time interval between dose escalations to ensure that no adverse effects have occurred at lower doses.
- Exclude persons who have a greatly increased risk for adverse events.
- Carry out additional tests and assays to monitor adverse events.
- Check whether a vector or transgene is present in unintended tissues.

STUDY 27.2   **(Continued).**

As information about cases of leukemia emerged from the X-SCID trials, the clinical trials were put on hold twice and then allowed to resume after protocols were modified to reduce risks. The trials in the United States were restricted to children who were not eligible for a haplotype-matched bone marrow transplant or who had failed previous transplantation. Furthermore, monitoring was increased for early signs of abnormal proliferation of lymphocyte clones. Parents were carefully informed of the risk of leukemia.

STUDY 27.3 (Continued).

Although the participant's death in Study 27.3 was not attributed to the study intervention, this tragedy suggests several additional safeguards that should be taken with any clinical trial of a new immune-modifying agent, including interventions that involve gene transfer. First, it would be prudent to exclude participants with a history of opportunistic infections. Researchers and IRBs should also consider whether to exclude persons who have evidence of previous subclinical infections that might be reactivated. Second, when new immune-modifying agents are intermittently administered, a dose should be given only after the participant has been screened for fever and symptoms that suggest infection, and relevant laboratory tests have been checked. By analogy, a cycle of cancer chemotherapy is administered only after laboratory values are checked. Study 27.3 was criticized because the investigator drew blood for lab tests but did not check the results before administering the study drug.

TAKE HOME POINTS

1. In biobank and genomics research, researchers should pay attention to ethical issues regarding informed consent, confidentiality, and sharing of genome-wide sequence data.
2. Disclosing individual results of research genomics tests is problematic if the analytic and clinical validity of the tests has not been established. If results are offered, researchers should provide interpretation and counseling.
3. In gene transfer clinical trials, researchers should not overstate the benefits or understate the risks, and should take steps to protect participants from adverse events.

ANNOTATED BIBLIOGRAPHY

Bookman EB, Langehorne AA, Eckfeldt JH, et al. Reporting genetic results in research studies: summary and recommendations of an NHLBI working group. *Am J Med Genet A* 2006;140:1033–1040.
　　Discusses whether and how to offer participants individual results from genomic research tests.
Cambon-Thomsen A, Rial-Sebbag E, Knoppers BM. Trends in ethical and legal frameworks for the use of human biobanks. *Eur Respir J* 2007;30:373–382.
　　Analysis of ethical issues regarding biobanks that combine genomic sequence data and extensive clinical data.
Caulfield T, McGuire AL, Cho M, et al. Research ethics recommendations for whole-genome research: consensus statement. *PLoS Biol* 2008;6:e73.
　　Overview of ethical issues in whole-genome research.
Greely HT. The uneasy ethical and legal underpinnings of large-scale genomic biobanks. *Annu Rev Genomics Hum Genet* 2007;8:343–364.
　　Analysis of ethical issues regarding biobanks that combine genomic sequence data and extensive clinical data.
Lowrance WW, Collins FS. Ethics. Identifiability in genomic research. *Science* 2007;317:600–602.
　　Analyzes the ethical implications of the potential to re-identify participants in genome-wide association studies.

REFERENCES

1. Arnason V. Coding and consent: moral challenges of the database project in Iceland. *Bioethics* 2004;18:27–49.
2. Merz JF, McGee GE, Sankar P. "Iceland Inc." On the ethics of commercial population genomics. *Soc Sci Med* 2004;58:1201–1209.
3. Cambon-Thomsen A, Rial-Sebbag E, Knoppers BM. Trends in ethical and legal frameworks for the use of human biobanks. *Eur Respir J* 2007;30:373–382.
4. Greely HT. The uneasy ethical and legal underpinnings of large-scale genomic biobanks. *Annu Rev Genomics Hum Genet* 2007;8:343–364.
5. Rose H. From hype to mothballs in four years: troubles in the development of large-scale DNA biobanks in Europe. *Community Genet* 2006;9:184–189.
6. Hausman D. Protecting groups from genetic research. *Bioethics* 2008;22:157–165.
7. McGregor JL. Population genomics and research ethics with socially identifiable groups. *J Law Med Ethics* 2008; 36:356–370.

8. Annas GJ. Privacy rules for DNA databanks. Protecting coded 'future diaries.' *JAMA* 1993;270:2346–2350.
9. Kevles DJ. *In the Name of Eugenics*. Berkeley: University of California Press; 1985:96–112.
10. Gould SJ. *The Mismeasure of Man*. New York: W.W. Norton & Company; 1981.
11. Nuffield Council on Bioethics. *Genetics and Human Behavior: the Ethical Concerns*. London: Nuffield Council on Bioethics; 2002.
12. The President's Council on Bioethics. Beyond therapy: biotechnology and the pursuit of happiness. 2003. Available at: http://www.bioethics.gov/reports/beyondtherapy/index.html. Accessed October 19, 2007.
13. Reilly PR. Rethinking risks to human subjects in genetic research. *Am J Hum Genet* 1998;63:682–685.
14. Rothstein MA. Expanding the ethical analysis of biobanks. *J Law Med Ethics* 2005;33:89–101.
15. Lowrance WW, Collins FS. Ethics. Identifiability in genomic research. *Science* 2007;317:600–602.
16. McGuire AL, Gibbs RA. Genetics. No longer de-identified. *Science* 2006;312:370–371.
17. Lin Z, Owen AB, Altman RB. Genetics. Genomic research and human subject privacy. *Science* 2004;305:183.
18. Lowrance WW. Access to collections of data and materials for health research. 2006. Available at: http://www.wellcome.ac.uk/stellent/groups/corporatesite/@msh_grants/documents/web_document/wtx030842.pdf. Accessed May 17, 2008.
19. National Institutes of Health. Policy for sharing of data obtained in NIH supported or conducted genome-wide association studies (GWAS). 2007. Available at: http://grants.nih.gov/grants/guide/notice-files/NOT-OD-07-088.html. Accessed May 17, 2008.
20. Mailman MD, Feolo M, Jin Y, et al. The NCBI dbGaP database of genotypes and phenotypes. *Nat Genet* 2007; 39:1181–1186.
21. McGuire AL, Caulfield T, Cho MK. Research ethics and the challenge of whole-genome sequencing. *Nat Rev Genet* 2008;9:152–156.
22. Caulfield T, McGuire AL, Cho M, et al. Research ethics recommendations for whole-genome research: consensus statement. *PLoS Biol* 2008;6:e73.
23. National Bioethics Advisory Commission. *Research on Human Stored Biologic Materials*. Rockville, MD: National Bioethics Advisory Commission; 1999.
24. National Research Council. *Reaping the Benefits of Genomic and Proteonomic Research: Intellectual Property Rights, Innovation, and Public Health*. Washington, DC: National Academies Press; 2005.
25. Weijer C, Emanuel EJ. Protecting communities in biomedical research. *Science* 2000;289:1142–1144.
26. Lo B, O'Connell ME, eds. *Ethical Considerations for Research on Housing-Related Health Hazards Involving Children*. Washington, DC: National Academies Press; 2005.
27. Bookman EB, Langehorne AA, Eckfeldt JH, et al. Reporting genetic results in research studies: summary and recommendations of an NHLBI working group. *Am J Med Genet A* 2006;140:1033–1040.
28. Renegar G, Webster CJ, Stuerzebecher S, et al. Returning genetic research results to individuals: points-to-consider. *Bioethics* 2006;20:24–36.
29. Lo B. *Resolving Ethical Dilemmas: A Guide for Clinicians*. 4th ed. Philadelphia: Lippincott Williams & Wilkins; 2009.
30. Secretary's Advisory Committee on Genetics, Health, and Society. Realizing the potential of pharmacogenomics: opportunities and challenges. 2008. Available at: http://www4.od.nih.gov/oba/sacghs.htm. Accessed May 16, 2008.
31. Recombinant DNA Advisory Committee. Minutes of meeting September 17–18, 2007. Available at: http://www4.od.nih.gov/oba/rac/meeting.html. Accessed August 3, 2008.
32. Reason JT. Understanding adverse events: the human factor. In: Vincent C, ed. *Clinical Risk Management: Enhancing Patient Safety*. 2nd ed. London: BMJ Books; 2001:9–30.
33. Henderson GE, Davis AM, King NM, et al. Uncertain benefit: investigators' views and communications in early phase gene transfer trials. *Mol Ther* 2004;10:225–231.
34. King NM, Henderson GE, Churchill LR, et al. Consent forms and the therapeutic misconception: the example of gene transfer research. *IRB* 2005;27:1–8.
35. Scharschmidt T, Lo B. Clinical trial design issues raised during recombinant DNA advisory committee review of gene transfer protocols. *Hum Gene Ther* 2006;17:448–454.

Stem Cell Research

Pluripotent stem cells perpetuate themselves in culture and can differentiate into all types of specialized cells. Scientists plan to differentiate pluripotent cells into specialized cells that can be used for transplantation in patients with such conditions as diabetes, spinal cord injury, Parkinson disease, and myocardial infarction (1). Pluripotent stem cell lines whose nuclear DNA matches a specific person have several scientific advantages. Stem cell lines matched to persons with specific diseases can serve as in vitro models of diseases, and can be used to elucidate the pathophysiology of diseases and screen potential new therapies. Lines matched to specific individuals also offer the promise of personalized autologous stem cell transplantation.

However, stem cell research has also given rise to sharp ethical and political disputes. The derivation of pluripotent stem cell lines from oocytes and embryos is fraught with controversies regarding the onset of human personhood and reproduction, and problems with informed consent. Several other methods of deriving stem cells raise fewer ethical or scientific concerns. Reprogramming of somatic cells to produce induced pluripotent stem (iPS) cells avoids most of the ethical problems associated with embryonic stem cells.

MULTIPOTENT STEM CELLS

Adult stem cells and cord blood stem cells do not raise insurmountable ethical concerns and are widely used in research and clinical care. However, these cells cannot be expanded in vitro and have not been definitively shown to be pluripotent.

CORD BLOOD STEM CELLS

Hematopoietic stem cells from cord blood can be banked and are widely used for allogenic and autologous stem cell transplantation in pediatric hematological diseases as an alternative to bone marrow transplantation.

ADULT STEM CELLS

Adult stem cells are found in many tissues and can both differentiate into specialized cells in their tissue of origin and transdifferentiate into specialized cells characteristic of other tissues. For example, hematopoietic stem cells can differentiate into not only all three blood cell types but also into neural stem cells, cardiomyocytes, and liver cells.

Adult stem cells can be isolated through plasmapheresis. They are already used to treat hematological malignancies and to modify the side effects of cancer chemotherapy. However, uses for other conditions are unvalidated or experimental, despite claims to the contrary (2). For example, autologous stem cells are being used in clinical trials in patients who have suffered myocardial infarction.

EMBRYONIC STEM CELLS

Pluripotent stem cell lines can be derived from the inner cell mass of a 5- to 7-day-old blastocyst. However, human embryonic stem cell (hESC) research is ethically and politically controversial because it involves the destruction of human embryos. Clearly, embryos are potential human beings: if implanted into a woman's uterus during the appropriate hormonal phase, an embryo may develop into a fetus and become a live-born child. Some people go further and believe that an embryo is a person with the same moral status as an adult or a live-born child. In their view, research to derive a new stem cell line from human embryos is tantamount to murder. The view that a fertilized egg should be accorded the moral status of a person is usually based on deeply held religious beliefs and is unlikely to be altered by scientific arguments or evidence. Opposition to hESC research is often associated with opposition to abortion. However, opposition to stem cell research is not monolithic. A number of pro-life leaders support using such frozen embryos for stem cell research, including former First Lady Nancy Reagan and Senator Orrin Hatch. On his senate website, Sen. Hatch states (3):

> *"The support of embryonic stem cell research is consistent with pro-life, pro-family values."*

> *"I believe that human life begins in the womb, not a Petri dish or refrigerator . . . To me, the morality of the situation dictates that these embryos, which are routinely discarded, be used to improve and save lives. The tragedy would be in not using these embryos to save lives when the alternative is that they would be discarded."*

EXISTING EMBYRONIC STEM CELL LINES

In 2001, President Bush, who holds staunch pro-life views, allowed federal NIH funding to be used for stem cell research using embryonic stem cell lines already in existence at the time. As of October 2008, 22 hESC lines were eligible for NIH funding, but some were no longer suitable for research use. Federal funds may not be used to derive new embryonic stem cell lines or to work with hESC lines that are not on the approved NIH list. This ban includes the use of NIH-funded equipment and laboratory space to work on nonapproved hESC lines. Both the derivation of new hESC lines and research with hESC lines not approved by the NIH under nonfederal funding are permitted.

President Bush's rationale was that the embryos from which these lines were produced had already been destroyed. Allowing research to be carried out on the stem cell lines might allow some good to come out of their destruction. However, using only existing embryonic stem cell lines is scientifically problematic. Many of the lines originally listed turned out to be not pluripotent or not usable. Furthermore, these lines may not be safe for transplantation into humans. Long-standing lines have been shown to accumulate mutations, including several known to predispose to cancer. In addition, concerns have been raised about the consent process for the derivation of some lines (4). The vast majority of scientific experts, including the director of the NIH, believe that not deriving new pluripotent stem cell lines hinders progress toward stem cell-based transplantation.

Because of these restrictions on NIH funding, a number of states have established programs to fund stem cell research, including the derivation of new embryonic stem cell lines. California has allocated $3 billion over 10 years to stem cell research.

STEM CELL LINES DERIVED FROM FROZEN EMBRYOS

Women and couples who undergo infertility treatment often have frozen embryos remaining after they complete their infertility treatment. The disposition of these frozen embryos is a difficult decision for them. Some choose to donate these remaining embryos to research rather than destroy them or give them to another couple for reproductive purposes.

Embryo research involves additional dilemmas about informed consent because frozen embryos may be created with sperm or oocytes from donors who will not participate in childrearing. Some people argue that consent from gamete donors is not required for embryo research because they have ceded their right to direct further usage of their gametes to the woman or couple in infertility treatment. However, gamete donors who are willing to help women and couples bear children may object to the use of their genetic materials for research. To respect gamete donors, their wishes regarding stem cell derivation should be determined and respected (5).

SOMATIC CELL NUCLEAR TRANSFER

The same techniques that produced Dolly the sheep might also be used with human cells. In somatic cell nuclear transfer (SCNT), nuclear DNA from a donor is transferred into an oocyte from which the nucleus has been removed. However, not only has creating human SCNT stem cell lines been impossible to date, it also is ethically controversial (6,7).

Ethical Concerns About SCNT

Objections to creating embryos specifically for research. Some object that creating embryos with the intention of using them for research and destroying them in that process violates respect for nascent human life. Some people who support deriving stem cell lines from frozen embryos that would otherwise be discarded reject the intentional creation of research embryos.

Ethical concerns about donating oocytes for research. The donation of fresh oocytes for research raises additional ethical concerns regarding the medical risks of oocyte retrieval (8) and payment. In the United States, women can be paid several thousand dollars to donate oocytes for in vitro fertilization (IVF). However, paying donors of oocytes for research in excess of reimbursement for reasonable expenses is controversial because of concerns about undue influence and commodification (9). Finally, sharing oocytes between a woman in IVF treatment with researchers may raise concerns about compromising the reproductive goals of the IVF patient (10).

Concerns about oocyte donation for research are particularly serious in light of the Hwang scandal in South Korea, in which widely hailed claims of deriving human SCNT lines were found to be fabricated. In addition to scientific fraud, the scandal involved inappropriate payments to oocyte donors, serious deficiencies in the informed consent process, undue influence on staff and junior scientists to serve as donors, and an unacceptably high rate of medical complications (11–13).

California has adopted innovative regulations to protect women who donate oocytes for research funded by the state (10). Oocyte donors must be asked questions to ensure that they comprehend the key features of the research. In addition, donors must receive free medical treatment for short-term direct medical complications. Furthermore, when oocytes from a woman undergoing infertility treatment are shared with researchers, the reproductive interests of the woman must not be compromised. However, very few women are willing to donate oocytes for research without payment.

Objections to human reproduction using SCNT. There are several compelling objections to the use of SCNT for human reproduction. First, because of errors that occur during reprogramming of genetic material, cloned animal embryos fail to activate key embryonic genes, and newborn clones misexpress hundreds of genes (14,15). The risk of severe congenital defects would be prohibitively high in humans. Second, even if SCNT could be carried out safely in humans, some object that it would violate human dignity and undermine traditional, fundamental moral, religious, and cultural values (6). A cloned child would have only one genetic parent and would be the genetic twin of that parent. In this view, cloning would lead children to be regarded more as "products of a designed manufacturing process than 'gifts' whom their parents are prepared to accept as they are" (6). Furthermore, cloning would violate "the natural boundaries between generations" (6). For these reasons, cloning for reproductive purposes is widely considered morally wrong and is illegal in a number of states.

Use of animal oocytes to create SCNT lines using human DNA. Because of the shortage of human oocytes for SCNT research, some scientists wish to use nonhuman oocytes to derive lines using human nuclear DNA. These so-called "cytoplasmic hybrid embryos" raise a number of ethical concerns.

Some fear the creation of chimeras, mythical beasts that appear part human and part animal and have characteristics of both humans and animals (16). Opponents may feel deep moral unease or repugnance, without articulating their concerns in more specific terms. Some people view such hybrid embryos as contrary to the moral order embodied in the natural world and in natural law. In this view, each species has a particular moral purpose or goal, which mankind should not try to change. Others view such research as an inappropriate crossing of species barriers, which should be an immutable part of natural design. Finally, some are concerned that there may be attempts to implant these embryos for reproductive purposes.

In rebuttal, supporters of such research point out that biological definitions of species are not natural and immutable, but empirical and pragmatic (17). Animal-animal hybrids of various sorts, such as the mule, exist and are not considered morally objectionable. Moreover, in medical research, human cells are commonly injected into nonhuman animals and incorporated into their functioning tissue. Indeed, this is widely done in research with all types of stem cells to demonstrate that cells are pluripotent or have differentiated into the desired type of cell. In addition, some concerns can be addressed through strict oversight (17). For example, reproductive uses of these embryos should be prohibited. In vitro development should be limited to 14 days or the development of the primitive streak—limits that are widely accepted for hESC research. Finally, repugnance per se is an unconvincing guide for making ethical judgments. People disagree over what is repugnant, and their views may change over time. Blood transfusion and cadaveric organ transplantation were originally viewed as repugnant but are now widely accepted. Furthermore, after public discussion and education, many people overcome their initial concerns.

FETAL STEM CELLS

Pluripotent stem cells can be derived from fetal tissue after abortion. However, the use of fetal tissue is ethically controversial because it is associated with abortion, which many people object to. Under federal regulations, research with fetal tissue is permitted provided that the donation of tissue for research is considered only after the decision to terminate pregnancy has been made. This requirement minimizes the possibility that a woman's decision to terminate pregnancy might be influenced by the prospect of contributing tissue to research. Currently, a Phase I clinical trial in Batten's disease, a lethal degenerative disease that affects children, is being conducted using neural stem cells derived from fetal tissue.

INDUCED PLURIPOTENT STEM CELLS

Somatic cells can be reprogrammed to form pluripotent stem cells (18,19), called induced pluripotential stem (iPS) cells. These iPS cell lines will have DNA matching that of the somatic cell donors and will be useful as disease models and potentially for allogenic transplantation. Because this technique does not produce an embryo, it avoids concerns about the destruction of potential human life or about the use of somatic cell nuclear transfer. Furthermore, because a skin biopsy to obtain somatic cells is relatively noninvasive, there are fewer concerns about risks to donors.

Early iPS cell lines were derived by inserting genes encoding for transcription factors, using retroviral vectors. Researchers are trying to eliminate safety concerns about inserting oncogenes and insertional mutagenesis. Reprogramming has been successfully accomplished without known oncogenes, and in animals advenovirus vectors have been used instead of retrovirus vectors. The ultimate goal is to induce pluripotentiality without genetic manipulation by using chemicals and small molecules that promote reprogramming.

However, some ethical concerns about future downstream research need to be addressed (20). iPS cells will be shared widely among researchers who will carry out a variety of studies. Certain kinds of future research may be regarded as sensitive by some donors. For instance, some people may not want to donate cells that will be injected into nonhuman animals or undergo whole-genome sequencing. However, these techniques are fundamental to basic stem cell research. Other donors may not want cells derived from them to be patented as a step toward developing new tests and therapies. It would be unfortunate if iPS lines—or other types of stem cell lines—that turned out to be extremely useful scientifically (for example, because of robust growth in tissue culture) could not be used in additional research because the somatic cell donor objected to such use. One approach is to use preferentially somatic cells from donors who are willing to allow all such basic research and to be contacted for future sensitive research that cannot be anticipated (20). Donors should also be offered the option of consenting to additional downstream research, such as allogenic transplantation into other humans and reproductive research involving the creation of totipotent entities.

STEM CELL CLINICAL TRIALS

Transplantation of cells derived through the manipulation of pluripotent stem cells offers the promise of effective new treatments. However, it may involve great uncertainty and the possibility of serious risks. Such transplantation should be allowed in clinical practice only after clinical trials demonstrate efficacy and safety. These clinical trials should follow the same ethical principles that guide all clinical research. Additional ethical requirements are also warranted to strengthen trial designs, coordinate scientific and ethics reviews, verify that participants understand key features of the trial, and ensure publication of negative findings (21,22). These measures are necessary because of the highly innovative nature of the intervention, the limited experience in humans, and the high hopes of patients who have no effective treatments.

OVERSIGHT OF STEM CELL RESEARCH

Human stem cell research raises some ethical issues that are beyond the mission or expertise of IRBs. For example, there must be a sound scientific justification for using human oocytes and embryos to derive new human stem cell lines. Some ethical concerns go beyond human subjects protection, for example, transplantation of human stem cells into nonhuman animals in ways that might result in the transfer of human characteristics or appearance.

THE STEM CELL RESEARCH OVERSIGHT COMMITTEE

A Stem Cell Research Oversight Committee (SCRO) that includes members with appropriate scientific and ethical expertise, as well as public members, should be convened at each institution to review, approve, and oversee stem cell research (23–25). The SCRO will need to work closely with the IRB and, in cases of animal research, with the Institutional Animal Care and Use Committee (IACUC). Because each institution will have different procedures for review of stem cell research, investigators need to know and follow the requirements at their institution.

USE OF STEM CELL LINES DERIVED AT ANOTHER INSTITUTION

Sharing of stem cells across institutions facilitates scientific progress and minimizes the number of oocytes, embryos, and somatic cells that need to be used. However, ethical concerns arise if researchers work with lines that were derived in other jurisdictions under conditions that would not be permitted at their home institution. Researchers and SCROs need to distinguish core ethical standards that are accepted by international consensus, such as informed consent, from issues on which different jurisdictions and cultures might reasonably disagree. Using lines whose derivation violated core standards would erode the ethical conduct of research by providing incentives to others to violate those standards.

The review process should focus on those types of hSC derivation that raise heightened levels of ethical concern. hSC lines derived using fresh oocytes and embryos require in-depth review because of concerns about the medical risks of oocyte donation, undue influence, and setbacks to the reproductive goals of a woman undergoing infertility treatment.

Dilemmas occur when donors of research oocytes receive payments that would not be permitted in the jurisdiction where the hSC cells will be used. For example, after public consultation and debate, the United Kingdom enacted an explicit policy to allow such payments and provided reasons to justify its decision (26–29). Even jurisdictions that ban payments should accept such carefully considered policies as embodying a reasonable difference of opinion on a complex issue. Concerns about payment are lower when lines are derived from frozen embryos that remain after IVF treatment and donors were paid in the reproductive context. Such payments are not an inducement for hESC research.

Other dilemmas arise from the use of hESC lines derived from embryos using gamete donors. As discussed above, explicit consent for the use of reproductive materials in hESC or SCNT research should be obtained from both gamete and embryo donors (5,30). An exception may be made to "grandparent" in older lines derived from embryos created before such explicit consent became the standard of care—for example, before the National Academy of Sciences 2005 guidelines were published (30). It would be unreasonable to expect physicians to comply with standards that have not yet been established. It is reasonable for such older lines to accept consent for unspecified future research without explicit mention of hSC derivation. However, the derivation should be consistent with the ethical and legal standards in place at the time.

TAKE HOME POINTS

1. hESC research raises ethical issues regarding informed consent and the destruction of embryos.
2. The use of iPS cells does not raise concerns regarding embryos, but does raise concerns about consent for future downstream research.
3. The use of stem cell lines derived at another institution requires some verification that the lines were derived under ethically appropriate circumstances.

ANNOTATED BIBLIOGRAPHY

Hyun I. Fair payment or undue inducement? *Nature* 2006;442:629–630.
    Lucid analysis of controversial issues regarding payment for research oocytes.
Lo B, Kriegstein A, Grady D. Clinical trials in stem cell transplantation: guidelines for scientific and ethical review. *Clin Trials* 2008;5:517–522.
    Analysis of ethical issues in stem cell clinical trials.
Hyun I, Lindvall O, Ahrlund-Richter L, et al. New ISSCR guidelines underscore major principles for responsible translational stem cell research. *Cell Stem Cell* 2008;3:607–609.
    Consensus guidelines for clinical trials involving stem cells.
Lomax GP, Hall ZH, Lo B. Responsible oversight of human stem cell research: the California Institute for Regenerative Medicine's medical and ethical standards. *PLoS Med* 2007;4:e114.
    Describes innovative requirements for stem cell research funded by the state of California, particularly for derivation of hESC lines.
National Research Council and Institute of Medicine. *Guidelines for Human Embryonic Stem Cell Research.* Washington, DC: National Academies Press; 2005.
National Research Council and Institute of Medicine. *2008 Amendments to the National Academies' Guidelines for Human Embryonic Stem Cell Research*. Washington, DC: National Academies Press; 2008.
    Consensus guidelines for human pluripotent stem cell research.
Zettler P, Wolf LE, Lo B. Establishing procedures for institutional oversight of stem cell research. *Acad Med* 2007;82:6–10.
    Recommendations for institutions setting up stem cell research oversight committees.

REFERENCES

1. National Research Council and Institute of Medicine. *Stem Cells and the Future of Regenerative Medicine.* Washington, DC: National Academies Press; 2002.
2. Smith S, Neaves W, Teitelbaum S. Adult versus embryonic stem cells: treatments. *Science* 2007;316:1422–1423; author reply 1422–1423.
3. Statement of Senator Orrin G. Hatch on stem cell research. July 17, 2001. Available at: http://hatch.senate.gov/public/index.cfm?FuseAction=PressReleases.Print&PressRelease_id=fca0c5e3-40c8-4cd3-822e-efff0f2633de&suppresslayouts=true&IsTextOnly=True. Accessed December 18, 2008.
4. Streiffer R. Informed consent and federal funding for stem cell research. *Hastings Cent Rep* 2008;38:40–47.
5. Lo B, Chou V, Cedars M, et al. Consent from donors for embryo and stem cell research. *Science* 2003;301:921.
6. The President's Council on Bioethics. *Human Cloning and Human Dignity: An Ethical Inquiry.* Washington, DC; 2002.
7. National Bioethics Advisory Commission. *Cloning Human Beings.* Rockville, MD: National Bioethics Advisory Commission; 1997.
8. National Research Council and Institute of Medicine. *Assessing the Medical Risks of Human Oocyte Donation for Stem Cell Research.* Washington, DC: National Academies Press; 2007.
9. Hyun I. Fair payment or undue inducement? *Nature* 2006;442:629–630.
10. Lomax GP, Hall ZH, Lo B. Responsible oversight of human stem cell research: the California Institute for Regenerative Medicine's medical and ethical standards. *PLoS Med* 2007;4:e114.
11. Holden C. Korean stem cell scandal. Schatten: Pitt panel finds 'misbehavior' but not misconduct. *Science* 2006;311:928.
12. Chong S. Scientific misconduct. Investigations document still more problems for stem cell researchers. *Science* 2006;311:754–755.
13. Chong S, Normile D. Stem cells. How young Korean researchers helped unearth a scandal. *Science* 2006;311:22–25.
14. Jaenisch R. Human cloning—the science and ethics of nuclear transplantation. *N Engl J Med* 2004;351:2787–2791.
15. National Research Council and Institute of Medicine. *Scientific and Medical Aspects of Human Reproductive Cloning.* Washington, DC: National Academies Press; 2002.
16. The President's Council on Bioethics. *White Paper: Alternative Sources of Human Pluripotent Stem Cells.* Washington, DC; 2005.
17. Human Fertilisation and Embryology Authority. Hybrids and chimeras: findings of the consultation. 2007. Available at: http://www.hfea.gov.uk/en/1581.html. Accessed September 22, 2007.
18. Takahashi K, Tanabe K, Ohnuki M, et al. Induction of pluripotent stem cells from adult human fibroblasts by defined factors. *Cell* 2007;131:861–872.
19. Park IH, Arora N, Huo H, et al. Disease-specific induced pluripotent stem cells. *Cell* 2008;134:877–886.
20. Aalto-Setala K, Conklin BR, Lo B. Informed consent for future research with induced pluripotent cells. *PLoS Biology* (in press).
21. Hyun I, Lindvall O, Ahrlund-Richter L, et al. New ISSCR guidelines underscore major principles for responsible translational stem cell research. *Cell Stem Cell* 2008;3:607–609.
22. Lo B, Kriegstein A, Grady D. Clinical trials in stem cell transplantation: guidelines for scientific and ethical review. *Clin Trials* 2008;5:517–522.
23. National Research Council and Institute of Medicine. *Guidelines for Human Embryonic Stem Cell Research.* Washington, DC: National Academies Press; 2005.
24. Zettler P, Wolf LE, Lo B. Establishing procedures for institutional oversight of stem cell research. *Acad Med* 2007;82:6–10.
25. National Research Council and Institute of Medicine. *2008 Amendments to the National Academies' Guidelines for Human Embryonic Stem Cell Research.* Washington, DC: National Academies Press; 2008.
26. Human Fertilisation and Embryology Authority. The code of practice: 7th edition. 2007. Available at: http://www.hfea.gov.uk/en/371.html. Accessed October 16, 2008.
27. Human Fertilisation and Embryology Authority. Donating eggs for research: safeguarding donors. 2007. Available at: http://www.hfea.gov.uk/en/1417.html. Accessed October 18, 2008.
28. Human Fertilisation and Embryology Authority. The regulation of donor-assisted conception: a consultation on policy and regulatory measures affecting sperm, egg and embryo donation in the United Kingdom. 2006. Available at: http:// www.hfea.gov.uk/en/492.html. Accessed October 18, 2008.
29. Human Fertilisation and Embryology Authority. HFEA statement on donating eggs for research. 2007. Available at: http://www.hfea.gov.uk/cps/rde/xchg/SID-3F57D79B-EF42B079/hfea/hs.xsl/1491.html. Accessed March 8, 2007.
30. National Academy of Sciences. *Guidelines for Human Embryonic Stem Cell Research.* Washington, DC: National Academies Press; 2005.

INDEX

Page numbers followed by *f* or *t* indicate material in figures or tables, respectively.

data sharing and, 122–123, 259
funding by, 4, 13
gene transfer trials and, 267
genomic research and, 257, 259
patent policy of, 130
on racial representation, 183
research misconduct and, 109–111, 114
stem cell research and, 271
Native Americans, 180, 182, 184
Nazi "experiments," 3, 46, 178
NCI. *See* National Cancer Institute
Negative results, withholding of, 5, 5*t*, 113, 119,
  134–136, 253–254
Nephropathy prevention trial, in diabetes, 241–242, 246,
  248
New England Journal of Medicine, 196
NHLBI. *See* National Heart, Lung, and Blood Institute
Nigeria, meningococcal meningitis study in, 205–207
NIH. *See* National Institutes of Health
No Child Left Behind Act of 2002, 163–164
Nonsteroidal antiinflammatory drugs (NSAIDs), miscon-
  duct in research on, 112–113

O

Objective response, 34
Observational studies, 225–231. *See also specific types*
Office for Human Research Protection (OHRP), 21, 23,
  30, 56, 174–175, 222
Office of Research Integrity (ORI), 110, 115
OHRP. *See* Office for Human Research Protection
Omega-3 fatty acids, prison study of, 191–193
Oocytes, research use of, 63–64, 111–112, 125–126,
  219–220, 271–273
Opting out, of specimen use, 221
Opt-in strategy, 84
Opt-out strategy, 84–85
Oral cancer, NSAIDs and, misconduct in research on,
  112–113
ORI. *See* Office of Research Integrity
Outcome research, HIPAA and, 74
Outcomes
  offering results to participants, 97–107, 228, 262–264
  unknown nature of, 43
Out-of-pocket expenses, reimbursement for, 88
Oversight. *See also* Data monitoring; Institutional Review
    Boards
  in conflicts of interest, 138–140
  general requirements for, 21
  in recruitment, 84–85
  in stem cell research, 274–275
  systems approach to, 16
  in U.S., criticism of, 15–16

P

Parent(s)
  payment to, 86–87, 164–165
  permission from, 161–164
    for adolescents, 168, 169–170
    best interests of child and, 157–158

in educational settings, 62–63, 163–164
passive, 62–63, 162
reason for requiring, 161–162
waiver or modification of, 162
Paroxetine, information withheld on, 5*t*, 135
Participants
  equitable selection of, 22, 90
  identification and recruitment of, 81–85
  payment to, 35, 52, 53, 86–92
  research results for, offering, 97–107, 228, 262–264
  vs. subjects, 18
  vulnerable. *See* Vulnerable participants
Passive consent, 62–63, 162, 221
Patents, 125–131
  access to products developed from, 130–131
  advocacy groups and, 130
  burdens on researchers imposed by, 127
  conflicts of interest and, 132
  criteria for, 126
  donors of materials and, 130
  ethical concerns about, 126–127
  for human embryonic stem cells, 125–126
  for human life, 126–127
  inventing around, inability of, 127
  nonprofit funders of research and, 130–131
  purpose of system, 126
  reform of system, 129–130
  research deterred by, 127
  research exemption from restrictions of, 129–130
  tests and therapies unaffordable under, 127–129
Pathology samples. *See* Biological specimens
Patient rights, in HIPAA, 71
Payment
  to participants, 86–92
    appreciation model of, 88–89
    as benefit, 35
    vs. compensation, 86
    conflicts of interest and, 87
    ethical concerns about, 89–90, 164–165
    fairness in, 89–90
    to increase enrollment, 88
    Institute of Medicine on, 91, 164–165
    IRB policies on, 90–91, 165
    levels of, 90–91
    lottery tickets as, 91
    market model of, 88
    in pediatric studies, 86–87, 164–165
    practical considerations in, 91
    reasons for, 87–88
    reimbursement model of, 88
    risk and, 87
    as undue influence, 52, 53, 86–87, 89
    wage-payment model of, 88
  to physicians, as incentive, 85
Pediatric research. *See* Adolescents; Children
Peer review
  confidentiality during, 77
  for equipoise in clinical trials, 243
  of innovative clinical care, 8
  research misconduct and, 111–112
  of research with ethnic/minority populations, 185